T0293404

Metabolic Diseases: A Case-Based Approach

Metabolic Diseases: A Case-Based Approach

Editor: Bryan Glover

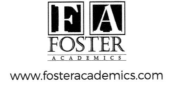

www.fosteracademics.com

www.fosteracademics.com

Cataloging-in-Publication Data

Metabolic diseases : a case-based approach / edited by Bryan Glover.
    p. cm.
Includes bibliographical references and index.
ISBN 978-1-64646-593-4
1. Metabolism--Disorders. 2. Metabolism--Disorders--Case studies. 3. Diseases.
4. Metabolic syndrome. I. Glover, Bryan.
RC627.54 .M48 2023
616.39--dc23

© Foster Academics, 2023

Foster Academics,
118-35 Queens Blvd., Suite 400,
Forest Hills, NY 11375, USA

ISBN 978-1-64646-593-4 (Hardback)

This book contains information obtained from authentic and highly regarded sources. Copyright for all individual chapters remain with the respective authors as indicated. All chapters are published with permission under the Creative Commons Attribution License or equivalent. A wide variety of references are listed. Permission and sources are indicated; for detailed attributions, please refer to the permissions page and list of contributors. Reasonable efforts have been made to publish reliable data and information, but the authors, editors and publisher cannot assume any responsibility for the validity of all materials or the consequences of their use.

Trademark Notice: Registered trademark of products or corporate names are used only for explanation and identification without intent to infringe.

Contents

Preface

Metabolism refers to the process through which a human body produces energy from food. In this process, food is broken down into sugars and acids with the help of chemicals in the digestive system. These acids and sugars provide the energy or fuel for the body, which is used to perform various functions by the body. Metabolic diseases are a group of diseases that cause a disruption in the metabolic process due to abnormal chemical reactions within the body. These diseases affect the parts of the cells that function to produce energy. The most common sign of metabolic diseases is diabetes along with increased circumference of the waist. The causes include obesity and physical inactivity. Metabolic diseases are linked with the complications related to heart and vessel disease. Preventive methods, such as limiting saturated fat and salt in diet, consuming sufficient vegetables and fruits, and avoiding smoking, can help in the management and control of conditions that lead to metabolic diseases. The topics included in this book on metabolic diseases are of utmost significance and bound to provide incredible insights to readers. Those in search of information to further their knowledge will be greatly assisted by it.

The researches compiled throughout the book are authentic and of high quality, combining several disciplines and from very diverse regions from around the world. Drawing on the contributions of many researchers from diverse countries, the book's objective is to provide the readers with the latest achievements in the area of research. This book will surely be a source of knowledge to all interested and researching the field.

In the end, I would like to express my deep sense of gratitude to all the authors for meeting the set deadlines in completing and submitting their research chapters. I would also like to thank the publisher for the support offered to us throughout the course of the book. Finally, I extend my sincere thanks to my family for being a constant source of inspiration and encouragement.

Editor

Dietary Strategies for Metabolic Syndrome

Sara Castro-Barquero [1,2,3], Ana María Ruiz-León [2,3], Maria Sierra-Pérez [1], Ramon Estruch [1,2,3] and Rosa Casas [1,2,3,*]

1 Department of Medicine, Faculty of Medicine and Life Sciences, University of Barcelona, 08036 Barcelona, Spain; sara.castro@ub.edu (S.C.-B.); mariasipe4@gmail.com (M.S.-P.); restruch@clinic.cat (R.E.)
2 Institut d'Investigacions Biomèdiques August Pi I Sunyer (IDIBAPS), 08036 Barcelona, Spain; amruiz@clinic.cat
3 Centro de Investigación Biomédica en Red, Fisiopatología de la Obesidad y la Nutrición (CIBEROBN), Instituto de Salud Carlos III, 28029 Madrid, Spain
* Correspondence: rcasas1@clinic.cat

Abstract: Metabolic syndrome is a cluster of metabolic risk factors, characterized by abdominal obesity, dyslipidemia, low levels of high-density lipoprotein cholesterol (HDL-c), hypertension, and insulin resistance. Lifestyle modifications, especially dietary habits, are the main therapeutic strategy for the treatment and management of metabolic syndrome, but the most effective dietary pattern for its management has not been established. Specific dietary modifications, such as improving the quality of the foods or changing macronutrient distribution, showed beneficial effects on metabolic syndrome conditions and individual parameters. On comparing low-fat and restricted diets, the scientific evidence supports the use of the Mediterranean Dietary Approaches to Stop Hypertension (DASH) diet intervention as the new paradigm for metabolic syndrome prevention and treatment. The nutritional distribution and quality of these healthy diets allows health professionals to provide easy-to-follow dietary advice without the need for restricted diets. Nonetheless, energy-restricted dietary patterns and improvements in physical activity are crucial to improve the metabolic disturbances observed in metabolic syndrome patients.

Keywords: metabolic syndrome; dietary pattern; Mediterranean diet; plant-based diet; DASH diet; low-carbohydrate diet; high-protein diet; low-fat diet

1. Introduction

Following unhealthy dietary patterns and sedentary lifestyles has led to a notable increase in the prevalence of overweight and obesity worldwide. Non-communicable chronic diseases (NCDs) related to unhealthy dietary patterns and weight gain have expanded in parallel, being the major cause of morbidity and mortality both in developed and underdeveloped countries [1]. Among NCDs, cardiovascular diseases (CVD) and type 2 diabetes mellitus (T2DM) are public health priorities, not only for their high prevalence and outcomes but also for the huge economic burden imposed on the health system [2,3].

Metabolic syndrome (MetS) is a clinical condition characterized by a clustering of metabolic risk factors, which is defined by the simultaneous occurrence of at least three of the following components: central obesity, dyslipidemia, impaired glucose metabolism, elevated blood pressure (BP), and low levels of high-density lipoprotein cholesterol (HDL-c), according to the consensual definition of the International Diabetes Federation, the American Heart Association, and the National Heart, Lung and

Blood Institute [4]. In developed countries, the prevalence of MetS has risen up to 20–25% in the adult population, and its incidence continues to increase over time [5–8]. In Spain, the prevalence of MetS is currently reaching epidemic proportions, affecting approximately 22.7% of the population, taking into account that its incidence increases with age [5]. In addition, MetS increases the risk of T2DM onset and major cardiovascular events by two-fold and five-fold, respectively, and other chronic disease such as cancer, neurodegenerative diseases, non-alcoholic fatty liver disease, the risk of reproductive, lipid and circulatory disorders, atherosclerosis, and all cause-mortality are also increased [8–13].

Recent evidence has demonstrated the association between the incidence and prevention of MetS and modifiable lifestyle factors, especially dietary habits. Steckhan et al. analyzed the positive effects of different dietary approaches on MetS inflammatory markers [14]. Regarding the prevention of MetS, Godos et al. also conducted a meta-analysis to demonstrate the preventive role of the promotion of healthy dietary patterns to reduce the prevalence of MetS [15]. Furthermore, some sub-studies from the PREDIMED-Plus cohort showed associations between some dietary components of the traditional Mediterranean Diet (MedDiet) and improvement in MetS components [16–20]. The aim of the present review was to analyze the potential benefits of different dietary approaches on MetS status and their use as efficient strategies to prevent and treat MetS and its comorbidities.

Dietary Patterns

A single-nutrient dietary intervention has several limitations, and dietary advice must be focused on the overall dietary pattern as part of MetS treatment. Recent evidence supports the implementation of healthy food-based dietary interventions instead of calorie or isolated nutrient restriction [1,21] diets. The health benefits, regarding MetS, of dietary macronutrient patterns and different dietary approaches are summarized in Table 1.

Table 1. Dietary strategies and potential health benefits for Metabolic Syndrome (MetS).

Dietary Pattern	Nutritional Distribution	Improvements in MetS Criteria	Ref.
Mediterranean diet	▪ 35–45% kcal/d from total fat (mainly MUFA [1], EVOO and nuts being the principal source) ▪ 35–45% kcal/d from CH ▪ 15–18% kcal/d from protein	Reduction of CVD incidence and outcomes Decreased BP (systolic and diastolic) Inverse association with mortality Improvements in dyslipemia Decreased incidence of T2DM	[22–29] [15,26] [24,30] [26] [12,22,23,29,31]
DASH diet	▪ Total fats 27% kcal/d ▪ Saturated fats 6% kcal/d ▪ Dietary cholesterol ▪ CH 55% kcal/d ▪ Proteins 18% kcal/d	Reduction of BP (systolic and diastolic) Reduction in BMI and waist circumference Improvement in cardiometabolic profile Reduction in T2DM incidence	[32,33] [34,35] [36–39] [40]
Plant-based diets	▪ Reduction or restriction of animal-derived foods ▪ High intake of plant-source foods ▪ Fat profile rich in UFAs	Reduction of BP (systolic and diastolic) Decreased body weight and risk of obesity Reduction of the risk of CVD Decreased all-cause mortality Decreased risk of T2DM	[41,42] [43–45] [46] [43,47,48] [43,47,48]
Low CH diets and very low CH diets (ketogenic diets)	▪ <50% kcal/d from carbohydrates and <10% kcal/d from CH in ketogenic diets ▪ High protein (20–30% kcal/d) ▪ High fat intake (30–70% kcal/d)	Weight-loss and weight-loss maintenance Reduction of DBP Reduction of LDL-c and triglycerides levels Increase of HDL-c levels Improvements in insulin resistance Reduction of HbA1c levels	[49–52] [52] [49–51] [49–51] [53,54] [49,51]
Low-fat diet	▪ <30% kcal/d from total fat (<10% of saturated fat) ▪ 15–17% kcal/d from protein ▪ 50–60% kcal/d from CH	Reduction of BP (systolic and diastolic) Short-term improvement of cholesterol profile Short-term weight loss Reduced risk of all-cause mortality	[33,55] [33,55] [55] [56]
High protein diet	▪ High protein (20–30% kcal/d) or 1.34–1.50 g/Kg body weight/d from protein ▪ Low CH (40–50% kcal/d)	Reduction of triglycerides levels	[57,58]

Table 1. *Cont.*

Dietary Pattern		Nutritional Distribution	Improvements in MetS Criteria	Ref.
	Nordic diet	■ High content of whole-grain high-fibre products	Reduction of BP (systolic and diastolic)	[59]
		■ Low in meat and processed foods	Increase of HDL-c levels	[59]
Other dietary patterns and strategies	Intermittent fasting	■ Fasting for a long period of time	Weight loss	[60–62]
			Improvements in insulin resistance	[60–62]
			Improvements in dyslipidaemia	[60–62]
			Reduction of BP (systolic and diastolic)	[60–62]
			Decreased risk of T2DM	[63]
			Decreased risk of CVD	[63]

[1] Monounsaturated fatty acids, MUFA; extra virgin olive oil, EVOO; carbohydrates, CH; cardiovascular disease, CVD; blood pressure, BP; type 2 diabetes mellitus, T2DM; Dietary Approaches to Stop Hypertension, DASH; unsaturated fatty acids, UFAs; body mass index, BMI; diastolic blood pressure, DBP; low-density lipoprotein cholesterol, LDL-c; high-density lipoprotein cholesterol, HDL-c; glycated hemoglobin, HbA1c; monounsaturated fatty acids, MUFA.

2. Mediterranean Diet

The MedDiet refers to the dietary pattern, culture and culinary techniques adhering to countries and populations living in the Mediterranean Sea basin [64]. This dietary pattern has stimulated a great deal of scientific evidence, demonstrating the potential health benefits associated with adherence, and the primary and secondary prevention of many health outcomes, such as CVD, T2DM, and MetS [10,22]. Recent scientific evidence concluded that the MedDiet not only has beneficial effects on health but also has beneficial effects on sustainability and culture [22,65]. Additionally, the MedDiet has been recognized by UNESCO as an Intangible Cultural Heritage of Humanity [66] and the 2015–2020 American Dietary guidelines referred to the MedDiet as an example of a healthy dietary pattern [21]. The MedDiet is a plant-based diet characterized by a high intake of vegetables including leafy green vegetables, fruits, whole-grain cereals, pulses, legumes, nuts, and extra virgin (cold pressed) olive oil (EVOO) as the main source of fat. Moreover, classical recipes are seasoned with sauces such as *sofrito*, whose main ingredients are olive oil, tomato, garlic, onion or leek, rich in phenolic compounds and carotenoids, such as naringenin, hydroxy-tyrosyl, lycopene and β-carotene [67]. Moderate alcohol intake of fermented alcoholic beverages such as red wine, mainly during meals, is also characteristic of the MedDiet, which also comprises a low to moderate intake of fish and poultry, and low consumption of red meat, butter, sweets, pastries and soft drinks [12,23,68]

The traditional MedDiet is a high fat and low-carbohydrate (CH) dietary pattern, which provides a 35–45% of total daily energy intake from fat, about 15% from protein, and 40–45% energy from CH [12,68]. However, the profile of this fat is mainly one of monounsaturated (MU) and polyunsaturated (PU) fatty acids (FA) and the main food sources of total fat intake are EVOO and nuts. EVOO is one of the key foods of the MedDiet and is the main contributor of monounsaturated fatty acids (MUFAs) in MedDiet countries. Oleic acid is the major component of EVOO and many studies have linked MUFA intake to improvements in insulin resistance, one of the main risk factors for MetS, and in blood lipid profile, and a reduction in both systolic and diastolic BP levels [12,24,69]. EVOO is also rich in polyphenols, which present anti-inflammatory and antioxidant effects and contribute to improving the lipid profile and endothelial function [70] Besides the beneficial effects of unsaturated fats, the whole dietary pattern characterized by the high intake of fruits and vegetables together with moderate red wine consumption provides wide nutritional components, such as antioxidant vitamins (vitamin C, E and β-carotene), phytochemicals (such as polyphenols), folates and minerals, which may exert beneficial effects [31,70].

Considering the effects of the MedDiet on MetS, Di Daniele et al. conducted a review addressing the impact of MedDiet adherence on MetS criteria, obesity and adipose tissue dysfunction [10]. The authors reported that prescription of the MedDiet can be used as a possible therapy for MetS, as it prevents the excess of adiposity and obesity-related inflammatory response. Franquesa et al. concluded that there is a strong evidence for the effect of the MedDiet on obesity and on MetS prevention in healthy or high-CVD risk individuals, as well as on the risk of mortality in overweight or obese individuals [22]. As previously cited, a meta-analysis of 12 cross-sectional and prospective cohorts showed that higher adherence to the MedDiet was associated with a 19% lower risk of developing MetS (relative risk (RR): 0.81 (95% confidence interval (CI) 0.71 to 0.92)), and individual components, such as waist circumference and BP, were also improved (RR: 0.82 (95% CI 0.70 to 0.96); RR: 0.87 (95% CI 0.77 to 0.97), respectively) [15]. Several prospective studies observed the same protective effects in Mediterranean and non-Mediterranean countries [25–27]. The CARDIA (Coronary Artery Risk Development in Young Adults) study is a prospective study including 4713 individuals which evaluated the evolution of CVD risk factors in black and white populations in the United States [28]. They observed a lower incidence of MetS in individuals with a higher adherence to the MedDiet (Hazard ratio (HR): 0.67 (95% CI 0.49 to 0.90)) compared to those with lower adherence, showing a linear trend according to the five score categories (p for trend = 0.005) [25]. Kesse-Guyot et al. conducted a prospective 6-year follow-up with 3232 subjects in the SU.VI.MAX study to evaluate the association between different MedDiet adherence scores and the incidence of MetS. They found that participants with higher adherence had a 53% lower risk compared to the lowest tertile of the MedDiet score (odds ratio (OR): 0.47 (95% CI 0.32 to 0.69) and 0.50 (95% CI 0.32 to 0.77 for each MedDiet score) [26]. In addition, MedDiet adherence scores were associated with improvements in some individual criteria for MetS, such as waist-circumference, BP, triglycerides and HDL-c levels [26]. Moreover, lower MetS prevalence was observed in Korean adults with medium to high MedDiet adherence (OR: 0.73 (95% CI 0.56 to 0.96) and 0.64 (95% CI 0.46 to 0.89), respectively) [30].

MedDiet adherence has been inversely associated with the incidence of CVD and mortality, as well as cancer and degenerative diseases [23,71]. In the case of CVD, the MedDiet is associated with clinically meaningful reductions in the risk of developing the main CVD outcomes, including coronary heart disease and stroke [72]. In a prospective cohort study with 25,994 healthy women from the US Women's Health Study, Ahmad et al. observed an inverse association between the highest MedDiet adherence score and the incidence of CVD compared to the lowest score (HR: 0.72 (95% CI 0.61 to 0.86), p for trend < 0.001) [73]. Among the health effects observed, MedDiet interventions have shown improvements in body composition by reducing total and segmental fat, which might have an effect on metabolic profile [10]. Furthermore, the MedDiet has contributed to a decrease in the incidence of T2DM and CVD, while lessening severity and associated complications in individuals who have already been diagnosed [12,22,23,29,31]. Due to the health benefits associated with this easy-to-follow dietary pattern, the MedDiet should be considered as one of the first treatment strategies for the prevention and management of MetS.

3. DASH Diet

In 1997, the Dietary Approaches to Stop Hypertension (DASH) diet became a promising strategy for the treatment of high BP [74], and subsequent randomized clinical trials (RCTs) have supported this evidence [32]. This eating pattern promotes vegetables, fruits, whole grains, low- or free-fat dairy products, legumes and nuts intake, while restricting the intake of red and processed meat and sugar-sweetened beverages [74,75]. The DASH diet is characterized by a low-fat content (27% of daily calorie intake from fat), especially saturated fats (6% of energy) and dietary cholesterol (150 mg/d approximately), and reduced sodium content (from 1500 to 2300 mg/day), but it is rich in fiber (>30 g/day), potassium, magnesium and calcium compared to other dietary patterns [55,76]. The DASH diet has proven to be a useful strategy for the treatment of hypertension [32,33,55,77], and several epidemiological studies have associated higher adherence to the DASH diet with a better cardiometabolic profile [34,36–39,78–80]. In a meta-analysis of several cohort studies, Schwingshackl et al. reported that higher adherence to the DASH diet was associated with a significant reduction in the risk of all-cause mortality (RR: 0.78 (95% CI 0.77 to 0.80), the incidence of or mortality by CVD and cancer (RR: 0.78 (95% CI 0.76 to 0.80); RR: 0.84 (95% CI 0.82 to 0.87), respectively) and the incidence of T2DM (RR: 0.82 (95% CI 0.78 to 0.85)) [40].

Regarding the use of DASH diet as an approach for the treatment of hypertension, a recent meta-analysis of 30 RCT with 5545 hypertensive and non-hypertensive participants concluded that the DASH diet together with lifestyle interventions significantly decreased systolic and diastolic BP measurements compared with a control diet (mean differences: −3.2 mm Hg (95% CI −4.2 to −2.3) and −2.5 mm Hg (95% CI −3.5 to −1.5), respectively) [32]. This effect was more pronounced when sodium intake was lower than 2400 mg/d, in subjects under the age of 50, and in participants with hypertension but without antihypertensive medication [32]. Moreover, on comparing the antihypertensive effects of the DASH diet with 13 other eating patterns (including low-fat diet, Nordic diet, MedDiet, Paleolithic diet and low-sodium diet), the DASH diet was the most effective, especially in comparison with low-fat diets [33]. In contrast, Ge et al. identified the Paleolithic and Atkins diets as the most effective dietary patterns for both systolic and diastolic BP management after six months of intervention compared to usual dietary advice, although this effect was not observed after one year of intervention [55].

The DASH diet intervention has also shown potential effects against excess body weight and abdominal obesity [35]. Middle-term dietary interventions have shown a significant reduction in body mass index (BMI) (weighted mean difference: −0.42 kg/m2 (95% CI −0.64 to −0.20)) and waist circumference (−1.05 cm (95% CI −1.61 to −0.49)) [35]. Nevertheless, in overweight or obese individuals, DASH dietary approaches showed significant weight loss compared to other dietary patterns (−3.63 kg (95% Credible Interval −2.52 to −4.76)) whereas this weight loss was lower after one year of intervention (−3.08 kg (95% Credible Interval −0.48 to −5.66)) [55].

The results are not consistent in the case of blood lipoproteins [55,77]. Ge et al. did not observe significant differences in HDL-c or low-density lipoprotein-cholesterol (LDL-c) levels after a DASH dietary intervention versus usual diet [55], whereas in a meta-analysis of 1917 participants with some CVD risk factors, Siervo et al. observed a reduction in total cholesterol and LDL-c levels after the DASH intervention (mean differences: −0.20 mmol/L (95% CI −0.31 to −0.10) and −0.10 mmol/L (95% CI −0.20 to 0.01), respectively), but reported no significant differences in HDL-c and triglyceride levels [77]. Similar results were obtained in a recently published controlled trial in 80 T2DM patients after 12 weeks following the DASH diet compared to an antidiabetic diet based on American Diabetes Association guidelines [81]. Both dietary interventions significantly reduced triglycerides, total cholesterol and very-low-density lipoproteins.

Epidemiological evidence suggests an association between higher adherence to the DASH diet and a better cardiometabolic profile and lower risk of CVD [36–39]. A cross-sectional study of 1493 adults showed that higher adherence to the DASH diet was associated with 48% less risk of developing MetS, whereas BMI, waist circumference, pro-inflammatory markers and adiposity measures were significantly lower compared to individuals with lower adherence [34]. Interestingly, Ashari et al. observed that higher adherence to the DASH diet was associated with a 64% lower risk of MetS in 425 healthy children and adolescents from 6–18 years of age [82]. In addition, the authors also observed inverse associations among adherence to the DASH diet and BP, fasting plasma glucose levels and abdominal obesity [82]. In this sense, adaptation of the DASH diet to type 1 diabetes glucose requirements (a reduction in CH of around 10% and 15% increase in fat content) resulted in better glucose control and improved the quality of the whole diet, showing a higher intake of fruits, vegetables, fiber and protein compared to the usual intake [83].

The health benefits associated with the DASH diet are probably due to its nutritional quality and distribution. The DASH diet is rich in vegetables and fruits, which translate into high potassium, magnesium and fiber intake, and these nutrients have shown to have a role in BP control, glucose metabolism and insulin response [84]. Furthermore, vegetables and fruits are the main food source of antioxidants and polyphenols, which have been linked to better glucose and insulin blood levels [84]. Moreover, it is limited in sodium and fat, mainly saturated fatty acids (SFA), which are closely related to CVD [84]. Nonetheless, Pickering et al. suggested that the potential health effects of the DASH diet are dependent on eating pattern adherence, with subjects with lower adherence to the DASH diet showing greater benefit from DASH dietary interventions in BP control than those with higher adherence before the dietary intervention [85]. Nonetheless, the commitment and implication of the patient are critical in all life-style interventions based on dietary modifications [86,87].

4. Plant-Based Diets

Plant-based diets include a wide variety of dietary patterns, which are characterized by a reduction or restriction in animal-derived food intake and the promotion of plant-source food intake, such as fruits, vegetables, nuts, legumes, and grains. Among plant-based diets, strict vegetarian diets, also known as vegan diets, are defined by the exclusion of all animal-derived products, including dairy products, eggs and honey; lacto-vegetarian diets restrict animal food intake except for dairy products; lacto-ovo-vegetarian diets exclude meat, seafood and poultry but include eggs and dairy products; and pesco-vegetarians or pescatarians are similar to lacto-ovo-vegetarian but include fish [88]. Despite the fact that plant-based diets are defined by the exclusion of some or all animal products, recent evidence defines plant-based diets as dietary patterns that promote a reduction in animal-source food intake along with an increase in plant-based food intake, such as the MedDiet [41,88–90].

Plant-based diets have consistently been associated with beneficial cardiometabolic effects, specifically with a lower risk of developing MetS and all of its components [91]. Moreover, these dietary patterns are associated with decreased all-cause mortality and a decreased risk of obesity, T2DM and CVD [43,47,48]. Some studies have found a lower risk of mortality from ischemic heart disease in vegetarians compared with non-vegetarians [43]. Additionally, recent systematic reviews and meta-analyses found significant associations between adherence to the MedDiet and DASH diets and a 38% and 20% lower risk of CVD, respectively, while a 28% reduction in the risk of coronary heart disease was observed following a vegetarian diet [46].

Regarding BP, a meta-analysis of seven RCTs reported a mean reduction of 4.8 mmHg in systolic BP (95% CI −3.1 to −6.6; $p < 0.001$) and a 2.2 mmHg reduction in diastolic BP (95% CI −1.0 to −3.5; $p < 0.001$) in participants following a vegetarian diet compared to an omnivorous diet [42]. These results were confirmed by the same authors in a meta-analysis of 32 observational studies including 604 participants, in which an association was observed between vegetarian diets and reductions in systolic and diastolic BP (−6.9 mmHg (95% CI −9.1 to −4.7; $p < 0.01$) and −4.7 mmHg (95% CI −6.3 to −3.1; $p < 0.01$), respectively) [41,42].

The effects of plant-based diets on blood lipid concentrations are controversial. Wang et al. conducted a meta-analysis of 11 RCTs to evaluate the effects of vegetarian diet on triglycerides, LDL-c, HDL-c and non-HDL-c levels [92]. Total cholesterol levels, LDL-c and HDL-c, were significantly reduced after following a vegetarian diet compared to an omnivorous control diet (0.36 mmol/L (95% CI 0.55 to 0.17; $p < 0.001$), 0.34 mmol/L (95% CI 0.57 to 0.11; $p < 0.001$) and 0.10 mmol/L (95% CI 0.14 to 0.06; $p < 0.001$), respectively). No significant effects were observed for triglyceride levels. This study also described a significant weight-loss in participants who followed the vegetarian compared to the omnivorous diet (−2.88 kg (95% CI −3.56 to −2.20; $p < 0.001$)). Similar results were observed in another meta-analysis of 12 RCTs involving 1151 individuals, in which subjects randomized to the vegetarian diet intervention group showed significant weight loss compared to the non-vegetarian group (mean difference −2.02 kg (95% CI −2.80 to −1.23; $p < 0.001$)) [44]. Other studies assessing plant-based dietary patterns, such as the MedDiet, have also described positive effects on body weight and waist circumference [45].

The health benefits observed are mainly explained by the nutritional quality of plant-based diets as they promote the intake of a wide variety of plant-based foods while cutting down the intake of animal-derived products, such as red and processed meat, which have been associated with a higher risk of developing T2DM, CVD and certain types of cancer [93]. However, it is important to consider that the term "plant-based" does not necessary mean "healthy", as there is evidence supporting adverse health effects of the excessive intake of some plant-derived foods, such as refined grains, snacks, pastries or sugar-sweetened beverages [41,88,94]. A healthy plant-based diet promotes the intake of whole grains, fruits, vegetables, legumes, and non-hydrogenated vegetable oils, such as EVOO. Thus, plant-based diets have low-energy density and high fiber content, which may contribute to CVD prevention, weight loss and long-term body weight maintenance [41,44,88]. Moreover, the profile of fat is mainly MUFA and polyunsaturated fatty acids (PUFA), while SFA intake is lower compared to other dietary patterns. Replacing SFA by MUFA and PUFA has been linked with anti-inflammatory effects and improvements in insulin sensitivity [88]. Among plant-derived foods, the antioxidant effect exerted by several nutrients and bioactive compounds such as vitamin C and E, β-carotenes and polyphenols has been linked to the prevention of CVD and MetS [41,88,95]. Finally, the replacement of some animal-derived foods implies intake restriction of the harmful components mainly present in red and processed meat, such as excessive sodium, heme iron, nitrates and nitrites, which have been linked to CVD outcomes [41,88,96].

In conclusion, recent evidence has demonstrated the protective effect of plant-based diets against MetS, CVD and their individual risk factors. However, healthy plant-derived food choices are crucial to ensure these beneficial effects. Thus, dietary guidelines should consider healthy plant-based dietary patterns as a potential dietary strategy for the prevention and treatment of MetS.

5. Low-Carbohydrate Diet

Low-CH dietary patterns are characterized by a reduction of total CH intake (<50% of daily calorie intake from CH). This type of diet implies a restriction in the intake of several ultra-processed foods, refined grains, starches and foods rich in simple or added sugars [1]. The association between CH intake and the prevalence and management of the MetS is discrepant [97]. In a meta-analysis of 18 studies with 69,554 MetS patients, Lui et al. concluded that the risk of developing MetS was increased in individuals with higher CH intake (2.5% increase in the risk of MetS per 5% energy from CH intake (95% CI 0.4 to 4.8)) [97]. Moreover, some effects on lipid profile were observed in individuals with high CH intake, such as elevated BP, triglycerides and LDL-c and reduced HDL-c levels [98,99]. The mechanisms underlying the health benefits observed in low-CH diets are the avoidance of the rapid absorption associated with some types of CH, such as glucose and refined grains, which leads to an increase in insulin resistance and insulin demand [53,54]. Therefore, in the case of T2DM, recent clinical guidelines do not recommend a specific CH distribution or restriction, and dietary individualization must be prioritized in the treatment and management of this condition [49]. Bazzano et al. conducted a RCT to analyze the effect of a low-CH diet (<40% of total energy intake from CH) compared with a low-fat diet (<30% of total energy from fat, <7% SFA) without energy restriction or physical activity advice in obese adults (BMI 30 to 45 kg/m^2) [50]. After 1 year of intervention, subjects on the low-CH diet without energy restriction showed greater weight loss (−3.5 kg (95% CI −5.6 to −1.4 kg)), specifically in fat mass (−1.5% (CI −2.6% to −0.4%)). Moreover, some cardiovascular risk factors were improved in the low-CH group, such as triglycerides, HDL-c and total cholesterol to HDL-c ratio [50]. Regarding the management of T2DM, low-CH compared to low-fat dietary interventions (<30% of total energy from fat) showed higher reductions of body weight, glycosylated hemoglobin (HbA1c), triglycerides and BP levels and increased HDL-c concentrations and, consequently, a modification in glucose-lowering medications was observed [49,51].

Recent evidence has shown an association between dietary CH intake and the risk of mortality. The Prospective Urban Rural Epidemiology (PURE) study is a cohort study of 135,335 individuals aged 35–70 years from 18 countries from five continents [98]. The aim of this study was to assess the association of dietary fat and CH intake and total mortality and CVD, differentiating this intake according to the profile of FA and CH. The findings of this study suggest the need for an update in dietary guidelines, with emphasis on fat restriction to promote low-fat and CH dietary patterns (around 50–55% of daily energy intake from CH) rich in PUFA and whole-grain CH. Other studies have also observed an association between refined CH intake and a higher risk of cardiovascular events, such as stroke or myocardial infarction [100,101]. However, there is insufficient scientific evidence on low-CH diets (<50–55% of total energy intake) and metabolic improvements have not been demonstrated in order to support or recommend very-low CH diets [98]. Seidelmann et al. observed that with high (>70% of total energy intake) and low (<40%) CH diets the total mortality increased, with 50–55% showing the lowest risk of mortality, representing a U-shaped association [102]. The replacement of CH with other nutrients has shown different effects on total mortality, which was increased in low-CH diets rich in animal-derived fat and/or protein. By definition, low-CH diets promote the restriction of foods rich in CH, such as vegetables, fruits, whole-grain cereals, legumes, etc. Consequently, low-CH diets, compared to diets with 50–55% of energy from CH, showed lower amounts of bioactive compounds such as fiber, PUFAs, polyphenols, vitamins and minerals [103]. Therefore, the use of very low-CH diets as a dietary approach for MetS should promote plant-based fat and/or protein food sources [102].

Among low-CH diets, it has been postulated that very low CH ketogenic diets have a therapeutic role in several NCDs, including overweight and obesity, CVD and MetS [104]. Although there is no standardized definition of the ketogenic diet, it is characterized by a reduction in CH to less than 10% of daily energy intake, which means around 30 to 50 g of CH per day, and a relative increase of fat intake (fat to CH and protein intake ratio of 3:1 to 4:1) [105]. This restrictive dietary pattern has shown protective effects for obesity and CVD by reducing body weight and improving the lipid profile [104,106–108]. The meta-analysis of Bueno et al. observed greater weight loss (weighted mean difference −0.91 kg (95% CI −1.65 to −0.17 kg)), and reduced triglyceride (−0.18 mmol/L (95% CI −0.27 to −0.08)) and diastolic BP levels (−1.43 mmHg (CI −2.49 to −0.37)), while HDL-c levels increased (0.09 mmol/L (95% CI 0.06 to 0.12)) after following a ketogenic diet compared to a low-fat diet [52]. The mechanisms of action underlying these protective effects are as follows: the absence of dietary CH intake leads to a decrease in insulin secretion, which is translated into an inhibition of lipogenesis and fat accumulation and an increase in lipolysis; a satiety effect of protein intake and its effect on appetite control hormones, such as leptin and ghrelin; and the modulation of insulin secretion and ketone body production which might lead to metabolic improvements, especially in insulin signaling [104,109]. Moreover, CH restriction and the glycogen depletion characteristic of this type of diet lead to the use of ketone bodies as the main source of energy. Nevertheless, energy restriction is necessary to maintain ketone body production. Thus, recent evidence suggests that body weight and CVD benefits observed with ketogenic dietary interventions are due to energy restriction, in spite of the macronutrient distribution of the diet [104,110]. However, health care professionals should consider the difficulties in following a ketogenic diet and the absence of healthy foods such as vegetables, fruits and whole-grain cereals, the intake of which is associated with a lower risk of developing chronic diseases such as CVD, T2DM and some types of cancer.

6. Low-Fat Diet

By definition, the fat content of the low-fat diet comprises less than 30% of total energy, of which <10% are SFA, with a moderate PUFA content and limited *trans* FA [111,112]. In proportion, CH intake is higher and protein intake is moderate (around 15–17% of total energy intake). Low-fat diets usually include foods and products with reduced total fat content, such as low-fat dairy products instead of whole-fat products and derivatives. Low fat diets in weight-loss oriented dietary interventions showed a reduction in the risk of premature mortality in obese adults [56]. In this sense, a meta-analysis of 34 RCTs observed an 18% lower risk of all-cause mortality in weight-loss oriented dietary interventions in obese adults (95% CI 0.71 to 0.95), while no significant effects were observed in CVD mortality or incidence [56]. Recently, a network meta-analysis described the effectiveness of the low-fat diet for body weight reduction compared to the usual dietary advice and dietary patterns after short-term intervention (6 months), with this effect being attenuated after one year [55].

Clinical trials evaluating the effect of a low-fat diet on the prevalence of MetS have shown conflicting results [113–116]. Dietary interventions based on low-fat intake (around 20% of total energy intake from fat) slightly reduced MetS components, but no significant effects were observed for CVD or the incidence of coronary heart disease in postmenopausal women compared to the usual diet [113,114]. Nevertheless, following a low-fat diet was not associated with a lower prevalence of MetS in older subjects at high CVD risk [115]. In this sense, Veum et al. compared the effect of a low-fat, high-CH diet (around 30% of total energy intake from fat) vs. a very high-fat, low-CH diet (around 73% total energy intake from fat) on MetS components [117]. No significant differences were observed in MetS components, body weight and body composition in the medium-term [117]. Similar findings were described by Gardner et al. in the DIETFITS trial, in which both low-fat and low-CH dietary approaches showed significant weight loss with no differences between the two interventions [118].

Regarding BP and blood lipoproteins, a low-fat diet showed beneficial effects on systolic and diastolic BP management, and improved HDL-c and LDL-c levels in the short term compared to usual diet, but these effects were reduced in long-term interventions [33,55]. However, in a meta-analysis of RCTs including 17,230 hypertensive and pre-hypertensive participants, Schwingshackl et al. suggested that the MedDiet and the DASH diet are more effective in long-term BP management compared to low-fat diets [33]. Likewise, low-CH diets showed greater effects on the control of glycated hemoglobin and blood lipid levels than low-fat diets in a short to medium term intervention [52,112,119,120]. In the case of glucose metabolism and insulin control, some RCTs have not identified significant effects of low-fat dietary interventions versus other dietary approaches, while higher triglyceride levels were observed, mostly when simple CH proportion is increased [121–125]. In the case of T2DM management,

Basterra-Gortari et al. found that a low-fat diet did not have an effect on glucose-lowering medication management while the MedDiet supplemented with EVOO could delay its requirement in older people at high CVD risk [126].

MetS is associated with a pro-inflammatory state, and it has been proposed that a low-fat dietary intervention inducing weight loss slightly reduces inflammatory biomarkers such as high-sensitive c-reactive protein (CRP), interleukin−6 (IL) and tumor necrosis factor alpha (TNF-α) levels [16,127–129]. These results are inconclusive, and the effects observed depend on weight loss and diet composition, particularly dietary fiber, fruits and vegetables [16,128]. Additionally, some studies observed that low-fat dietary interventions could improve the microbiome dysbiosis linked to MetS by increasing α-diversity [130,131]. However, limited results are available and more evidence regarding long-term response is needed [132]. Furthermore, nutrigenetic interactions have been described between dietary fat content and metabolic response [133].

Based on the evidence available, current dietary guidelines, such as the 2015–2020 American and European Dietary Guidelines, should avoid stating upper limits of total fat intake, mainly from healthy unsaturated FA. Moreover, this recommendation should include not exceeding 10% of total energy intake from SFA and the replacement of SFA by MUFA and PUFA [22,134].

7. High-Protein Diet

Recent evidence suggests that a high-protein dietary pattern leads to greater weight-loss and CVD improvements than standard protein diets (0.8 g protein/kg body weight). High-protein diets are characterized by a 20–30% of daily energy intake from protein, which means around 1.34 to 1.5 g protein/kg body weight [57]. Currently, the use of high-protein dietary interventions has been postulated for the treatment of obesity, MetS and glycemic control [58,93]. The effect of high-protein dietary strategies for weight management is controversial. A meta-analysis of 18 studies on the effect of a high-protein diet in T2DM patients showed that a high-protein diet did not significantly decrease body weight compared to a regular protein diet [135]. Moreover, no significant effects where observed for glycemic control parameters, such as fasting glucose, insulin and HbA1c, blood lipid profile or BP levels. Nevertheless, a significant reduction of triglyceride levels was observed in participants who followed a high-protein diet. In the case of MetS, high-protein diets with CH restriction have shown effective weight-loss in obese adults with MetS [57,58]. Campos-Nonato et al. performed a RCT in 118 adults with MetS to evaluate the effect of a hypocaloric high-protein diet compared to a hypocaloric standard protein diet (500 kcal/day less than the metabolic rate and 1.34 g protein/kg body weight or 0.8 g protein/kg body weight, respectively) [57]. Weight-loss after 6 months of the dietary interventions was significantly higher in participants who followed a high-protein diet (−7.0 kg ± 3.7; p-value = 0.046) compared to the standard protein diet (−5.1 kg ± 3.6; p-value = 0.157) [57]. MetS criteria, including fasting blood glucose, insulin, homeostatic model assessment for insulin resistance (HOMA-IR) index, and triglyceride, and cholesterol levels, improved in both intervention arms, but non-significant differences were observed in the comparison between groups. The Optimal Macronutrient Intake Trial to Prevent Heart Disease (OmniHeart) study was a randomized, controlled, three-period, crossover nutritional study with 164 participants with overweight or obesity and prehypertension or stage 1 hypertension free of T2DM [136]. This study aimed to evaluate insulin sensitivity with the quantitative insulin sensitivity check index among three dietary interventions: a high-CH diet (58% of daily kcal from CH; 15% from protein and 27% from fat); a protein diet (replacement of 10% of total CH to protein, 25% of daily kcal intake from protein, mainly from plant-based protein sources); and an unsaturated diet (replacement of 10% of total CH to unsaturated fat, 37% of daily kcal intake from fat, mainly from seeds and oils such as olive, canola and safflower oils and nuts). The protein and high-CH dietary patterns did not affect insulin sensitivity, while the unsaturated diet showed improvements in insulin sensitivity, suggesting that the replacement of CH by unsaturated fat, such as in the MedDiet patterns, are alternative dietary approaches to improve insulin sensitivity. The mechanism underlying the potential health benefits of a high-protein diet is that protein induces satiety, which is translated into reduced energy intake in the next meals [137,138]. Furthermore, high protein intake avoids muscle mass loss during energy-restrictive dietary interventions for weight loss [139].

Among protein food sources, meat and meat derived products have been associated with a higher risk of developing T2DM, CVD and MetS [12,13,140]. Dietary guidelines recommend prioritizing plant-based protein food sources such as soy, legumes, beans, nuts and seeds instead of meat and processed meat [21]. Plant-based protein food sources are rich in fibre, phenolic compounds and PUFA, while cholesterol, trans or SFA are in lower proportions [141]. In a recent meta-analysis of 36 RCTs, red meat consumption had no effect on the blood lipid profile or BP, while after analyses stratified by the type of comparison diet, the substitution of red meat with plant-based protein foods showed a reduction in total cholesterol and LDL-c levels [93]. Thus, strong evidence promotes the intake of plant-based protein food sources, and this should also be recommended to promote environmental sustainability.

8. Other Dietary Patterns and Strategies

Other dietary alterations have been shown to improve the MetS condition, such as the Nordic Diet, which is characterized by a high content of whole-grain high-fiber products (such as rye, barley, oat, rice, vegetables, fruits and nuts), with rapeseed oil as the main source of dietary fat and a high intake of fish and shellfish [142,143]. Similar to the DASH and the MedDiet, the Nordic diet is considered to be a healthy dietary pattern in that it promotes the intake of vegetables, fruits, fish, poultry, nuts, and is low in sodium, red meat and processed foods. A recent meta-analysis of 5 RCTs including 513 participants demonstrated the effectiveness of the Nordic diet in improving some MetS criteria, mainly systolic and diastolic BP (weighted mean differences −3.97 mmHg (95% CI −6.40 to −1.54; $p < 0.001$); −2.08 mmHg (95% CI −3.43 to −0.72; $p = 0.003$), respectively) [59]. Moreover, improvements in LDL-c (0.30 mmol/l (95% CI −0.54 to −0.06; $p = 0.013$)), but not in HDL-c and TG levels, were observed compared to control diets [59]. Further studies are needed to evaluate the beneficial effects of the Nordic diet on MetS management and prevention.

Among dietary strategies, intermittent fasting has shown benefits for CVD, T2DM, metabolic disturbances and cancer, mainly because of the daily caloric restriction involved [63]. The main cardiometabolic effects observed after an intermittent-fasting intervention are weight loss and improvements in insulin resistance, dyslipidemia, BP levels and inflammation [60–62]. Despite the evidence and potential health benefits of intermittent fasting, the applicability of this dietary strategy is complex and trained health care providers are needed to avoid side effects. Furthermore, De la Iglesia et al. postulated other potential dietary approaches for the prevention and treatment of MetS, such as diets rich in omega−3 FA, low glycemic index, high antioxidant capacity or high meal frequency dietary interventions [144].

Thus, dietary intervention based on energy restriction, independently of the distribution of macronutrients, might influence BP and CVD. Accordingly, most scientific evidence highlights the relevance of dietary quality rather than quantity, especially in the management and prevention of MetS [8,145–147]. Moreover, the effectiveness of every dietary intervention is associated with the previous metabolic state (e.g., presence of insulin resistance, T2DM, altered fasting glucose levels, etc.) [148,149]. While multifaceted lifestyle interventions focus on weight-loss and the promotion of physical activity, adherence is the key factor in achieving the beneficial effects observed in each dietary pattern, with intervention adherence being decisive in the results observed independently of the type of diet [150–152].

9. Conclusions

The protective effects of healthy dietary patterns on MetS seem to be due to the sum of small dietary changes rather than the restriction of any single nutrient. On comparing low-fat diets and very-restricted diets, the scientific evidence supports the use of the MedDiet intervention as the new paradigm for MetS prevention and treatment. The nutritional distribution and quality of the MedDiet allows health professionals to provide easy-to-follow dietary advice without the need for a restricted diet. Nonetheless, RCTs on the effects of a low-CH MedDiet style diet, promoting the intake of whole grain and plant-based protein food sources in patients with MetS, are needed to demonstrate the efficacy of this dietary pattern.

Author Contributions: Conceptualization, R.C. and S.C.-B.; writing—original draft preparation, S.C.-B.; A.M.R.-L.; M.S.-P.; writing—review and editing, R.E. and R.C.; supervision, R.C. All authors have read and agreed to the published version of the manuscript.

Acknowledgments: This work has been partially supported by PIE14/00045, PI16/00381 and PI19/01226 from the Instituto de Salud Carlos III, Spain. CIBER OBN is an initiative of the Instituto de Salud Carlos III, Spain. S.C.-B. thanks the Spanish Ministry of Science Innovation and Universities for the Formación de Profesorado Universitario (FPU17/00785) contract.

References

1.   Mozaffarian, D. Dietary and Policy Priorities for Cardiovascular Disease, Diabetes, and Obesity: A Comprehensive Review. *Circulation* **2016**, *133*, 187–225. [CrossRef] [PubMed]

2.   Seuring, T.; Archangelidi, O.; Suhrcke, M. The Economic Costs of Type 2 Diabetes: A Global Systematic Review. *Pharmacoeconomics* **2015**, *33*, 811–831. [CrossRef] [PubMed]

3.   Gheorghe, A.; Griffiths, U.; Murphy, A.; Legido-Quigley, H.; Lamptey, P.; Perel, P. The economic burden of cardiovascular disease and hypertension in low- and middle-income countries: A systematic review. *BMC Public Health* **2018**, *18*, 975. [CrossRef] [PubMed]

4.   Alberti, K.G.M.M.; Eckel, R.H.; Grundy, S.M.; Zimmet, P.Z.; Cleeman, J.I.; Donato, K.A.; Fruchart, J.C.; Loria, C.M.; Smith, S.C., Jr. Harmonizing the metabolic syndrome: A joint interim statement of the international diabetes federation task force on epidemiology and prevention; National heart, lung, and blood institute; American heart association; World heart federation; International atherosclerosis society; and international association for the study of obesity. *Circulation* **2009**, *120*, 1640–1645. [CrossRef]

5.   Cano-Ibáñez, N.; Gea, A.; Martínez-González, M.A.; Salas-Salvadó, J.; Corella, D.; Zomeño, M.D.; Romaguera, D.; Vioque, J.; Aros, F.; Wärnberg, J.; et al. Dietary diversity and nutritional adequacy among an older Spanish population with metabolic syndrome in the PREDIMED-plus study: A cross-sectional analysis. *Nutrients* **2019**, *11*, 958. [CrossRef]

6.   Garralda-Del-Villar, M.; Carlos-Chillerón, S.; Diaz-Gutierrez, J.; Ruiz-Canela, M.; Gea, A.; Martínez-González, M.A.; Bes-Restrollo, M.; Ruiz-Estigarribia, L.; Kales, S.N.; Fernández-Montero, A. Healthy lifestyle and incidence of metabolic syndrome in the SUN cohort. *Nutrients* **2018**, *11*, 65. [CrossRef]

7.   Saklayen, M.G. The Global Epidemic of the Metabolic Syndrome. *Curr. Hypertens. Rep.* **2018**, *20*, 12. [CrossRef]

8.   Julibert, A.; Bibiloni, M.D.M.; Mateos, D.; Angullo, E.; Tur, J.A. Dietary Fat Intake and Metabolic Syndrome in Older Adults. *Nutrients* **2019**, *11*, 1901. [CrossRef]

9.   Wang, H.H.; Lee, D.K.; Liu, M.; Portincasa, P.; Wang, D.Q. Novel Insights into the Pathogenesis and Management of the Metabolic Syndrome. *Pediatr. Gastroenterol. Hepatol. Nutr.* **2020**, *23*, 189–230. [CrossRef]

10.   Di Daniele, N.D.; Noce, A.; Vidiri, M.F.; Moriconi, E.; Marrone, G.; Annicchiarico-Petruzzelli, M.; D'Urso, G.; Tesauro, M.; Rovella, V.; De Lorenzo, A. Impact of Mediterranean diet on metabolic syndrome, cancer and longevity. *Oncotarget* **2017**, *8*, 8947–8979. [CrossRef]

11.   Mendrick, D.L.; Diehl, A.M.; Topor, L.S.; Dietert, R.R.; Will, Y.; La Merrill, M.A.; Bouret, S.; Varma, V.; Hastings, K.L.; Schug, T.T.; et al. Metabolic Syndrome and Associated Diseases: From the Bench to the Clinic. *Toxicol. Sci.* **2018**, *162*, 36–42. [CrossRef] [PubMed]

12.   Pérez-Martínez, P.; Mikhailidis, D.P.; Athyros, V.G.; Bullo, M.; Couture, P.; Covas, M.I.; de Koning, L.; Delgado-Lista, J.; Díaz-López, A.; Drevon, C.A.; et al. Lifestyle recommendations for the prevention and management of metabolic syndrome: An international panel recommendation. *Nutr. Rev.* **2017**, *75*, 307–326. [CrossRef] [PubMed]

13.   Worm, N. Beyond Body Weight-Loss: Dietary Strategies Targeting Intrahepatic Fat in NAFLD. *Nutrients* **2020**, *12*, 1316. [CrossRef] [PubMed]

14. Steckhan, N.; Hohmann, C.D.; Kessler, C.; Dobos, G.; Michalsen, A.; Cramer, H. Effects of different dietary approaches on inflammatory markers in patients with metabolic syndrome: A systematic review and meta-analysis. *Nutrition* **2016**, *32*, 338–348. [CrossRef]

15. Godos, J.; Zappalà, G.; Bernardini, S.; Giambini, I.; Bes-Rastrollo, M.; Martinez-Gonzalez, M. Adherence to the Mediterranean diet is inversely associated with metabolic syndrome occurrence: A meta-analysis of observational studies. *Int. J. Food Sci. Nutr.* **2017**, *68*, 138–148. [CrossRef]

16. Tresserra-Rimbau, A.; Castro-Barquero, S.; Vitelli-Storelli, F.; Becerra-Tomas, N.; Vázquez-Ruiz, Z.; Díaz-López, A.; Corella, D.; Castañer, O.; Romaguera, D.; Vioque, J.; et al. Associations between dietary polyphenols and type 2 diabetes in a cross-sectional analysis of the PREDIMED-Plus trial: Role of body mass index and sex. *Antioxidants* **2019**, *8*, 537. [CrossRef]

17. Castro-Barquero, S.; Tresserra-Rimbau, A.; Vitelli-Storelli, F.; Doménech, M.; Salas-Salvadó, J.; Martín-Sánchez, V.; Rubín-García, M.; Buil-Cosiales, P.; Corella, D.; Fitó, M.; et al. Dietary Polyphenol Intake is Associated with HDL-Cholesterol and A Better Profile of other Components of the Metabolic Syndrome: A PREDIMED-Plus Sub-Study. *Nutrients* **2020**, *12*, 689. [CrossRef]

18. Sayón-Orea, C.; Razquin, C.; Bulló, M.; Corella, D.; Fitó, M.; Romaguera, D.; Vioque, J.; Alonso-Gómez, Á.M.; Wärnberg, J.; Martínez, J.A.; et al. Effect of a Nutritional and Behavioral Intervention on Energy-Reduced Mediterranean Diet Adherence Among Patients with Metabolic Syndrome: Interim Analysis of the PREDIMED-Plus Randomized Clinical Trial. *JAMA* **2019**, *322*, 1486–1499. [CrossRef]

19. Julibert, A.; Bibiloni, M.D.M.; Bouzas, C.; Martínez-González, M.Á.; Salas-Salvadó, J.; Corella, D.; Zomeño, M.D.; Romaguera, D.; Vioque, J.; Alonso-Gómez, Á.M.; et al. Total and Subtypes of Dietary Fat Intake and Its Association with Components of the Metabolic Syndrome in a Mediterranean Population at High Cardiovascular Risk. *Nutrients* **2019**, *11*, 1493. [CrossRef]

20. Alvarez-Alvarez, I.; Toledo, E.; Lecea, O.; Salas-Salvadó, J.; Corella, D.; Buil-Cosiales, P.; Zomeño, M.D.; Vioque, J.; Martínez, J.A.; Konieczna, J.; et al. Adherence to a priori dietary indexes and baseline prevalence of cardiovascular risk factors in the PREDIMED-Plus randomised trial. *Eur. J. Nutr.* **2020**, *59*, 1219–1232. [CrossRef]

21. McGuire, S. Scientific Report of the 2015 Dietary Guidelines Advisory Committee. Washington, DC: US Departments of Agriculture and Health and Human Services, 2015. *Adv. Nutr.* **2016**, *7*, 202–204. [CrossRef] [PubMed]

22. Franquesa, M.; Pujol-Busquets, G.; García-Fernández, E.; Rico, L.; Shamirian-Pulido, L.; Aguilar-Martínez, A.; Medina, F.X.; Serra-Majem, L.; Bach-Faig, A. Mediterranean Diet and Cardiodiabesity: A Systematic Review through Evidence-Based Answers to Key Clinical Questions. *Nutrients* **2019**, *11*, 655. [CrossRef] [PubMed]

23. Finicelli, M.; Squillaro, T.; Di Cristo, F.; Di Salle, A.; Melone, M.A.B.; Galderisi, U.; Peluso, G. Metabolic syndrome, Mediterranean diet, and polyphenols: Evidence and perspectives. *J. Cell Physiol.* **2019**, *234*, 5807–5826. [CrossRef] [PubMed]

24. Gaforio, J.J.; Visioli, F.; Alarcón-De-la-lastra, C.; Castañer, O.; Delgado-Rodríguez, M.; Fitó, M.; Hernánedez, A.F.; Huertas, J.R.; Martínez-González, M.A.; Menendez, J.A.; et al. Virgin Olive Oil and Health: Summary of the III International Conference on Virgin Olive Oil and Health Consensus Report, JAEN (Spain) 2018. *Nutrients* **2019**, *11*, 2039. [CrossRef] [PubMed]

25. Steffen, L.M.; Van Horn, L.; Daviglus, M.L.; Zhou, X.; Reis, J.P.; Loria, C.M.; Jacobs, D.R.; Duffey, K.J. A modified Mediterranean diet score is associated with a lower risk of incident metabolic syndrome over 25 years among young adults: The CARDIA (Coronary Artery Risk Development in Young Adults) study. *Br. J. Nutr.* **2014**, *112*, 1654–1661. [CrossRef]

26. Kesse-Guyot, E.; Ahluwalia, N.; Lassale, C.; Hercberg, S.; Fezeu, L.; Lairon, D. Adherence to Mediterranean diet reduces the risk of metabolic syndrome: A 6-year prospective study. *Nutr. Metab. Cardiovasc. Dis.* **2013**, *23*, 677–683. [CrossRef]

27. Mirmiran, P.; Moslehi, N.; Mahmoudof, H.; Sadeghi, M.; Azizi, F. A Longitudinal Study of Adherence to the Mediterranean Dietary Pattern and Metabolic Syndrome in a Non-Mediterranean Population. *Int. J. Endocrinol. Metab.* **2015**, *13*, e26128. [CrossRef]

28. Friedman, G.D.; Cutter, G.R.; Donahue, R.P.; Hughes, G.H.; Hulley, S.B.; Jacobs, D.R.; Liu, K.; Savage, P.J. CARDIA: Study design, recruitment, and some characteristics of the examined subjects. *J. Clin. Epidemiol.* **1988**, *41*, 1105–1116. [CrossRef]

29. Sleiman, D.; Al-Badri, M.R.; Azar, S.T. Effect of mediterranean diet in diabetes control and cardiovascular risk modification: A systematic review. *Front. Public Health* **2015**, *3*, 69. [CrossRef]

30. Kim, Y.; Je, Y. A modified Mediterranean diet score is inversely associated with metabolic syndrome in Korean adults. *Eur. J. Clin. Nutr.* **2018**, 1682–1689. [CrossRef]

31. Tosti, V.; Bertozzi, B.; Fontana, L. Health Benefits of the Mediterranean Diet: Metabolic and Molecular Mechanisms. *J. Gerontol. A Biol. Sci. Med. Sci.* **2018**, *73*, 318–326. [CrossRef] [PubMed]

32. Filippou, C.D.; Tsioufis, C.P.; Thomopoulos, C.G.; Mihas, C.C.; Dimitriadis, K.S.; Sotiropoulou, L.I.; Chrysochoou, C.A.; Nihoyannopoulos, P.I.; Tousoulis, D.M. Dietary Approaches to Stop Hypertension (DASH) Diet and Blood Pressure Reduction in Adults with and without Hypertension: A Systematic Review and Meta-Analysis of Randomized Controlled Trials. *Adv. Nutr.* **2020**. [CrossRef] [PubMed]

33. Schwingshackl, L.; Chaimani, A.; Schwedhelm, C.; Toledo, E.; Pünsch, M.; Hoffmann, G.; Boeing, H. Comparative effects of different dietary approaches on blood pressure in hypertensive and pre-hypertensive patients: A systematic review and network meta-analysis. *Crit. Rev. Food Sci. Nutr.* **2019**, *59*, 2674–2687. [CrossRef] [PubMed]

34. Phillips, C.M.; Harrington, J.M.; Perry, I.J. Relationship between dietary quality, determined by DASH score, and cardiometabolic health biomarkers: A cross-sectional analysis in adults. *Clin. Nutr.* **2019**, *38*, 1620–1628. [CrossRef] [PubMed]

35. Soltani, S.; Shirani, F.; Chitsazi, M.J.; Salehi-Abargouei, A. The effect of dietary approaches to stop hypertension (DASH) diet on weight and body composition in adults: A systematic review and meta-analysis of randomized controlled clinical trials. *Obes. Rev.* **2016**, *17*, 442–454. [CrossRef]

36. Drehmer, M.; Odegaard, A.O.; Schmidt, M.I.; Duncan, B.B.; De Oliveira Cardoso, L.; Matos, S.M.A.; Molina, M.C.B.; Barreto, S.M.; Pereira, M.A. Brazilian dietary patterns and the dietary approaches to stop hypertension (DASH) diet-relationship with metabolic syndrome and newly diagnosed diabetes in the ELSA-Brasil study. *Diabetol. Metab. Syndr.* **2017**, *9*, 13. [CrossRef] [PubMed]

37. Gibson, R.; Eriksen, R.; Singh, D.; Vergnaud, A.-C.; Heard, A.; Chan, Q.; Elliott, P.; Frost, G. A cross-sectional investigation into the occupational and socio-demographic characteristics of British police force employees reporting a dietary pattern associated with cardiometabolic risk: Findings from the Airwave Health Monitoring Study. *Eur. J. Nutr.* **2018**, *57*, 2913–2926. [CrossRef]

38. Jones, N.R.V.; Forouhi, N.G.; Khaw, K.T.; Wareham, N.J.; Monsivais, P. Accordance to the Dietary Approaches to Stop Hypertension diet pattern and cardiovascular disease in a British, population-based cohort. *Eur. J. Epidemiol.* **2018**, *33*, 235–244. [CrossRef]

39. Mertens, E.; Markey, O.; Geleijnse, J.M.; Lovegrove, J.A.; Givens, D.I. Adherence to a healthy diet in relation to cardiovascular incidence and risk markers: Evidence from the Caerphilly Prospective Study. *Eur. J. Nutr.* **2018**, *57*, 1245–1258. [CrossRef]

40. Schwingshackl, L.; Bogensberger, B.; Hoffmann, G. Diet Quality as Assessed by the Healthy Eating Index, Alternate Healthy Eating Index, Dietary Approaches to Stop Hypertension Score, and Health Outcomes: An Updated Systematic Review and Meta-Analysis of Cohort Studies. *J. Acad. Nutr. Diet.* **2018**, *118*, 74–100.e11. [CrossRef]

41. Hemler, E.C.; Hu, F.B. Plant-Based Diets for Cardiovascular Disease Prevention: All Plant Foods Are Not Created Equal. *Curr. Atheroscler. Rep.* **2019**, *21*, 18. [CrossRef] [PubMed]

42. Yokoyama, Y.; Nishimura, K.; Barnard, N.D.; Takegami, M.; Watanabe, M.; Sekikawa, A.; Okamura, T.; Miyamoto, Y. Vegetarian diets and blood pressure: A meta-analysis. *JAMA Intern. Med.* **2014**, *174*, 577–587. [CrossRef] [PubMed]

43. Crowe, F.L.; Appleby, P.N.; Travis, R.C.; Key, T.J. Risk of hospitalization or death from ischemic heart disease among British vegetarians and nonvegetarians: Results from the EPIC-Oxford cohort study. *Am. J. Clin. Nutr.* **2013**, *97*, 597–603. [CrossRef] [PubMed]

44. Huang, R.Y.; Huang, C.C.; Hu, F.B.; Chavarro, J.E. Vegetarian Diets and Weight Reduction: A Meta-Analysis of Randomized Controlled Trials. *J. Gen. Intern Med.* **2016**, *31*, 109–116. [CrossRef] [PubMed]

45. Konieczna, J.; Romaguera, D.; Pereira, V.; Fiol, M.; Razquin, C.; Estruch, R.; Asensio, E.M.; Babio, N.; Fitó, M.; Gómez-Gracia, E.; et al. Longitudinal association of changes in diet with changes in body weight and waist circumference in subjects at high cardiovascular risk: The PREDIMED trial. *Int. J. Behav. Nutr. Phys. Act.* **2019**, *16*, 139. [CrossRef]

46. Kahleova, H.; Salas-Salvadó, J.; Rahelić, D.; Kendall, C.W.; Rembert, E.; Sievenpiper, J.L. Dietary Patterns and Cardiometabolic Outcomes in Diabetes: A Summary of Systematic Reviews and Meta-Analyses. *Nutrients* **2019**, *11*, 2209. [CrossRef]

47. Orlich, M.J.; Singh, P.N.; Sabaté, J.; Jaceldo-Siegl, K.; Fan, J.; Knutsen, S.; Beeson, W.L.; Fraser, G.E. Vegetarian dietary patterns and mortality in Adventist Health Study 2. *JAMA Intern. Med.* **2013**, *173*, 1230–1238. [CrossRef]

48. Kim, H.; Caulfield, L.E.; Rebholz, C.M. Healthy Plant-Based Diets Are Associated with Lower Risk of All-Cause Mortality in US Adults. *J. Nutr.* **2018**, *148*, 624–631. [CrossRef]

49. Evert, A.B.; Dennison, M.; Gardner, C.D.; Timothy Garvey, W.; Karen Lau, K.H.; MacLeod, J.; Mitri, J.; Pereira, R.F.; Rawlings, K.; Robinson, S.; et al. Nutrition Therapy for Adults with Diabetes or Prediabetes: A Consensus Report. *Diabetes Care* **2019**, *42*, 731–754. [CrossRef]

50. Bazzano, L.A.; Hu, T.; Reynolds, K.; Yao, L.; Bunol, C.; Liu, Y.; Chen, C.S.; Klag, M.J.; Whelton, P.K.; He, J. Effects of low-carbohydrate and low-fat diets: A randomized trial. *Ann. Intern. Med.* **2014**, *161*, 309–318. [CrossRef]

51. Van Zuuren, E.J.; Fedorowicz, Z.; Kuijpers, T.; Pijl, H. Effects of low-carbohydrate- compared with low-fat-diet interventions on metabolic control in people with type 2 diabetes: A systematic review including GRADE assessments. *Am. J. Clin. Nutr.* **2018**, *108*, 300–331. [CrossRef] [PubMed]

52. Bueno, N.B.; de Melo, I.S.; de Oliveira, S.L.; da Rocha Ataide, T. Very-low-carbohydrate ketogenic diet v. low-fat diet for long-term weight loss: A meta-analysis of randomised controlled trials. *Br. J. Nutr.* **2013**, *110*, 1178–1187. [CrossRef] [PubMed]

53. Augustin, L.S.A.; Kendall, C.W.C.; Jenkins, D.J.A.; Willett, W.C.; Astrup, A.; Barclay, A.W.; Björck, I.; Brand-Miller, J.C.; Brighenti, F.; Buyken, A.E.; et al. Glycemic index, glycemic load and glycemic response: An International Scientific Consensus Summit from the International Carbohydrate Quality Consortium (ICQC). *Nutr. Metab. Cardiovasc. Dis.* **2015**, *25*, 795–815. [CrossRef] [PubMed]

54. Livesey, G.; Taylor, R.; Livesey, H.F.; Buyken, A.E.; Jenkins, D.J.A.; Augustin, L.S.A.; Sievenpiper, J.L.; Barclay, A.W.; Liu, S.; Wolever, T.M.S.; et al. Dietary Glycemic Index and Load and the Risk of Type 2 Diabetes: A Systematic Review and Updated Meta-Analyses of Prospective Cohort Studies. *Nutrients* **2019**, *11*, 1280. [CrossRef]

55. Ge, L.; Sadeghirad, B.; Ball, G.D.C.; Da Costa, B.R.; Hitchcock, C.L.; Svendrovski, A.; Kiflen, R.; Quadri, K.; Kwon, H.Y.; Karamouzian, M.; et al. Comparison of dietary macronutrient patterns of 14 popular named dietary programmes for weight and cardiovascular risk factor reduction in adults: Systematic review and network meta-analysis of randomised trials. *BMJ* **2020**, *369*, m696. [CrossRef]

56. Ma, C.; Avenell, A.; Bolland, M.; Hudson, J.; Stewart, F.; Robertson, C.; Sharma, P.; Fraser, C.; MacLennan, G. Effects of weight loss interventions for adults who are obese on mortality, cardiovascular disease, and cancer: Systematic review and meta-analysis. *BMJ* **2017**, *359*, j4849. [CrossRef]

57. Campos-Nonato, I.; Hernandez, L.; Barquera, S. Effect of a High-Protein Diet versus Standard-Protein Diet on Weight Loss and Biomarkers of Metabolic Syndrome: A Randomized Clinical Trial. *Obes. Facts* **2017**, *10*, 238–251. [CrossRef]

58. Rock, C.L.; Flatt, S.W.; Pakiz, B.; Taylor, K.S.; Leone, A.F.; Brelje, K.; Heath, D.D.; Quintana, E.L.; Sherwood, N.E. Weight loss, glycemic control, and cardiovascular disease risk factors in response to differential diet composition in a weight loss program in type 2 diabetes: A randomized controlled trial. *Diabetes Care* **2014**, *37*, 1573–1580. [CrossRef]

59. Ramezani-Jolfaie, N.; Mohammadi, M.; Salehi-Abargouei, A. The effect of healthy Nordic diet on cardio-metabolic markers: A systematic review and meta-analysis of randomized controlled clinical trials. *Eur. J. Nutr.* **2019**, *58*, 2159–2174. [CrossRef]

60. Lefevre, M.; Redman, L.M.; Heilbronn, L.K.; Smith, J.V.; Martin, C.K.; Rood, J.C.; Greenway, F.L.; Williamson, D.A.; Smith, S.R.; Ravussin, E.; et al. Caloric restriction alone and with exercise improves CVD risk in healthy non-obese individuals. *Atherosclerosis* **2009**, *203*, 206–213. [CrossRef]

61. Most, J.; Gilmore, L.A.; Smith, S.R.; Han, H.; Ravussin, E.; Redman, L.M. Significant improvement in cardiometabolic health in healthy nonobese individuals during caloric restriction-induced weight loss and weight loss maintenance. *Am. J. Physiol. Endocrinol. Metab.* **2018**, *314*, E396–E405. [CrossRef] [PubMed]

62. Wan, R.; Camandola, S.; Mattson, M.P. Intermittent food deprivation improves cardiovascular and neuroendocrine responses to stress in rats. *J. Nutr.* **2003**, *133*, 1921–1929. [CrossRef] [PubMed]

63.   de Cabo, R.; Mattson, M.P. Effects of Intermittent Fasting on Health, Aging, and Disease. *N. Engl. J. Med.* **2019**, *381*, 2541–2551. [CrossRef] [PubMed]

64.   Lăcătuşu, C.M.; Grigorescu, E.D.; Floria, M.; Onofriescu, A.; Mihai, B.M. The Mediterranean Diet: From an Environment-Driven Food Culture to an Emerging Medical Prescription. *Int. J. Environ. Res. Public Health* **2019**, *16*, 942. [CrossRef]

65.   Dernini, S.; Berry, E.M.; Serra-Majem, L.; La Vecchia, C.; Capone, R.; Medina, F.X.; Aranceta-Bartrina, J.; Belahsen, R.; Burlingame, B.; Calabrese, G.; et al. Med Diet 4.0: The Mediterranean diet with four sustainable benefits. *Public Health Nutr.* **2017**, *20*, 1322–1330. [CrossRef]

66.   Xavier Medina, F. Mediterranean diet, culture and heritage: Challenges for a new conception. *Public Health Nutr.* **2009**, *12*, 1618–1620. [CrossRef]

67.   Storniolo, C.E.; Sacanella, I.; Mitjavila, M.T.; Lamuela-Raventos, R.M.; Moreno, J.J. Bioactive Compounds of Cooked Tomato Sauce Modulate Oxidative Stress and Arachidonic Acid Cascade Induced by Oxidized LDL in Macrophage Cultures. *Nutrients* **2019**, *11*, 1880. [CrossRef]

68.   Davis, C.; Bryan, J.; Hodgson, J.; Murphy, K. Definition of the Mediterranean Diet; a Literature Review. *Nutrients* **2015**, *7*, 9139–9153. [CrossRef]

69.   Widmer, R.J.; Flammer, A.J.; Lerman, L.O.; Lerman, A. The Mediterranean diet, its components, and cardiovascular disease. *Am. J. Med.* **2015**, *128*, 229–238. [CrossRef]

70.   Chiva-Blanch, G.; Badimon, L. Effects of Polyphenol Intake on Metabolic Syndrome: Current Evidences from Human Trials. *Oxid Med. Cell Longev.* **2017**, *2017*, 5812401. [CrossRef]

71.   Soltani, S.; Jayedi, A.; Shab-Bidar, S.; Becerra-Tomás, N.; Salas-Salvadó, J. Adherence to the Mediterranean Diet in Relation to All-Cause Mortality: A Systematic Review and Dose-Response Meta-Analysis of Prospective Cohort Studies. *Adv. Nutr.* **2019**, *10*, 1029–1039. [CrossRef]

72.   Martínez-González, M.A.; Gea, A.; Ruiz-Canela, M. The Mediterranean Diet and Cardiovascular Health. *Circ. Res.* **2019**, *124*, 779–798. [CrossRef] [PubMed]

73.   Ahmad, S.; Moorthy, M.V.; Demler, O.V.; Hu, F.B.; Ridker, P.M.; Chasman, D.I.; Mora, S. Assessment of Risk Factors and Biomarkers Associated with Risk of Cardiovascular Disease Among Women Consuming a Mediterranean Diet. *JAMA Netw. Open* **2018**, *1*, e185708. [CrossRef] [PubMed]

74.   Appel, L.J.; Moore, T.J.; Obarzanek, E.; Vollmer, W.M.; Svetkey, L.P.; Sacks, F.M.; Bray, G.A.; Vogt, T.M.; Cutler, J.A.; Windhauser, M.M.; et al. A clinical trial of the effects of dietary patterns on blood pressure. DASH Collaborative Research Group. *N. Engl. J. Med.* **1997**, *336*, 1117–1124. [CrossRef] [PubMed]

75.   Fung, T.T.; Chiuve, S.E.; McCullough, M.L.; Rexrode, K.M.; Logroscino, G.; Hu, F.B. Adherence to a DASH-style diet and risk of coronary heart disease and stroke in women. *Arch. Intern. Med.* **2008**, *168*, 713–720. [CrossRef]

76.   U.S. Department of Health and Human Services. Dash Diet. In *Handbook of Disease Burdens and Quality of Life Measures*; National Institute of Health, National Heart, Lung and Blood Institute: Bethesda, MD, USA, 2010.

77.   Siervo, M.; Lara, J.; Chowdhury, S.; Ashor, A.; Oggioni, C.; Mathers, J.C. Effects of the Dietary Approach to Stop Hypertension (DASH) diet on cardiovascular risk factors: A systematic review and meta-analysis. *Br. J. Nutr.* **2015**, *113*, 1–15. [CrossRef]

78.   Farhadnejad, H.; Darand, M.; Teymoori, F.; Asghari, G.; Mirmiran, P.; Azizi, F. The association of Dietary Approach to Stop Hypertension (DASH) diet with metabolic healthy and metabolic unhealthy obesity phenotypes. *Sci. Rep.* **2019**, *9*, 18690. [CrossRef] [PubMed]

79.   Djoussé, L.; Ho, Y.; Nguyen, X.T.; Gagnon, D.R.; Wilson, P.W.F.; Cho, K.; Gaziano, J.M.; The VA Million Veteran Program; Halasz, I.; Federman, D.; et al. DASH Score and Subsequent Risk of Coronary Artery Disease: The Findings From Million Veteran Program. *J. Am. Heart Assoc.* **2018**, *7*, e008089. [CrossRef]

80.   Kang, S.H.; Cho, K.H.; Do, J.Y. Association between the Modified Dietary Approaches to Stop Hypertension and Metabolic Syndrome in Postmenopausal Women Without Diabetes. *Metab. Syndr. Relat. Disord.* **2018**, *16*, 282–289. [CrossRef]

81.   Hashemi, R.; MehdizadehKhalifani, A.; Rahimlou, M.; Manafi, M. Comparison of the effect of Dietary Approaches to Stop Hypertension diet and American Diabetes Association nutrition guidelines on lipid profiles in patients with type 2 diabetes: A comparative clinical trial. *Nutr. Diet.* **2020**, *77*, 204–211. [CrossRef]

82.   Asghari, G.; Yuzbashian, E.; Mirmiran, P.; Hooshmand, F.; Najafi, R.; Azizi, F. Dietary Approaches to Stop Hypertension (DASH) Dietary Pattern Is Associated with Reduced Incidence of Metabolic Syndrome in Children and Adolescents. *J. Pediatr.* **2016**, *174*, 178–184.e1. [CrossRef] [PubMed]

83. Peairs, A.D.; Shah, A.S.; Summer, S.; Hess, M.; Couch, S.C. Effects of the dietary approaches to stop hypertension (DASH) diet on glucose variability in youth with Type 1 diabetes. *Diabetes Manag.* **2017**, *7*, 383–391.

84. Akhlaghi, M. Dietary Approaches to Stop Hypertension (DASH): Potential mechanisms of action against risk factors of the metabolic syndrome. *Nutr. Res. Rev.* **2019**, 1–18. [CrossRef]

85. Pickering, R.T.; Bradlee, M.L.; Singer, M.R.; Moore, L.L. Baseline diet modifies the effects of dietary change. *Br. J. Nutr.* **2020**, *123*, 951–958. [CrossRef]

86. Dudum, R.; Juraschek, S.P.; Appel, L.J. Dose-dependent effects of lifestyle interventions on blood lipid levels: Results from the PREMIER trial. *Patient Educ. Couns.* **2019**, *102*, 1882–1891. [CrossRef] [PubMed]

87. Steinberg, D.; Kay, M.; Burroughs, J.; Svetkey, L.P.; Bennett, G.G. The Effect of a Digital Behavioral Weight Loss Intervention on Adherence to the Dietary Approaches to Stop Hypertension (DASH) Dietary Pattern in Medically Vulnerable Primary Care Patients: Results from a Randomized Controlled Trial. *J. Acad. Nutr. Diet.* **2019**, *119*, 574–584. [CrossRef]

88. Satija, A.; Hu, F.B. Plant-based diets and cardiovascular health. *Trends Cardiovasc. Med.* **2018**, *28*, 437–441. [CrossRef]

89. Lynch, H.; Johnston, C.; Wharton, C. Plant-Based Diets: Considerations for Environmental Impact, Protein Quality, and Exercise Performance. *Nutrients* **2018**, *10*, 1841. [CrossRef]

90. Sterling, S.R.; Bowen, S.A. The Potential for Plant-Based Diets to Promote Health among Blacks Living in the United States. *Nutrients* **2019**, *11*, 2915. [CrossRef]

91. Kahleova, H.; Levin, S.; Barnard, N. Cardio-Metabolic Benefits of Plant-Based Diets. *Nutrients* **2017**, *9*, 848. [CrossRef]

92. Wang, F.; Zheng, J.; Yang, B.; Jiang, J.; Fu, Y.; Li, D. Effects of Vegetarian Diets on Blood Lipids: A Systematic Review and Meta-Analysis of Randomized Controlled Trials. *J. Am. Heart Assoc.* **2015**, *4*, e002408. [CrossRef] [PubMed]

93. Guasch-Ferré, M.; Satija, A.; Blondin, S.A.; Janiszewski, M.; Emlen, E.; O'Connor, L.E.; Campbell, W.W.; Hu, F.B.; Willet, W.C.; Stampfer, M.J. Meta-Analysis of Randomized Controlled Trials of Red Meat Consumption in Comparison with Various Comparison Diets on Cardiovascular Risk Factors. *Circulation* **2019**, *139*, 1828–1845. [CrossRef] [PubMed]

94. Satija, A.; Bhupathiraju, S.N.; Spiegelman, D.; Chiuve, S.E.; Manson, J.A.E.; Willett, W.; Rexrode, K.M.; Rimm, E.B.; Hu, F.B. Healthful and Unhealthful Plant-Based Diets and the Risk of Coronary Heart Disease in U.S. Adults. *J. Am. Coll. Cardiol.* **2017**, *70*, 411–422. [CrossRef] [PubMed]

95. Tresserra-Rimbau, A.; Arranz, S.; Vallverdu-Queralt, A. New Insights into the Benefits of Polyphenols in Chronic Diseases. *Oxid. Med. Cell Longev.* **2017**, *2017*, 1432071. [CrossRef] [PubMed]

96. Hever, J. Plant-Based Diets: A Physician's Guide. *Perm. J.* **2016**, *20*, 15–82. [CrossRef]

97. Liu, Y.S.; Wu, Q.J.; Xia, Y.; Zhang, J.Y.; Jiang, Y.T.; Chang, Q.; Zhao, Y.H. Carbohydrate intake and risk of metabolic syndrome: A dose-response meta-analysis of observational studies. *Nutr. Metab. Cardiovasc. Dis.* **2019**, *29*, 1288–1298. [CrossRef]

98. Dehghan, M.; Mente, A.; Zhang, X.; Swaminathan, S.; Li, W.; Mohan, V.; Iqbal, R.; Kumar, R.; Wentzel-Viljoen, E.; Rosengren, A.; et al. Associations of fats and carbohydrate intake with cardiovascular disease and mortality in 18 countries from five continents (PURE): A prospective cohort study. *Lancet* **2017**, *390*, 2050–2062. [CrossRef]

99. Hoogeveen, R.C.; Gaubatz, J.W.; Sun, W.; Dodge, R.C.; Crosby, J.R.; Jiang, J.; Couper, D.; Virani, S.S.; Kathiresan, S.; Boerwinkle, E.; et al. Small dense low-density lipoprotein-cholesterol concentrations predict risk for coronary heart disease: The Atherosclerosis Risk In Communities (ARIC) study. *Arterioscler. Thromb. Vasc. Biol.* **2014**, *34*, 1069–1077. [CrossRef]

100. Puska, P. Fat and heart disease: Yes we can make a change—The case of North Karelia (Finland). *Ann. Nutr. Metab.* **2009**, *54*, 33–38. [CrossRef]

101. Yu, E.; Rimm, E.; Qi, L.; Rexrode, K.; Albert, C.M.; Sun, Q.; Willet, W.C.; Hu, F.B.; Manson, J.E. Diet, Lifestyle, Biomarkers, Genetic Factors, and Risk of Cardiovascular Disease in the Nurses' Health Studies. *Am. J. Public Health* **2016**, *106*, 1616–1623. [CrossRef]

102. Seidelmann, S.B.; Claggett, B.; Cheng, S.; Henglin, M.; Shah, A.; Steffen, L.M.; Folsom, A.R.; Rimm, E.B.; Willet, W.C.; Solomon, S.D. Dietary carbohydrate intake and mortality: A prospective cohort study and meta-analysis. *Lancet Public Health* **2018**, *3*, e419–e428. [CrossRef]

103. Budhathoki, S.; Sawada, N.; Iwasaki, M.; Yamaji, T.; Goto, A.; Kotemori, A.; Ishihara, J.; Takachi, R.; Charvat, H.; Mizoure, T.; et al. Association of Animal and Plant Protein Intake with All-Cause and Cause-Specific Mortality in a Japanese Cohort. *JAMA Intern Med.* **2019**, *179*, 1509–1518. [CrossRef] [PubMed]

104. Paoli, A.; Rubini, A.; Volek, J.S.; Grimaldi, K.A. Beyond weight loss: A review of the therapeutic uses of very-low-carbohydrate (ketogenic) diets. *Eur. J. Clin. Nutr.* **2013**, *67*, 789–796. [CrossRef]

105. Jensen, M.D.; Ryan, D.H.; Apovian, C.M.; Ard, J.D.; Comuzzie, A.G.; Donato, K.A.; Hu, F.B.; Hubbard, V.S.; Jakicic, J.M.; Fushner, R.F.; et al. 2013 AHA/ACC/TOS guideline for the management of overweight and obesity in adults: A report of the American College of Cardiology/American Heart Association Task Force on Practice Guidelines and The Obesity Society. *Circulation* **2014**, *129*, S102–S138. [CrossRef] [PubMed]

106. Moreno, B.; Bellido, D.; Sajoux, I.; Goday, A.; Saavedra, D.; Crujeiras, A.B.; Casanueva, F.F. Comparison of a very low-calorie-ketogenic diet with a standard low-calorie diet in the treatment of obesity. *Endocrine* **2014**, *47*, 793–805. [CrossRef]

107. Hu, T.; Mills, K.T.; Yao, L.; Demanelis, K.; Eloustaz, M.; Yancy, W.S.; Kelly, T.N.; He, J.; Bazzano, L.A. Effects of low-carbohydrate diets versus low-fat diets on metabolic risk factors: A meta-analysis of randomized controlled clinical trials. *Am. J. Epidemiol.* **2012**, *176* (Suppl. 7), S44–S54. [CrossRef]

108. Choi, H.R.; Kim, J.; Lim, H.; Park, Y.K. Two-Week Exclusive Supplementation of Modified Ketogenic Nutrition Drink Reserves Lean Body Mass and Improves Blood Lipid Profile in Obese Adults: A Randomized Clinical Trial. *Nutrients* **2018**, *10*, 1895. [CrossRef]

109. Corpeleijn, E.; Saris, W.H.; Blaak, E.E. Metabolic flexibility in the development of insulin resistance and type 2 diabetes: Effects of lifestyle. *Obes. Rev.* **2009**, *10*, 178–193. [CrossRef]

110. Westerterp-Plantenga, M.S.; Nieuwenhuizen, A.; Tomé, D.; Soenen, S.; Westerterp, K.R. Dietary protein, weight loss, and weight maintenance. *Annu. Rev. Nutr.* **2009**, *29*, 21–41. [CrossRef]

111. Schwingshackl, L.; Dias, S.; Hoffmann, G. Impact of long-term lifestyle programmes on weight loss and cardiovascular risk factors in overweight/obese participants: A systematic review and network meta-analysis. *Syst. Rev.* **2014**, *3*, 130. [CrossRef]

112. Ajala, O.; English, P.; Pinkney, J. Systematic review and meta-analysis of different dietary approaches to the management of type 2 diabetes. *Am. J. Clin. Nutr.* **2013**, *97*, 505–516. [CrossRef] [PubMed]

113. Prentice, R.L.; Aragaki, A.K.; Van Horn, L.; Thomson, C.A.; Beresford, S.A.A.; Robinson, J.; Snetselaar, L.; Anderson, G.L.; Manson, J.E.; Allison, M.A.; et al. Low-fat dietary pattern and cardiovascular disease: Results from the Women's Health Initiative randomized controlled trial. *Am. J. Clin. Nutr.* **2017**, *106*, 35–43. [CrossRef]

114. Neuhouser, M.L.; Howard, B.; Lu, J.; Tinker, L.F.; Van Horn, L.; Caan, B.; Rohan, T.; Stefanick, M.L.; Thomson, C.A. A low-fat dietary pattern and risk of metabolic syndrome in postmenopausal women: The Women's Health Initiative. *Metabolism* **2012**, *61*, 1572–1581. [CrossRef] [PubMed]

115. Babio, N.; Toledo, E.; Estruch, R.; Ros, E.; Martínez-González, M.A.; Castañer, O.; Bulló, M.; Corella, D.; Arós, F.; Gómez-Garcia, E.; et al. Mediterranean diets and metabolic syndrome status in the PREDIMED randomized trial. *CMAJ* **2014**, *186*, E649–E657. [CrossRef] [PubMed]

116. Paniagua, J.A.; Pérez-Martinez, P.; Gjelstad, I.M.F.; Tierney, A.C.; Delgado-Lista, J.; Defoort, C.; Blaak, E.E.; Risérus, U.; Drevon, C.A.; Kiec-Wilk, B.; et al. A low-fat high-carbohydrate diet supplemented with long-chain n-3 PUFA reduces the risk of the metabolic syndrome. *Atherosclerosis* **2011**, *218*, 443–450. [CrossRef] [PubMed]

117. Veum, V.L.; Laupsa-Borge, J.; Eng, Ø.; Rostrup, E.; Larsen, T.H.; Nordrehaug, J.E.; Nygård, O.K.; Sagen, J.V.; Gudbrandsen, O.A.; Dankel, S.N.; et al. Visceral adiposity and metabolic syndrome after very high-fat and low-fat isocaloric diets: A randomized controlled trial. *Am. J. Clin. Nutr.* **2017**, *105*, 85–99. [CrossRef] [PubMed]

118. Gardner, C.D.; Trepanowski, J.F.; Gobbo, L.C.D.; Hauser, M.E.; Rigdon, J.; Ioannidis, J.P.A.; Desai, M.; King, A.C. Effect of Low-Fat vs Low-Carbohydrate Diet on 12-Month Weight Loss in Overweight Adults and the Association with Genotype Pattern or Insulin Secretion: The DIETFITS Randomized Clinical Trial. *JAMA* **2018**, *319*, 667–679. [CrossRef]

119. Gjuladin-Hellon, T.; Davies, I.G.; Penson, P.; AmiriBaghbadorani, R. Effects of carbohydrate-restricted diets on low-density lipoprotein cholesterol levels in overweight and obese adults: A systematic review and meta-analysis. *Nutr. Rev.* **2019**, *77*, 161–180. [CrossRef]

120. Mansoor, N.; Vinknes, K.J.; Veierød, M.B.; Retterstøl, K. Effects of low-carbohydrate diets v. low-fat diets on body weight and cardiovascular risk factors: A meta-analysis of randomised controlled trials. *Br. J. Nutr.* **2016**, *115*, 466–479. [CrossRef]

121. Gulseth, H.L.; Gjelstad, I.M.F.; Tiereny, A.C.; McCarthy, D.; Lovegrove, J.A.; Defoort, C.; Blaak, E.E.; Lopez-Miranda, J.; Dembinska-Kiec, A.; Risérus, U.; et al. Effects of dietary fat on insulin secretion in subjects with the metabolic syndrome. *Eur. J. Endocrinol.* **2019**, *180*, 321–328. [CrossRef]

122. Fortin, A.; Rabasa-Lhoret, R.; Lemieux, S.; Labonté, M.E.; Gingras, V. Comparison of a Mediterranean to a low-fat diet intervention in adults with type 1 diabetes and metabolic syndrome: A 6-month randomized trial. *Nutr. Metab. Cardiovasc. Dis.* **2018**, *28*, 1275–1284. [CrossRef] [PubMed]

123. Mirza, N.M.; Palmer, M.G.; Sinclair, K.B.; McCarter, R.; He, J.; Ebbeling, C.B.; Ludwig, D.S.; Yanovski, J.A. Effects of a low glycemic load or a low-fat dietary intervention on body weight in obese Hispanic American children and adolescents: A randomized controlled trial. *Am. J. Clin. Nutr.* **2013**, *97*, 276–285. [CrossRef] [PubMed]

124. Petrisko, M.; Kloss, R.; Bradley, P.; Birrenkott, E.; Spindler, A.; Clayton, Z.S.; Kern, M. Biochemical, Anthropometric, and Physiological Responses to Carbohydrate-Restricted Diets Versus a Low-Fat Diet in Obese Adults: A Randomized Crossover Trial. *J. Med. Food* **2020**, *23*, 206–214. [CrossRef] [PubMed]

125. Lu, M.; Wan, Y.; Yang, B.; Huggins, C.E.; Li, D. Effects of low-fat compared with high-fat diet on cardiometabolic indicators in people with overweight and obesity without overt metabolic disturbance: A systematic review and meta-analysis of randomised controlled trials. *Br. J. Nutr.* **2018**, *119*, 96–108. [CrossRef] [PubMed]

126. Javier Basterra-Gortari, F.; Ruiz-Canela, M.; Martínez-González, M.A.; Babio, N.; Sorlí, J.V.; Fito, M.; Ros, E.; Gómez-Garcia, E.; Fiol, M.; Lapetra, J.; et al. Effects of a Mediterranean Eating Plan on the Need for Glucose-Lowering Medications in Participants with Type 2 Diabetes: A Subgroup Analysis of the PREDIMED Trial. *Diabetes Care* **2019**, *42*, 1390–1397. [CrossRef]

127. Monserrat-Mesquida, M.; Quetglas-Llabrés, M.; Capó, X.; Bouzas, C.; Mateos, D.; Pons, A.; Tur, J.A.; Sureda, A. Metabolic Syndrome is Associated with Oxidative Stress and Proinflammatory State. *Antioxidants* **2020**, *9*, 236. [CrossRef]

128. Pickworth, C.K.; Deichert, D.A.; Corroon, J.; Bradley, R.D. Randomized controlled trials investigating the relationship between dietary pattern and high-sensitivity C-reactive protein: A systematic review. *Nutr. Rev.* **2019**, *77*, 363–375. [CrossRef]

129. Smidowicz, A.; Regula, J. Effect of nutritional status and dietary patterns on human serum C-reactive protein and interleukin-6 concentrations. *Adv. Nutr.* **2015**, *6*, 738–747. [CrossRef]

130. Santos-Marcos, J.A.; Perez-Jimenez, F.; Camargo, A. The role of diet and intestinal microbiota in the development of metabolic syndrome. *J. Nutr. Biochem.* **2019**, *70*, 1–27. [CrossRef]

131. Wan, Y.; Wang, F.; Yuan, J.; Li, J.; Jiang, D.; Zhang, J.; Li, H.; Wang, R.; Tang, J.; Huang, T.; et al. Effects of dietary fat on gut microbiota and faecal metabolites, and their relationship with cardiometabolic risk factors: A 6-month randomised controlled-feeding trial. *Gut* **2019**, *68*, 1417–1429. [CrossRef]

132. Fragiadakis, G.K.; Wastyk, H.C.; Robinson, J.L.; Sonnenburg, E.D.; Sonnenburg, J.L.; Gardner, C.D. Long-term dietary intervention reveals resilience of the gut microbiota despite changes in diet and weight. *Am. J. Clin. Nutr.* **2020**, *111*, 1127–1136. [CrossRef] [PubMed]

133. Goni, L.; Qi, L.; Cuervo, M.; Milagro, F.I.; Saris, W.H.; MacDonald, I.A.; Langin, D.; Astrup, A.; Arner, P.; Oppert, J.M.; et al. Effect of the interaction between diet composition and the PPM1K genetic variant on insulin resistance and β cell function markers during weight loss: Results from the Nutrient Gene Interactions in Human Obesity: Implications for dietary guidelines (NUGENOB) randomized trial. *Am. J. Clin. Nutr.* **2017**, *106*, 902–908. [CrossRef]

134. Catapano, A.L.; Graham, I.; De Backer, G.; Wiklund, O.; Chapman, M.J.; Drexel, H.; Hoes, A.W.; Jennings, C.S.; Landmesser, U.; Pedersen, T.R.; et al. 2016 ESC/EAS Guidelines for the Management of Dyslipidaemias: The Task Force for the Management of Dyslipidaemias of the European Society of Cardiology (ESC) and European Atherosclerosis Society (EAS) Developed with the special contribution of the European Asscociation for Cardiovascular Prevention & Rehabilitation (EACPR). *Atherosclerosis* **2016**, *253*, 281–344. [CrossRef] [PubMed]

135. Zhao, W.T.; Luo, Y.; Zhang, Y.; Zhou, Y.; Zhao, T.T. High protein diet is of benefit for patients with type 2 diabetes: An updated meta-analysis. *Medicine* **2018**, *97*, e13149. [CrossRef] [PubMed]

136. Gadgil, M.D.; Appel, L.J.; Yeung, E.; Anderson, C.A.M.; Sacks, F.M.; Miller, E.R. The effects of carbohydrate, unsaturated fat, and protein intake on measures of insulin sensitivity: Results from the OmniHeart trial. *Diabetes Care* **2013**, *36*, 1132–1137. [CrossRef]

137. Astrup, A. The satiating power of protein-a key to obesity prevention? *Am. J. Clin. Nutr.* **2005**, *82*, 1–2. [CrossRef]

138. Li, J.; Armstrong, C.L.; Campbell, W.W. Effects of Dietary Protein Source and Quantity during Weight Loss on Appetite, Energy Expenditure, and Cardio-Metabolic Responses. *Nutrients* **2016**, *8*, 63. [CrossRef]

139. Wycherley, T.P.; Moran, L.J.; Clifton, P.M.; Noakes, M.; Brinkworth, G.D. Effects of energy-restricted high-protein, low-fat compared with standard-protein, low-fat diets: A meta-analysis of randomized controlled trials. *Am. J. Clin. Nutr.* **2012**, *96*, 1281–1298. [CrossRef]

140. Pan, A.; Sun, Q.; Bernstein, A.M.; Manson, J.E.; Willett, W.C.; Hu, F.B. Changes in red meat consumption and subsequent risk of type 2 diabetes mellitus: Three cohorts of US men and women. *JAMA Intern. Med.* **2013**, *173*, 1328–1335. [CrossRef]

141. Hu, F.B. Plant-based foods and prevention of cardiovascular disease: An overview. *Am. J. Clin. Nutr.* **2003**, *78*, 544S–551S. [CrossRef]

142. Fogelholm, M. New Nordic Nutrition Recommendations are here. *Food Nutr. Res.* **2013**, *57*. [CrossRef]

143. Uusitupa, M.; Hermansen, K.; Savolainen, M.J.; Schwab, U.; Kolehmainen, M.; Brader, L.; Mortensen, L.S.; Cloetens, L.; Johansson-Persson, A.; Önning, G.; et al. Effects of an isocaloric healthy Nordic diet on insulin sensitivity, lipid profile and inflammation markers in metabolic syndrome—A randomized study (SYSDIET). *J. Intern. Med.* **2013**, *274*, 52–66. [CrossRef] [PubMed]

144. de la Iglesia, R.; Loria-Kohen, V.; Zulet, M.A.; Martinez, J.A.; Reglero, G.; Ramirez de Molina, A. Dietary Strategies Implicated in the Prevention and Treatment of Metabolic Syndrome. *Int. J. Mol. Sci.* **2016**, *17*, 1877. [CrossRef] [PubMed]

145. Peña-Orihuela, P.; Camargo, A.; Rangel-Zuñiga, O.A.; Perez-Martinez, P.; Cruz-Teno, C.; Delgado-Lista, J.; Yubero-Serrano, E.M.; Paniagua, J.A.; Tinahones, F.J.; Malagon, M.M.; et al. Antioxidant system response is modified by dietary fat in adipose tissue of metabolic syndrome patients. *J. Nutr. Biochem.* **2013**, *24*, 1717–1723. [CrossRef] [PubMed]

146. Giardina, S.; Sala-Vila, A.; Hernández-Alonso, P.; Calvo, C.; Salas-Salvadó, J.; Bulló, M. Carbohydrate quality and quantity affects the composition of the red blood cell fatty acid membrane in overweight and obese individuals. *Clin. Nutr.* **2018**, *37*, 481–487. [CrossRef]

147. Chang, C.Y.; Kanthimathi, M.S.; Tan, A.T.; Nesaretnam, K.; Teng, K.T. The amount and types of fatty acids acutely affect insulin, glycemic and gastrointestinal peptide responses but not satiety in metabolic syndrome subjects. *Eur. J. Nutr.* **2018**, *57*, 179–190. [CrossRef]

148. Hjorth, M.F.; Ritz, C.; Blaak, E.E.; Saris, W.H.M.; Langin, D.; Poulsen, S.K.; Larsen, T.M.; Sørensen, T.I.; Zohar, Y.; Astrup, A. Pretreatment fasting plasma glucose and insulin modify dietary weight loss success: Results from 3 randomized clinical trials. *Am. J. Clin. Nutr.* **2017**, *106*, 499–505. [CrossRef]

149. Rock, C.L.; Flatt, S.W.; Pakiz, B.; Quintana, E.L.; Heath, D.D.; Rana, B.K.; Natarjan, L. Effects of diet composition on weight loss, metabolic factors and biomarkers in a 1-year weight loss intervention in obese women examined by baseline insulin resistance status. *Metabolism* **2016**, *65*, 1605–1613. [CrossRef]

150. Van Namen, M.; Prendergast, L.; Peiris, C. Supervised lifestyle intervention for people with metabolic syndrome improves outcomes and reduces individual risk factors of metabolic syndrome: A systematic review and meta-analysis. *Metabolism* **2019**, *101*, 153988. [CrossRef]

151. Tobias, D.K.; Chen, M.; Manson, J.E.; Ludwig, D.S.; Willett, W.; Hu, F.B. Effect of low-fat diet interventions versus other diet interventions on long-term weight change in adults: A systematic review and meta-analysis. *Lancet Diabetes Endocrinol.* **2015**, *3*, 968–979. [CrossRef]

152. Pirozzo, S.; Summerbell, C.; Cameron, C.; Glasziou, P. Should we recommend low-fat diets for obesity? *Obes. Rev.* **2003**, *4*, 83–90. [CrossRef] [PubMed]

Sex Differences in Risk Factors for Metabolic Syndrome in the Korean Population

Yunjeong Yi and Jiyeon An *

Department of Nursing, Kyungin Women's University, Incheon 21041, Korea; yinyis@kiwu.ac.kr
* Correspondence: jyan030@kiwu.ac.kr

Abstract: With an increase in the obese population, the prevalence of metabolic syndrome is increasing in Korea. This study aimed to identify sex- and age-specific risk factors for metabolic syndrome. A secondary data analysis was performed using the Korean National Health and Nutritional Examination Survey. Participants comprised 6144 adults aged 20–79 years. The prevalence of metabolic syndrome was high in the middle- and old-aged men (31.9% and 34.5%, respectively) and in old-aged women (39.1%). Risk factors for metabolic syndrome showed different patterns for men and women. In men, alcohol drinking was identified as the main risk factor for hypertension (odds ratio (OR); young = 3.3 vs. middle age = 2.0), high triglycerides (young = 2.4 vs. middle age = 2.2), and high fasting blood sugar (middle age = 1.6). In women, the main risk factors were household income and education level, showing different patterns in different age groups. In conclusion, the vulnerable groups at high risk of metabolic syndrome are those of middle-aged men and women. The pattern of risk factors is sex-specific.

Keywords: metabolic syndrome; obesity; lifestyle; health behavior; alcohol consumption; socioeconomic status

1. Background

Metabolic syndrome is a group of conditions, which together increase the risk of developing atherosclerotic cardiovascular disease, insulin resistance and diabetes mellitus, and vascular and neurological diseases. Metabolic syndrome is associated with high all-cause mortality as well as mortality due to cardiovascular disease [1]. The main causes of metabolic syndrome are abdominal obesity, high blood pressure, diabetes, and dyslipidemia. With an increase in the obese population worldwide, the prevalence of metabolic syndrome is increasing [2,3]. The global prevalence of metabolic syndrome varies slightly depending on the definition of each component and ranges from 24.3% to 45.5% [4,5].

Since metabolic syndrome is a cluster of factors, it is difficult to manage and treat this condition compared to other diseases. The pathogenesis of metabolic syndrome can be described by a complex mechanism. Overweight and obesity are central to the development of metabolic syndrome, predisposing to hypertension, insulin resistance, and dyslipidemia, all of which are risk factors of metabolic syndrome. Physical inactivity and fatty food intake are major causes of obesity [6]. The metabolic abnormality triggered by some intrauterine conditions is accompanied by epigenetic changes [7]. Studies showed that metabolic syndrome is caused by epigenetic modifications rather than genetic predisposition [8], suggesting that external environmental factors lead to changes in gene expression that cause metabolic syndrome.

The external environmental factors associated with metabolic syndrome have been identified as demographic and social characteristics, socio-economic factors, and health behavior and lifestyle [7]. Most countries have national health policies for the management of metabolic syndrome. The public policy for this condition aims to correct lifestyle habits, such as improving eating habits, increasing physical activity, encouraging smoking cessation, regulating alcohol drinking, and managing stress. Despite the implementation of the national health policy for metabolic syndrome, it is difficult to manage the risk factors associated with this condition during adulthood because health behavior and lifestyle are developed through the interaction of genetic, social, and environmental factors since childhood. Moreover, there are several barriers to lifestyle changes due to heterogeneity between different social groups [9]. Individual heterogeneity may be affected by behavioral or environmental effects, but biological sex differences are affected by environmental influences with aging, resulting in more remarkable differences [10]. Therefore, individual heterogeneity, associated with metabolic syndrome development, is primarily explained by sex and age. As people age, they face increasingly complex and often interrelated problems, including physical, psychological, and social problems. Sex differences in metabolic syndrome, in addition to age differences, increase individual heterogeneity. Sex- and age-related factors of metabolic syndrome are sensitive to biological, environmental, and psychosocial conditions [11]. For this reason, sex and age are statistically treated as control variables or used as mediating variables. In previous studies, the hypothesis that the pattern of eating habits directly affects the components of the metabolic syndrome was rejected, and in the end, it was explained that sex differences influenced the linear relationship between the pattern of eating habits and metabolic syndrome [12]. Moreover, sex differences in risk factors for metabolic syndrome are caused by age differences; consequently, sex differences in metabolic syndrome prevalence are due to physiological differences such as hormones, differences in social and psychological stressors, and differences in lifestyle. This is formed integrally [13]. Differences in sex or age appear not only as risk factors for metabolic syndrome but also for mortality from metabolic syndrome.

According to a recent meta-analysis on metabolic syndrome, low high-density lipoprotein cholesterol (HDL-C), hyperglycemia, and elevated blood pressure have higher association with all-cause mortality and cardiovascular mortality in women [14]. Differences in sex and age in the incidence of and mortality from metabolic syndrome can be explained by differences in risk factors. As Korea quickly transitions from being a developing to a developed country, studies on obesity and metabolic syndrome are increasing due to westernized dietary habits and increased sedentary lifestyle. With ongoing research on the risk factors for metabolic syndrome, accumulated knowledge on metabolic syndrome risk factors is still a necessity. Most previous studies only investigated differences according to sex or restricted their investigation to the elderly population only [15,16]. As such, when determining the risk factors for metabolic syndrome, it is necessary to comprehensively consider the influence of sex and age; thus, national policies for metabolic syndrome management may be more specific. Herein, we aimed to identify the sex- and age-specific risk factors for metabolic syndrome in the Korean population and attempted to determine whether any pattern exists among the risk factors.

2. Materials and Methods

2.1. Research Design

This study used the 2017 survey data of the Korea National Health and Nutrition Examination Survey (KNHANES). It was a secondary data analysis study to determine how the factors influencing each variable of metabolic syndrome vary with sex and age.

2.2. Setting

The KNHANES has been conducted since 1998, and the sampling frame of the survey used the most recent census data and public prices of apartments available at the point of sampling. The sampling method was a two-stage stratified cluster sampling method in which the primary extraction unit was a survey unit and the secondary extraction unit a household. In the 2017 survey, 192 households were surveyed, and 23 sample households were selected using the system extraction method. All subjects aged 1 year and above were selected for the survey.

2.3. Participants

This study used the 2017 survey data with 3580 households participating and 8127 participants (proportion of men, 46.3%). In total, 6144 people were analyzed, with age between 20 and 79 years, and the proportion of men was 45.1%.

2.4. Variables

2.4.1. Dependent Variable

The dependent variables in this study were the five variables used in diagnosing metabolic syndrome: waist circumference, blood pressure, triglycerides, fasting blood sugar, and HDL-C. These standards were announced by the American Heart Association/National Heart, Lung, and Blood Institute Scientific Statement [17].

This clinical definition of metabolic syndrome required the presence of three or more of the following five criteria: (1) waist circumference over 90 cm for men and over 85 cm for women; (2) blood pressure above 130 mmHg for systolic or 85 mmHg for diastolic blood pressure; (3) triglyceride levels of 150 mg/dL or higher; (4) fasting blood sugar level of 100 mg/dL or higher; (5) HDL-cholesterol level less than 40 mg/dL for men and less than 50 mg/dL for women.

2.4.2. Independent Variables

The independent variables included sex, age, household income, education level, subjective health status, monthly alcohol intake, stress recognition, smoking status, aerobic physical activity, number of "eating out" episodes per day, and living with spouse. The subjects were divided into young (20–39 years old), middle-aged (40–59 years old), and old-aged (60–79 years old), and income was divided into quintiles using the household income.

The level of education was classified into "below high school" and "above college." Regarding the subjective health status, the five-point scale from "very bad" to "very good" was divided into two categories: "under average" and "over good." Drinking status was categorized as "drunk more than once a month in the past year" or "drunk once per month".

Stress recognition was divided into two categories: "a lot" and "little" based on an unusual four-point scale of "how much stress you usually feel in your daily life?".

A smoker was defined as a person who smoked more than five packs (100 cigarettes) in his lifetime and at the same time, smokes daily. Aerobic physical activity was considered if a person engaged in more than 2.5 h of high-intensity physical activity per week, more than 1.25 h of moderate-intensity physical activity, or the time equivalent to each activity by mixing moderate- and high-intensity physical activity (1 min of high-intensity equates to 2 min of moderate-intensity physical activity). Based on dining out, people who eat out more than once a day and those who do not eat out were distinguished.

The analysis criteria of the KNHANES were used to categorize subjective health status, monthly alcohol intake, stress recognition, smoking, aerobic physical activity, and dining out. These criteria are used by the Ministry of Health and Welfare in its "annual statistics book" based on data from the KNHANES.

2.5. Data Measurement

The KNHANES collects data through household member confirmation surveys, health questionnaire surveys, examination surveys, and nutrition surveys. Health questionnaire surveys were divided into household surveys, health interview surveys, and health behavior surveys. The family survey was conducted in the form of an interview survey on one adult (over 19 years of age) in the household. The health interview survey investigated the level of education and physical activities by the interview survey method, whereas the health behavior survey investigated smoking, drinking, mental health, etc., by the self-reported survey method. The examination surveys consisted of physical measurement, blood pressure and pulse measurement, blood and urine test, oral examination, lung function test, eye test, and grip test.

2.6. Statistical Methods

Since the KNHANES data were from two-stage stratified cluster sampling rather than a full-scale survey, they were analyzed to reflect the complex sampling elements, which can be expanded to the target group, the Korean population. A complex sample analysis with strata, cluster, and weights was performed, and the missing values were valid, and the sex and age-group data were applied to the parent group. In frequency analysis, non-weighted frequencies were calculated as statistics, and odds ratios (ORs) were calculated through complex sample logistic regression.

2.7. Ethical Considerations

The KNHANES was performed without being reviewed by the Research Ethics Review Committee from 2015 under the provisions of the Bioethics Act, which falls under the research conducted directly by the state for public welfare. The raw data for this study were downloaded and analyzed after signing and submitting the "Statistics User's Compliance Statement" and "Security pledge" on the website of the National Health and Nutrition Survey.

3. Results

The general characteristics of the study subjects according to sex and age are shown in Table 1. The old-aged group had a lower income and a lower education level than that of the other age groups. The young age group had a higher monthly alcohol intake, stress recognition, aerobic physical activity, and number of instances of "dining out" per day than that of other age groups. Subjective health and smoking habits differed in the dominant age groups by sex (Table 1).

The prevalence of each variable of metabolic syndrome in men and women of different age groups is shown in Table 2. In women, the prevalence of all variables was highest in the old-aged group ($p < 0.001$), whereas in men, the prevalence of hypertension and high triglyceride level ($p < 0.001$) was highest in the middle-aged group; no difference in waist circumference was observed between different age groups (Table 2). In men, the prevalence of metabolic syndrome was more than 30% in middle-aged and old-aged groups ($p < 0.001$), whereas in women, the prevalence was more than 30% in the middle-aged group only ($p < 0.001$).

The factors influencing each component of the metabolic syndrome in males and in females of different age groups are presented in Tables 3–5. In men, subjective health status and monthly alcohol drinking were the main variables of all ages (Table 3). Alcohol drinking was a risk factor for hypertension (OR = 2.0, $p < 0.001$), high triglyceride levels (OR = 2.2, $p < 0.001$), and increased fasting blood sugar (OR = 1.6, $p < 0.05$) in middle-aged men.

More variables affected women than men and included household income, education level, monthly alcohol drinking, and subjective health status (Table 4). Factors affecting each sex and different age groups were very different. Household income was identified as a prominent risk factor in women. The middle-aged group had the highest number of risk factors in both men and women. In males, the young age group was mainly affected by monthly alcohol drinking, the middle-aged group was affected by monthly alcohol drinking and subjective health status, and the old-aged group was affected by subjective health and smoking. In women, the middle-aged group was mainly affected by education levels and subjective health status, whereas the old-aged group was mainly affected by income levels. In both men and women, most of the variables affected the middle-aged group. In all age groups, women had more influencing variables than men (Table 5).

Table 1. General characteristics of subjects by sex and age groups (n, %).

		Male				Female			
		20–39 (n = 789)	40–59 (n = 1131)	60–79 (n = 852)	Chi-Square (p)	20–39 (n = 918)	40–59 (n = 1352)	60–79 (n = 1102)	Chi-Square (p)
Household income	Low	42 (6.7)	76 (5.9)	199 (22.0)	182.5 (<0.001)	29 (3.2)	81 (5.7)	370 (34.7)	328.7 (<0.001)
	Middle low	90 (12.5)	135 (12.4)	220 (26.1)		130 (14.7)	197 (15.2)	280 (25.1)	
	Middle	180 (25.5)	192 (19.5)	185 (23.5)		222 (27.5)	282 (20.9)	192 (17.8)	
	Middle high	206 (29.0)	284 (27.0)	113 (14.6)		253 (28.8)	332 (26.6)	117 (11.9)	
	High	207 (26.3)	362 (35.2)	106 (13.9)		221 (25.8)	408 (31.7)	107 (10.5)	
Education Level	Under high school	281 (42.4)	489 (48.9)	615 (77.4)	102.1 (<0.001)	252 (29.8)	737 (59.9)	938 (92.2)	282.1 (<0.001)
	Over college	411 (57.6)	483 (51.1)	159 (22.6)		566 (70.2)	499 (40.1)	73 (7.8)	
Subjective health status	Over good	251 (36.3)	273 (27.9)	222 (29.5)	11.9 (0.003)	255 (29.9)	338 (26.2)	136 (13.0)	64.4 (<0.001)
	Under average	443 (63.7)	706 (72.1)	560 (70.5)		565 (70.1)	904 (73.8)	879 (87.0)	
Monthly alcohol drinking	<1	169 (23.6)	251 (24.5)	297 (34.3)	22.5 (<0.001)	329 (38.0)	695 (53.1)	812 (76.9)	213.4 (<0.001)
	≥1	554 (76.4)	786 (75.5)	521 (65.7)		520 (62.0)	596 (46.9)	246 (23.1)	
Stress recognition	No	458 (64.1)	763 (73.6)	685 (83.4)	60.1 (<0.001)	534 (61.2)	938 (72.4)	786 (73.9)	37.3 (<0.001)
	Yes	265 (35.9)	274 (26.4)	132 (16.6)		315 (38.8)	351 (27.6)	267 (26.1)	
Smoking	No	433 (59.5)	605 (58.3)	621 (76.2)	54.4 (<0.001)	785 (92.1)	1237 (95.5)	1030 (97.5)	27.2 (<0.001)
	Yes	290 (40.5)	432 (41.7)	195 (23.8)		64 (7.9)	52 (4.5)	26 (2.5)	
Aerobic physical activity	No	290 (41.4)	516 (52.9)	510 (64.1)	48.8 (<0.001)	403 (47.2)	674 (55.2)	698 (68.3)	65.2 (<0.001)
	Yes	401 (58.6)	457 (47.1)	263 (35.9)		415 (52.8)	562 (44.8)	308 (31.7)	
Number of instances of dining out per day	<1	292 (49.6)	503 (58.0)	674 (88.1)	160.6 (<0.001)	557 (74.7)	1005 (85.8)	935 (96.0)	106.1 (<0.001)
	≥1	295 (50.4)	333 (42.0)	79 (11.9)		187 (25.3)	173 (14.2)	38 (4.0)	
Living with spouse	Yes	291 (98.7)	859 (92.1)	728 (90.5)	14.7 (0.001)	467 (96.8)	1104 (88.5)	671 (63.2)	209.0 (<0.001)
	No	5 (1.3)	80 (7.9)	84 (9.5)		17 (3.2)	151 (11.5)	390 (36.8)	

Table 2. Prevalence of metabolic syndrome components according to sex and age groups (n, %).

		Male				Female			
		20–39 (n = 789)	40–59 (n = 1131)	60–79 (n = 852)	Chi-Square (p)	20–39 (n = 918)	40–59 (n = 1352)	60–79 (n = 1102)	Chi-Square (p)
Waist circumference	No	482 (68.1)	674 (67.3)	491 (62.8)	4.6 (0.101)	739 (88.4)	991 (78.4)	578 (57.6)	133.4 (<0.001)
	Yes	225 (31.9)	329 (32.7)	294 (37.2)		104 (11.6)	279 (21.4)	441 (42.4)	
Hypertension	No	532 (73.1)	632 (60.0)	494 (61.4)	25.7 (<0.001)	81.2 (94.7)	998 (78.0)	558 (54.2)	241.9 (<0.001)
	Yes	195 (26.9)	420 (40.0)	330 (38.6)		48 (5.3)	303 (22.0)	511 (45.8)	
Triglyceride	No	456 (65.1)	556 (54.2)	515 (64.8)	25.2 (<0.001)	735 (89.5)	1007 (79.5)	711 (71.2)	61.7 (<0.001)
	Yes	254 (34.9)	472 (45.8)	283 (35.2)		93 (10.5)	257 (20.5)	292 (28.8)	
Fasting blood sugar	No	562 (80.8)	520 (50.9)	346 (44.2)	215.9 (<0.001)	760 (92.5)	913 (72.4)	515 (51.8)	237.4 (<0.001)
	Yes	148 (19.2)	508 (49.1)	452 (55.8)		67 (7.5)	351 (27.6)	488 (48.2)	
HDL cholesterol	No	570 (82.1)	752 (73.2)	548 (70.3)	24.9 (<0.001)	612 (75.4)	837 (67.1)	506 (51.0)	88.0 (<0.001)
	Yes	130 (17.9)	267 (26.8)	238 (29.7)		207 (24.6)	407 (32.9)	487 (49.0)	
Metabolic syndrome	No	547 (80.9)	662 (68.1)	489 (65.5)	43.4 (<0.001)	765 (95.6)	999 (82.9)	563 (60.9)	156.6 (<0.001)
	Yes	134 (19.1)	310 (31.9)	258 (34.5)		39 (4.4)	215 (17.1)	384 (39.1)	

Table 3. Factors affecting metabolic syndrome components in different male age groups.

Variables	Reference	Categories	Waist Circumference			Hypertension			Triglyceride			Fasting Blood Sugar			HDL Cholesterol			Metabolic Syndrome		
			20–39	40–59	60–79	20–39	40–59	60–79	20–39	40–59	60–79	20–39	40–59	60–79	20–39	40–59	60–79	20–39	40–59	60–79
Household income	High	Low	3.5	0.9	1.3	0.4	1.3	1.3	4.0	2.7*	1.0	0.1	1.4	1.4	0.0**	1.5	1.3	0.5	1.9	2.0
		Middle low	1.1	1.0	1.0	0.5	0.6	1.1	0.9	1.6	1.2	0.5	1.5	1.0	0.8	1.2	1.1	0.4	1.7	1.3
		Middle	0.8	1.2	1.0	0.7	0.9	1.2	1.0	1.0	1.0	0.5	0.8	1.0	1.3	1.1	1.3	0.5	1.4	1.2
		Middle high	0.5	1.1	1.3	0.8	0.9	1.2	1.3	1.0	1.3	0.4*	1.3	0.8	2.1	1.0	1.0	0.4	1.5	1.5
Education level	Over college	Under high school	1.0	1.4	1.0	0.6	1.2	0.7	1.7	0.8	0.9	0.9	1.3	2.0**	0.9	0.8	0.8	1.3	0.9	1.2
Subjective health status	Over good	Under average	1.6	1.3	1.3	1.4	1.6*	1.3	1.4	1.5*	1.7*	1.4	1.4	1.5*	2.4	1.1	1.1	1.4	1.7*	1.9*
Monthly alcohol drinking	<1	≥1	1.3	1.1	0.8	3.3*	2.0**	1.4	2.4*	2.2**	1.0	1.1	1.6*	1.4	0.6	0.7	0.4**	2.2	1.9*	0.9
Stress recognition	No	Yes	0.6	1.1	0.7	0.8	1.0	0.7	1.4	1.1	1.1	1.1	1.3	1.1	1.0	1.0	1.0	0.7	1.0	0.7
Smoking	No	Yes	1.0	0.7*	1.1	1.4	0.7*	1.1	1.4	1.4	1.6*	1.2	1.0	0.9	1.6	1.3	1.9**	1.7	1.0	1.2
Aerobic physical activity	No	Yes	0.6	0.7*	1.3	1.2	1.1	1.1	1.0	0.9	0.9	1.4	0.7	1.4	1.2	0.7	0.7	0.9	0.7	0.9
Number of instances of dining out per day	<1	≥1	1.0	0.9	1.3	1.0	0.9	1.0	1.1	0.9	0.9	1.1	0.6**	2.0*	0.9	0.7	0.8	1.0	0.6*	1.2
Living with spouse	Yes	No	3.6	0.7	1.0	2.5	1.1	0.7	1.1	0.7	1.0	1.3	1.0	0.8	2.3	1.3	1.9	1.2	0.5*	1.1

*p < 0.05; **p < 0.01.

Table 4. Factors affecting metabolic syndrome components in different female age groups.

Variables	Reference	Categories	Waist Circumstance			Hypertension			Triglyceride			Fasting Blood Sugar			HDL Cholesterol			Metabolic Syndrome		
			20–39	40–59	60–79	20–39	40–59	60–79	20–39	40–59	60–79	20–39	40–59	60–79	20–39	40–59	60–79	20–39	40–59	60–79
Household income	High	Low	4.3	1.1	1.9*	0.0**	2.0	1.1	1.4	1.1	2.3**	0.7	1.1	1.6	1.6	0.9	2.2*	1.7	1.0	2.1*
		Middle low	4.4*	2.1*	1.3	1.2	1.2	1.2	1.1	1.3	1.7	2.5	0.8	1.2	1.1	1.2	1.7	1.5	1.6	1.8
		Middle	3.4	1.4	1.4	1.3	1.1	1.2	1.2	0.9	1.0	1.1	0.6*	1.0	1.8	1.0	1.5	1.7	1.0	1.4
		Middle high	2.8	1.4	1.0	0.9	1.4	0.5*	1.9	0.7	1.1	1.0	0.8	1.2	2.1*	0.9	1.5	2.5	0.9	0.8
Education level	Over college	Under high school	1.7	2.0**	2.0	1.1	1.8**	1.0	1.4	1.5*	1.4	1.8	1.7**	1.4	1.4	1.4*	1.4	2.5	1.8**	1.6
Subjective health status	Over good	Under average	1.2	1.7*	1.5	1.0	1.9**	1.1	2.1	1.8*	1.0	0.7	1.3	1.1	1.1	1.2	1.0	1.8	2.2**	1.2
Monthly alcohol Drinking	<1	≥1	0.5	0.9	0.9	3.3*	1.1	0.7*	1.0	1.1	0.9	1.1	1.0	0.8	0.5*	0.7*	0.7*	0.7	0.8	0.7*
Stress recognition	No	Yes	1.1	1.4	0.9	0.9	1.2	1.4	0.8	1.0	1.1	0.8	0.8	0.9	1.0	1.1	0.8	1.5	1.3	0.8
Smoking	No	Yes	1.7	1.0	0.2*	1.0	1.1	1.4	1.4	2.0	0.3	2.9	0.5	1.1	4.0**	1.5	0.9	1.7	1.4	0.8
Aerobic physical activity	No	Yes	1.5	0.6**	0.9	1.4	1.0	0.9	0.9	0.7*	0.8	1.8	0.9	0.8	1.0	0.9	0.9	1.6	0.8	0.9
Number of instances of dining out per day	<1	≥1	0.8	1.0	0.5	0.7	0.4**	1.3	0.7	0.8	0.6	0.6	1.0	1.5	0.9	1.0	0.6	0.3	0.8	0.7
Living with spouse	Yes	No	1.0	1.1	1.3	15.1**	1.1	1.2	1.6	0.7	0.8	4.3*	0.9	1.5*	0.5	0.7	0.7*	3.4	1.0	0.8

*p < 0.05; **p < 0.01.

Table 5. The number of significant risk factors associated with different components of metabolic syndrome in the different age groups of both sexes.

Variables	Male															Female														
	20–39					40–59					60–79					20–39					40–59					60–79				
	WC	HT	TG	FBS	HDL-C	WC	HT	TG	FBS	HDL-C	WC	HT	TG	FBS	HDL-C	WC	HT	TG	FBS	HDL-C	WC	HT	TG	FBS	HDL-C	WC	HT	TG	FBS	HDL-C
Household income					−			+								+	−				+	+	+	−			−		+	+
Education level				−										+							+	+		+	+					+
Subjective health status							+	+				+	+	+		+	+				+	+	+							
Monthly alcohol drinking	+		+				+	+	+						−		+								−					−
Stress recognition					−																	−								
Smoking						−	−						+		+						−									
Aerobic physical activity						−																	−							
Number of instances of dining out per day									−					+								−								
Living with spouse		+															+		+							+				−
Number of significant factors	0	1	1	2	2	2	3	3	2	0	0	0	2	3	2	1	3	0	1	3	4	3	3	2	2	2	2	1	1	3

WC: Waist Circumstance; HT: Hypertension; TG: Triglyceride; FBS: Fasting Blood Sugar; HDL-C: HDL-Cholesterol. (−) protective factor; (+) risk factor.

4. Discussion

This study investigated risk factors for metabolic syndrome by considering sex and age differences. Unlike previous studies, the study subjects included both adults and the elderly. Regarding the prevalence rate of each component of metabolic syndrome, there were differences in frequency by sex and age, excluding waist circumference. Compared to men, women generally had a higher prevalence rate for each component of metabolic syndrome in the elderly than in young adults. These results support the existing research findings that women experience physiological changes that make them susceptible to metabolic syndrome with aging. Menopause, characterized by a decline in circulating estrogen levels, may increase cardiovascular risk through its effects on adiposity and lipid metabolism [18]. In fact, it is known that postmenopausal women have more than double the prevalence of metabolic syndrome compared to premenopausal women, especially with low HDL-C, high blood pressure, and high fast glucose levels [19].

The implications of the risk factors for metabolic syndrome by sex and age are as follows. The middle-aged people, regardless of sex, are exposed to more risk factors associated with metabolic syndrome than any other age group. Thus, the target risk group for managing metabolic syndrome is that of middle-aged people for both men and women. Compared to other age groups, middle-aged people spend a lot of time on economic activities; therefore, they neglect their own health care.

The risk factors for metabolic syndrome differed by sex. In middle-aged men, alcohol consumption was a risk factor for hypertension and high triglycerides, and in middle-aged women, education level was a risk factor for all five components of metabolic syndrome. The differences between men and women in risk factors related to metabolic syndrome may be due to differences in health behavior and lifestyle of men and women.

In general, excessive energy intake and concomitant obesity cause metabolic syndrome, resulting in atherosclerotic cardiovascular disorder and type 2 diabetes [20]. The main mechanism by which these complications arise from metabolic syndrome can be explained by vascular thickness and stiffness [21]. Among the pathological changes in blood vessels, vascular stiffness causes arteriosclerosis, and the blood vessels are narrowed due to fatty deposits. Thus, obesity-related diet and lifestyle are directly related to metabolic syndrome [22]. Among the obesity-related eating habits is alcohol consumption. Previous studies have identified that alcohol consumption cause metabolic syndrome because alcohol stimulates food consumption, resulting in an increase in total energy consumption [23]. In general, because the frequency and amount of alcohol intake is greater in men than in women, the negative effects of alcohol are more pronounced in men [24].

The association between the quantity of alcohol intake and metabolic syndrome is debatable. According to a previous study, considering both the quantity and the frequency of drinking, heavy alcohol consumption increases the risk of metabolic syndrome, while light alcohol consumption lowers the risk of metabolic syndrome [25,26]. Furthermore, it is reported that the link between drinking and metabolic syndrome is more pronounced in men than in women [27]. We observed that in men, alcohol consumption is a risk factor for metabolic syndrome, with relatively high OR values in young and middle-aged people. While alcohol consumption was identified as a risk factor in men, it was identified as a protective factor in women. This can be explained based on differences in the quantity and frequency of alcohol intake between men and women or due to interaction with other variables.

In middle-aged women, education level was identified as a risk factor in all five categories of metabolic syndrome. In women (young, middle-aged, and old) household income was shown as a risk factor for certain components of metabolic syndrome. Socioeconomic status, such as education level and household income, was reported to be a major risk factor for metabolic syndrome, especially in women.

The close association between socioeconomic status and metabolic syndrome, which is usually prominent in women, could be explained by the stress theory. In females, chronic psychosocial stress induces changes in the hypothalamus-pituitary-adrenal axis, resulting in increased insulin resistance or adipocyte proliferation, which ultimately causes metabolic syndrome. Stress influences health risk behaviors (smoking, low physical activity, drinking, and eating fat and sugar-rich products) leading to the development of metabolic syndrome [28]. Few studies suggest that low economic status is a specific barrier to change in lifestyle. Sparing time for physical activity or ensuring a budget to buy healthier food is not easy in the low-income group. Moreover, low-fat food or slow food is too expensive, and it is costly to use fitness centers to support lifestyle change [9].

In Korean women, education level and household income are associated with the risk of metabolic syndrome. With a low education level or low household income, they are likely to do domestic work as well as jobs for livelihood, which is a scenario known to cause metabolic syndrome due to increased stress and economic deprivation [29]. The study of the association between socioeconomic status (SES) and metabolic syndrome uses subjective SES. Subjective SES is known to increase the risk of central adiposity (waist-hip ratio), low HDL cholesterol, elevated serum triglycerides, and blood pressure in middle-aged women [30].

Our results are consistent between men and women. Physical activity has been shown to affect the waist circumference for both middle-aged men and women. The linear relationship between physical activity and obesity is already proven. According to a study conducted on twins, physical activity reduces the risk of developing high BMI and high waist circumference [31].

Obesity is a health issue that is most prominent in middle-aged people. A prospective study involving young adults aged 18–30 years who were not initially obese showed that more than 40%of these individuals developed overall and abdominal obesity during middle age and obesity was linked to the occurrence of subclinical heart disease [32]. It is the fact that obesity in adults lasts for a long time, which consequently leads to the development of atherosclerosis during middle age. Some researchers showed that the risk of metabolic syndrome increases after middle age because metabolic syndrome is affected by the aging process [33]. With aging, the risk of metabolic syndrome as well as the risk of cardiovascular disease increases. The management of metabolic syndrome in people of all age groups is necessary. However, in the middle-aged group, since the aging process is accelerated during this period, the management of metabolic syndrome needs to be focused [34]. Abdominal obesity management in middle-aged men and women is important healthcare that can prevent cardiovascular disease as well as metabolic syndrome.

In this study, we also investigated the association between the external environmental factors on different components of the metabolic syndrome in men and women of different age groups. Drinking is a risk factor in men; however, in women, it appears to be a protective factor for some components of metabolic syndrome. Regarding smoking, it was a protective factor for waist circumference; however, for dyslipidemia, it was found to be a risk factor. Smoking is known to be associated with low HDL-C and high triglyceride as well as with pathological changes in the blood vessels [35]. This study also showed that smoking was associated with high triglyceride and low HDL-C levels in older men, which is consistent with previous studies.

In summary, this study found that the prevalence of metabolic syndrome differs by sex and age and shows that the risk factors for metabolic syndrome that can be intervened also differ by sex and age. Although it is difficult to determine how risk factors cause metabolic changes in each sex and age group, this study suggests that the management of metabolic syndrome needs to integrate genetic and acquired influencing factors. Metabolic syndrome requires integrated treatment due to comorbidities. It is also a chronic and complex disease that increases the risk of cardiovascular disease and type 2 diabetes and is associated with high mortality. Since some individuals are predisposed to risk factors and the risk of complications associated with metabolic syndrome, some people require lifestyle modification, while others need direct pharmacological treatment [7]. Therefore, screening is required for high-risk groups, and customized guidelines are needed.

There are several limitations to our study. Although our study included a large sample, it does not include dietary-related variables related to metabolic syndrome and used some variables from the self-reporting survey. Unlike previous studies, our study analyzed factors affecting metabolic syndrome according to sex and age and identified patterns of related variables.

5. Conclusions

In summary, the target risk groups for metabolic syndrome are middle-aged men and women, and the risk factors for men and women are different. Middle-aged men are advised not to drink and smoke excessively, and women need to minimize unmet healthcare needs due to economic stress through preventive health service programs. For women, the risk factors of metabolic syndrome were higher than those in men. Women become more susceptible to metabolic syndrome with aging; hence, intensive interventions are needed after middle age to address the risk factors. Thus, different guidelines are required for men and women. These results will be applicable not only to the Korean population but also to people who have unhealthy health behaviors while living a competitive life globally. In particular, in all the countries with an increasing obese population, increasing interest in sex- and age-related risk factors for metabolic syndrome is required.

Author Contributions: Conceptualization, Y.Y. and J.A.; Methodology, Y.Y.; Writing—Original Preparation, Y.Y. and J.A.; Writing—Review and Editing, J.A. Both authors have read and agreed to the published version of the manuscript.

References

1. Ford, E.S. The metabolic syndrome and mortality from cardiovascular disease and all-causes: Findings from the National Health and Nutrition Examination Survey II Mortality Study. *Atherosclerosis* **2004**, *173*, 309–314. [CrossRef] [PubMed]

2. Mozumdar, A.; Liguori, G. Persistent increase of prevalence of metabolic syndrome among U.S. adults: NHANES III to NHANES 1999–2006. *Diabetes Care* **2011**, *34*, 216–219. [CrossRef] [PubMed]

3. Lim, S.; Shin, H.; Song, J.H.; Kwak, S.H.; Kang, S.M.; Yoon, J.W.; Choi, S.H.; Cho, S.I.; Park, K.S.; Lee, H.K.; et al. Increasing prevalence of metabolic syndrome in Korea: The Korean National Health and Nutrition Examination Survey for 1998–2007. *Diabetes Care* **2011**, *34*, 1323–1328. [CrossRef] [PubMed]

4. Saklayen, M.G. The Global Epidemic of the Metabolic Syndrome. *Curr. Hypertens. Rep.* **2018**, *20*, 12. [CrossRef] [PubMed]

5. Ranasinghe, P.; Mathangasinghe, Y.; Jayawardena, R.; Hills, A.P.; Misra, A. Prevalence and trends of metabolic syndrome among adults in the asia-pacific region: A systematic review. *BMC Public Health* **2017**, *17*, 101. [CrossRef]

6. O'Neill, S.; O'Driscoll, L. Metabolic syndrome: A closer look at the growing epidemic and its associated pathologies. *Obes. Rev.* **2015**, *16*, 1–12. [CrossRef]

7. Kassi, E.; Pervanidou, P.; Kaltsas, G.; Chrousos, G. Metabolic syndrome: Definitions and controversies. *BMC Med.* **2011**, *9*, 1–13. [CrossRef]

8. Smith, C.J.; Ryckman, K.K. Epigenetic and developmental influences on the risk of obesity, diabetes, and metabolic syndrome. *Diabetes Metab. Syndr. Obes.* **2015**, *8*, 295–302. [CrossRef]

9. Nielsen, J.P.; Leppin, A.; Gyrd-Hansen, D.E.; Jarbøl, D.E.; Søndergaard, J.; Larsen, P.V. Barriers to lifestyle changes for prevention of cardiovascular disease—A survey among 40–60-year old Danes. *BMC Cardiovasc. Disord.* **2017**, *17*, 245. [CrossRef]

10. Santos, A.C.; Ebrahim, S.; Barros, H. Gender, socio-economic status and metabolic syndrome in middle-aged and old adults. *BMC Public Health* **2008**, *62*, 1–8. [CrossRef]

11. Pucci, G.; Alcidi, R.; Tap, L.; Battista, F.; Mattace-Raso, F.; Schillaci, G. Sex-and gender-related prevalence, cardiovascular risk and therapeutic approach in metabolic syndrome: A review of the literature. *Pharmacol. Res.* **2017**, *120*, 34–42. [CrossRef] [PubMed]

12. Kang, Y.; Kim, J. Gender difference on the association between dietary patterns and metabolic syndrome in Korean population. *Eur. J. Nutr.* **2016**, *55*, 2321–2330. [CrossRef] [PubMed]

13. Tian, X.; Xu, X.; Zhang, K.; Wang, H. Gender difference of metabolic syndrome and its association with dietary diversity at different ages. *Oncotarget* **2017**, *8*, 73568–73575. [CrossRef] [PubMed]

14. Sergi, G.; Dianin, M.; Bertocco, A.; Zanforlini, B.M.; Curreri, C.; Mazzochin, M.; Simons, L.; Manzato, E.; Trevisan, C. Gender Differences in the impact of metabolic syndrome components on mortality in older people: A systematic review and meta-analysis. *Nutr. Metab. Cardiovasc. Dis.* **2020**, *30*, 1452–1464. [CrossRef] [PubMed]

15. Lee, S.J.; Ko, Y.; Kwak, C.Y.; Yim, E.S. Gender differences in metabolic syndrome components among the Korean 66-year-old population with metabolic syndrome. *BMC Geriatr.* **2016**, *16*. [CrossRef]

16. Cho, K.I.; Kim, B.H.; Je, H.G.; Jang, J.S.; Park, Y.H. Gender-specific association between socioeconomic status and psychological factors and metabolic syndrome in the Korean population: Findings from the 2013 Korean National and Nutrition Examination survey. *BioMed. Res. Int.* **2016**, 1–8. [CrossRef]

17. Grundy, S.M.; Cleeman, J.I.; Daniels, S.R.; Donato, K.A.; Eckel, R.H.; Franklin, B.A.; Gordon, D.J.; Krauss, R.M.; Savage, P.J.; Smith, S.C., Jr.; et al. Diagnosis and management of the metabolic syndrome: An American Heart Association/National Heart, Lung, and Blood Institute Scientific Statement. *Circulation* **2005**, *112*, 2735–2752. [CrossRef]

18. Schneider, J.G.; Tompkins, C.; Blumenthal, R.S.; Mora, S. The metabolic syndrome in women. *Cardiol. Rev.* **2006**, *14*, 286–291. [CrossRef]

19. March, R.; Dell'Agnolo, C.M.; Lopes, T.; Gravena, A.; Demitto, M.; Brischillari, S.; Borghesan, D.; Carvalho, M.; Pelloso, S. Prevalence of metabolic syndrome in pre-and postmenopausal women. *Arch. Endocrinol. Metab.* **2017**, *61*, 160–166. [CrossRef]

20. Grundy, S.M. Metabolic syndrome update. *Trends Cardiovasc. Med.* **2016**, *26*, 364–373. [CrossRef]

21. Scuteri, A.; Najjar, S.S.; Muller, D.C.; Andres, R.; Hougaku, H.; Metter, E.J.; Lakatta, E.G. Metabolic syndrome amplifies the age-associated increases in vascular thickness and stiffness. *J. Am. Coll. Cardiol.* **2004**, *43*, 1388–1395. [CrossRef] [PubMed]

22. Aroor, A.R.; Jia, G.; Sowers, J.R. Cellular mechanisms underlying obesity-induced arterial stiffness. *Am. J. Physiol. Regul. Integr. Comp. Physiol.* **2018**, *314*, R387–R398. [CrossRef] [PubMed]

23. Yeomans, M.R. Alcohol, appetite and energy balance: Is alcohol intake a risk factor for obesity? *Physiol. Behav.* **2010**, *100*, 82–89. [CrossRef] [PubMed]

24. Wilsnack, R.W.; Vogeltanz, N.D.; Wilsnack, S.C.; Harris, T.R. Gender differences in alcohol consumption and adverse drinking consequences: Cross-cultural patterns. *Addiction* **2000**, *95*, 251–265. [CrossRef] [PubMed]

25. Sun, K.; Ren, M.; Liu, D.; Wang, C.; Yang, C.; Yan, L. Alcohol consumption and risk of metabolic syndrome: A meta-analysis of prospective studies. *Clin. Nutr.* **2014**, *33*, 596–602. [CrossRef]

26. Alkerwi, A.; Boutsen, M.; Vaillant, M.; Barre, L.; Lair, M.L.; Albert, A.; Guillaume, M.; Dramaix, M. Alcohol consumption and the prevalence of metabolic syndrome: A meta-analysis of observational studies. *Atherosclerosis* **2009**, *204*, 624–635. [CrossRef]

27. Traversy, G.; Chaput, J.P. Alcohol consumption and obesity: An update. *Curr. Obes. Rep.* **2015**, *4*, 122–130. [CrossRef]

28. Bergmann, N.; Gyntelberg, F.; Faber, J. The appraisal of chronic stress and the development of the metabolic syndrome: A systematic review of prospective cohort studies. *Endocr. Connect.* **2014**, *3*, R55–R80. [CrossRef]

29. Seo, J.M.; Lim, N.K.; Lim, J.Y.; Park, H.Y. Gender difference in association with socioeconomic status and incidence of metabolic syndrome in Korean adults. *Korean J. Obes.* **2016**, *25*, 247–254. [CrossRef]

30. Manuck, S.B.; Phillips, J.E.; Gianaros, P.J.; Flory, J.D.; Muldoon, M.F. Subjective socioeconomic status and presence of the metabolic syndrome in midlife community volunteers. *Psychosom. Med.* **2010**, *72*, 35–45. [CrossRef]

31. Mustelin, L.; Silventoinen, K.; Pietiläinen, K.; Rissanen, A.; Kaprio, J. Physical activity reduces the influence of genetic effects on BMI and waist circumference: A study in young adult twins. *Int. J. Obes.* **2009**, *33*, 29–36. [CrossRef]

32. Reis, J.P.; Loria, C.M.; Lewis, C.E.; Powell-Wiley, T.M.; Wei, G.S.; Carr, J.J.; Terry, J.G.; Liu, K. Association between duration of overall and abdominal obesity beginning in young adulthood and coronary artery calcification in middle age. *JAMA* **2013**, *310*, 280–288. [CrossRef] [PubMed]

33. Bonomini, F.; Rodella, L.F.; Rezzani, R. Metabolic syndrome, aging and involvement of oxidative stress. *Aging Dis.* **2015**, *6*, 109–120. [CrossRef] [PubMed]

34. Hildrum, B.; Mykletun, A.; Hole, T.; Midthjell, K.; Dahl, A.A. Age-specific prevalence of the metabolic syndrome defined by the International Diabetes Federation and the National Cholesterol Education Program: The Norwegian HUNT 2 study. *BMC Public Health* **2007**, *7*, 220. [CrossRef] [PubMed]

35. Berlin, I.; Lin, S.; Lima, J.A.C.; Bertoni, A.G. Smoking status and metabolic syndrome in the multi-ethnic study of atherosclerosis. A cross-sectional study. *Tob. Induc. Dis.* **2012**, *10*, 9. [CrossRef] [PubMed]

3

PXR and 4β-Hydroxycholesterol Axis and the Components of Metabolic Syndrome

Janne Hukkanen [1],* and **Jukka Hakkola** [2],*

[1] Research Unit of Internal Medicine, Biocenter Oulu, Medical Research Center Oulu, University of Oulu and Oulu University Hospital, POB 5000, FI-90014 Oulu, Finland
[2] Research Unit of Biomedicine, Biocenter Oulu, Medical Research Center Oulu, University of Oulu and Oulu University Hospital, POB 5000, FI-90014 Oulu, Finland
* Correspondence: janne.hukkanen@oulu.fi (J.H.); jukka.hakkola@oulu.fi (J.H.)

Abstract: Pregnane X receptor (PXR) activation has been found to regulate glucose and lipid metabolism and affect obesity in response to high-fat diets. PXR also modulates vascular tone. In fact, PXR appears to regulate multiple components of metabolic syndrome. In most cases, the effect of PXR action is harmful to metabolic health, and PXR can be hypothesized to play an important role in metabolic disruption elicited by exposure to endocrine-disrupting chemicals. The majority of the data on the effects of PXR activation on metabolic health come from animal and cell culture experiments. However, randomized, placebo-controlled, human trials indicate that the treatment with PXR ligands impairs glucose tolerance and increases 24-h blood pressure and heart rate. In addition, plasma 4β-hydroxycholesterol (4βHC), formed under the control of PXR in the liver, is associated with lower blood pressure in healthy volunteers. Furthermore, 4βHC regulates cholesterol transporters in peripheral tissues and may activate the beneficial reverse HDL cholesterol transport. In this review, we discuss the current knowledge on the role of PXR and the PXR–4βHC axis in the regulation of components of metabolic syndrome.

Keywords: pregnane X receptor; 4β-hydroxycholesterol; metabolic syndrome; hypertension; reverse cholesterol transport; hyperglycemia; obesity

1. Introduction

Metabolic syndrome (MetS) is a cluster of risk factors that increases the risk of coronary heart disease, type 2 diabetes, and stroke [1,2]. Its prevalence has increased significantly in recent decades, with up to one third of the adult population having MetS [3,4]. The components of MetS include abdominal obesity, hyperglycemia, high blood pressure, low HDL cholesterol, and elevated triglycerides. MetS can be diagnosed if three or more of the following findings are present: a waist circumference of ≥94 cm in men and ≥80 cm in females, elevated triglyceride levels (≥1.7 mmol/L), low levels of HDL cholesterol (<1.0 mM in men, <1.3 mmol/L in women), high blood pressure (≥130/ ≥85 mmHg), and increased fasting glucose (≥5.6 mmol/L) [5]. Drug treatment for hypertension, low HDL cholesterol, hypertriglyceridemia, or hyperglycemia are included as alternate indicators.

The rising prevalence of MetS is largely attributed to the sedentary lifestyle and the obesity epidemic afflicting the global population. However, exposure to environmental pollutants has been suggested to be an additional risk factor for the development of MetS [6,7]. These metabolism-disrupting or endocrine-disrupting chemicals (EDCs) are especially linked to the incidence of type 2 diabetes and its preceding phenomena, namely insulin resistance and prediabetes [8,9]. In addition, a closely related environmental obesogen hypothesis has been proposed suggesting a causative role for EDCs in the pathogenesis of obesity [10,11]. There are also links between exposure to EDCs and the other components of MetS, i.e., hypertension, low HDL cholesterol (HDL-C), and elevated triglycerides [7].

Several molecular mechanisms mediating the effects of EDCs on metabolism have been proposed, including estrogen and other sex hormone receptors, glucocorticoid receptor, peroxisome proliferator-activated receptors, and xenobiotic-sensing receptors such as aryl hydrocarbon receptor (AhR), constitutive androstane receptor (CAR), and pregnane X receptor (PXR) [6,12]. In this review, we concentrate on the effects of PXR on MetS and discuss the possibility that, due to its roles as a xenosensor and a regulator of glucose and lipid metabolism as well as blood pressure [13,14], PXR activation could contribute to the development of MetS.

2. PXR and Obesity

Obesity is a major driver of MetS. The main cause of obesity is thought to be overnutrition, i.e., prolonged positive energy balance. Furthermore, certain chemicals have been shown to promote obesity. These so-called obesogens are considered a subclass of EDCs [11,15]. As a major xenosensor and a regulator of energy metabolism [13], PXR represents a putative target for the EDCs to mediate their weight-gain-promoting and other metabolic effects [16].

PXR has been reported to modulate the development of obesity in response to high-fat diets (HFDs). Several studies have observed reduced weight gain in *Pxr*-knockout (KO) mice under HFD, suggesting that PXR deficiency could protect against diet-induced obesity [17–19]. The *Pxr* KO did not affect the food intake [17,18], suggesting that energy expenditure must be altered. Indeed, He et al. observed increased oxygen consumption in *Pxr*-KO mice [18]. Furthermore, a recent study found increased fibroblast growth factor 15 (FGF15) expression, reduced serum bile acids level, and increased fecal lipid content in the HFD-fed *Pxr*-KO mice [19]. These findings suggest that *Pxr* KO reduces lipid absorption, possibly through FGF15-mediated regulation of bile acid synthesis [19].

While the results in the *Pxr*-KO models suggest that PXR plays an obesity-promoting role, there are also contradictory results. Ma and Liu reported that treatment of obesity-prone ARK/J mice with PXR ligand pregnenolone 16α-carbonitrile (PCN) inhibited weight gain under HFD and at the final time point of seven weeks, the weight of the PCN-treated mice was similar to the chow-fed mice [20]. The prevention of HFD-induced weight gain by PCN was due to reduced fat mass [20]. The PCN-treated mice ate less; however, the caloric intake ratio to the bodyweight was actually slightly increased [20]. The authors observed higher body temperature in the PCN-treated mice upon cold exposure and induction of thermogenesis genes in the brown adipose tissue, suggesting enhanced thermogenesis. Thus, although the oxygen consumption was not measured, these results suggest that the brown adipose tissue activity in response to PCN could cause increased energy expenditure. There was no *Pxr*-KO control in these experiments, and therefore some uncertainty about the molecular mediator remains; however, the majority of the PCN effects are mediated by PXR [20]. Together, these results appear to suggest a puzzling conclusion that both *Pxr* KO and PXR activation attenuate HFD-induced obesity. Clearly, more studies are still needed to fully characterize the effect of PXR on diet-induced obesity in mice.

The situation is even more complex when the *PXR*-humanized mouse model is studied. In males, *PXR* humanization inhibited HFD-induced weight gain [17]. In contrast, in females, the *PXR* humanization aggravated HFD-induced obesity [21]. Although these models have humanized *PXR*, it needs to be kept in mind that otherwise they still represent mouse physiology, and thus the results cannot be directly translated to humans. No data from controlled clinical studies exist on this subject. The current view of the PXR effect on obesity has been collected in Table 1.

Table 1. Summary of studies on PXR and obesity.

Study	Model	Observed Effect on Obesity	Suggested Mechanism
Ma and Liu 2012 [20]	Male obesity-prone ARK/J mice on HFD (60%) for 7 weeks, treated with PCN or vehicle twice weekly	PCN treatment inhibited weight gain	PCN treatment enhanced thermogenesis, reduced food intake
He et al. 2013 [18]	WT and *Pxr*-KO mice on HFD (60%) for 12 weeks	*Pxr* KO inhibited weight gain	*Pxr* KO increased energy expenditure
	Pxr-KO mouse line crossed with *Ob/Ob* mice and fed with chow diet	*Pxr* KO did not affect weight gain but the *Pxr* KO mice had decreased fat mass	
	Alb-VP-*Pxr* mouse line crossed with *Ob/Ob* mice and fed with chow diet	Transgenic activation of PXR reduced body weight	
Spruiell et al. 2014a [17]	Male WT and *Pxr*-KO mice on HFD (45%) for 16 weeks	*Pxr* KO inhibited weight gain	
	Male *PXR*-humanized mice on HFD (45%) for 16 weeks	*PXR* humanization inhibited weight gain	Reduced food intake, higher basal serum leptin level
Spruiell et al. 2014b [21]	Female *PXR*-humanized mice on HFD (45%) for 16 weeks	*PXR* humanization increased weight gain	Suppression of protective role of estrogen
Zhao et al. 2017 [19]	Male WT and *Pxr* KO mice on HFD (45%) for 4 weeks	*Pxr* KO inhibited weight gain	Induction of FGF15 expression in *Pxr*-KO mice, reduced lipid absorption

3. PXR and Glucose Homeostasis

Among the components of MetS, disruption of glucose metabolism is the one with the strongest evidence of being targeted by PXR activation. The harmful effect of PXR ligands on postprandial glucose metabolism has been established in two clinical intervention trials [22,23]. We performed a randomized, single-blind, placebo-controlled, crossover trial to investigate the effect of rifampicin, a well-established PXR agonist, on oral glucose tolerance [22]. Remarkably, relatively short, 7-day treatment with rifampicin impaired glucose tolerance as measured with oral glucose tolerance test, suggesting that PXR activation induces postprandial hyperglycemia. An analogous effect has been observed in rats with a structurally different, nonantibiotic rodent PXR ligand PCN, supporting the idea that PXR indeed mediates the effect [22,24]. Furthermore, four-day treatment of mice with PCN similarly impaired glucose tolerance [25]. The effect was abolished by *Pxr* KO, confirming the involvement of PXR. Studies in rats and humans indicated that the disruption of glucose tolerance by PXR agonists is not mediated by incretin hormones such as glucagon-like peptide-1 [26].

Stage et al. performed a clinical trial using 21-day treatment with St. John's wort, an herbal medicine with established PXR-activation property [23]. Comparison of the oral glucose tolerance test results before and after the treatment indicated that St. John's wort caused impairment of glucose tolerance. Strikingly, the impairment remained six weeks after cessation of the treatment, suggesting a long-lasting effect. However, the design of that study was not ideal as there was no control arm.

The mechanisms involved in the PXR-elicited glucose intolerance have been characterized in some detail and appear to be due to suppression of hepatic glucose uptake [25]. At the molecular level, PXR represses glucose transporter 2 (GLUT2) mRNA and protein expression in liver, both constitutively and in response to glucose [22,25]. Furthermore, immunohistochemistry of the PCN-treated and control mice livers suggested that the PXR activation promotes GLUT2 internalization from the plasma membrane to the cytosol [25]. Dysregulation of GLUT2 function may play an important role in the reduced hepatic glucose uptake. Additionally, the next step in the glucose uptake, phosphorylation by glucokinase (GCK), may also be repressed since the GCK mRNA expression tended to be downregulated in the mouse and rat liver by PXR activation, although the effect was not as consistent as that of the GLUT2 repression [22,25]. In HepG2 cells, PXR ligands rifampicin and atorvastatin, unlike the non-PXR-ligand pravastatin, repressed GLUT2 and GCK protein levels [24]. Knockdown of PXR had an opposite effect [24], supporting the in vivo results in rodents. Both *Glut2* and *Gck* KO mice have been shown to manifest mild hyperglycemia in a fed state, fitting with the theory that repression of these proteins involved in glucose utilization could result in postprandial hyperglycemia [27,28]. The current model of PXR's effect on hepatic glucose uptake is presented in Figure 1.

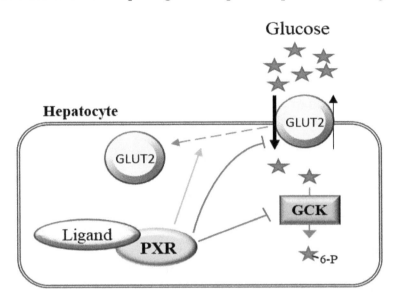

Figure 1. Mechanisms mediating the effect of PXR activation on hepatic glucose uptake. In the postprandial state, GLUT2 glucose transporter facilitates glucose uptake into the hepatocytes. In the next step of glucose utilization, glucose is phosphorylated by GCK. Ligand-activated PXR represses expression of both GLUT2 and GCK. PXR activation also relocates GLUT2 from the plasma membrane to the cytosol. Together, these alterations reduce postprandial hepatic glucose uptake.

In addition to the glucose uptake, PXR activation may affect gluconeogenesis. However, the effect may be species-specific. It is rather well established that PXR ligands repress the key gluconeogenic genes glucose-6-phosphatase (*G6Pase*) and phosphoenolpyruvate carboxykinase (*Pepck*) in mouse liver and mouse primary hepatocytes (for review, see [13] and the references therein). Mechanistically, this involves PXR-mediated transrepression through interaction with several key transcription factors regulating gluconeogenesis, including Forkhead box protein O1 (FOXO1) and cAMP response element-binding protein (CREB), or, in the case of hepatocyte nuclear factor 4 (HNF4), competition for the common coactivator PGC-1α (peroxisome proliferator-activated receptor gamma (PPARγ) coactivator 1α) [29–31].

Repression of the gluconeogenic genes is expected to result in the downregulation of gluconeogenesis and hepatic glucose output, i.e., beneficial effect in insulin resistance models. In some experimental settings, such an effect has been observed. Ma and Liu reported that PCN treatment of HFD-fed mice improved glucose tolerance [20]. As described above, this was associated with a beneficial effect on weight gain that may explain the finding. On the other hand, He et al. observed that transgenic activation of PXR with liver specific Alb-VP-*Pxr* allele worsened glucose tolerance and insulin sensitivity in the *Ob/Ob* mice [18]. In the same study, *Pxr*-KO improved glucose tolerance in the context of HFD-feeding or *Ob/Ob* genotype. Finally, Spruiell et al. reported that both *Pxr* KO and humanization aggravated HFD-induced impairment of glucose tolerance in male mice [17]. Surprisingly, in both cases, these genetic manipulations were associated with a beneficial effect on weight gain [17]. One explanation for the poor glucose tolerance in these models could have been impaired induction of GCK, possibly affecting glucose utilization [17]. At the moment, the reasons behind the different effects of *Pxr* KO on glucose tolerance observed in the studies of He et al. [18] and Spruiell et al. [17] are not clear. However, two different *Pxr* KO lines [32,33] were used in these studies, and there are reported differences between the lines, including a different effect of *Pxr* KO on basal CYP3A11 expression.

Some of the early observations on the repressive effect of PXR activation on gluconeogenesis were made in human hepatoma cell lines [29,30]. However, it has more recently been suggested that human hepatocytes may respond to PXR activation differently from mouse hepatocytes, and at least in some models, the gluconeogenic genes are induced [34,35]. The mechanism has been shown to involve serum/glucocorticoid regulated kinase 2 (SGK2). In response to pharmacological activation, demonstrated with simvastatin and rifampicin, PXR scaffolds the protein phosphatase 2C (PP2C), which dephosphorylates SGK2 [34,35]. Dephosphorylated SGK2 then acts as a coactivator for PXR in a complex binding directly or indirectly to the response elements regulating the *G6Pase* and *PEPCK* genes [35].

Interestingly, it has been reported that, in addition to ligand binding, VRK Serine/Threonine Kinase 1 (VRK1) mediated phosphorylation of PXR at Ser^{350} may initiate a cascade resulting in SGK2 dephosphorylation and *PEPCK* activation [36]. VRK1 was activated in low-glucose condition, and thus PXR would appear to be a part of the glucose level sensing apparatus regulating gluconeogenesis.

It has also been reported that PXR activity is induced under high-glucose conditions and that this is related to AMPK activity; AMPK activation exhibited an inverse relation to PXR activity [37]. However, these effects were mostly demonstrated with unphysiologically high glucose concentrations. As an additional demonstration of the nutritional regulation of PXR function, the PXR-regulated transcriptome was strongly modified, both qualitatively and quantitatively, by fasting and feeding status [38]. In general, glucose feeding of the fasted mice enhanced the induction of PXR-regulated genes. However, for some genes, there was a more dramatic effect and for *Cyp8b1*, involved in bile acid synthesis, and the glucose feeding switched the response from PXR-mediated repression to induction [38].

In conclusion, PXR appears be at the crossroad of glucose and xenobiotic metabolism. There are still many inconsistencies in the data describing the effect of PXR activation (and inactivation) on glucose metabolism. and the mechanisms have been only partially characterized. However, the clinical data in humans support the notion that PXR activation is harmful to glucose metabolism and promote the development of MetS. Mechanistically, this may involve reduced hepatic glucose uptake and activation of gluconeogenesis.

4. PXR-4β-Hydroxycholesterol Axis and Blood Pressure Regulation

Elevated blood pressure above 130/85 mmHg is one of the key features of MetS. We had noticed in our previous trial exploring the effect of rifampicin on glucose metabolism that rifampicin appeared to increase systolic and diastolic blood pressure [22]. The office systolic blood pressure (BP) was elevated by 4.8 mmHg ($p = 0.027$), diastolic BP by 3.5 mmHg ($p = 0.020$), and heart rate by 5.0 bpm ($p = 0.042$) after 1 week of rifampicin dosing compared with the placebo arm. Therefore, in our recent study, we set out to test the hypothesis that PXR activation by rifampicin elevates 24-h BP [14]. In a randomized, single-blind, placebo-controlled, and crossover trial, 22 healthy volunteers were given rifampicin 600 mg vs. placebo daily for a week, and 24 h ambulatory BP was measured at the end of the study arms. Study personnel were blinded; subjects were not blinded because rifampicin colors urine red, rendering blinding impossible. However, volunteers were not aware of the hypothesis that BP was expected to rise.

We showed that rifampicin elevated the mean systolic 24-hour BP by 4.7 mmHg ($p < 0.0001$) and diastolic BP by 3.0 mmHg ($p < 0.001$). The 24-h mean arterial pressure and pulse pressure were also elevated. In addition to BP indices, the mean 24 h heart rate was increased by 3.5 bpm ($p = 0.038$). Thus, we have evidence from two trials on healthy volunteers that PXR activation elevates office and 24 h ambulatory systolic and diastolic BP and heart rate [14,22].

There is no previous human study exploring the effect of PXR activation on blood pressure regulation, but a few animal studies have indicated that PXR is involved. Rifampicin treatment for 5 weeks increased plasma aldosterone in *PXR*-humanized mice [39]. Aldosterone is the adrenal mineralocorticoid regulating BP and an essential part of the renin–angiotensin–aldosterone system (RAAS). In our human study, serum renin concentration and plasma renin activity were increased by about 35%, while serum aldosterone concentration was not affected by rifampicin dosing.

In a study in spontaneously hypertensive rats and control Wistar-Kyoto rats, both BP and cytochrome P450 (CYP) 3A activity, measured as corticosterone 6β-hydroxylation, were higher in the hypertensive rats than in the control rats [40]. Crucially, BP was lowered with troleandomycin, a macrolide antibiotic and inhibitor of CYP3A. This study thus indicates that perhaps CYP3A activity and not PXR activation is the mechanism for elevated BP.

However, PXR is expressed in human and mice aorta and mice mesenteric arteries, and direct PXR-mediated effects on the vasculature have been described [41–44]. The 2-week administration of indole 3-propionic acid, an intestinal microbiota-derived metabolite of tryptophan and a PXR agonist, reduced the endothelium-dependent vasodilation in isolated and cultured aorta in wild-type mice but not in the *Pxr*-KO mice [44]. In contrast, 7-day treatment of pregnant mice with 5β-dihydroprogesterone, a PXR agonist, enhanced endothelium-dependent relaxation of mouse mesenteric arteries in the *Pxr+/+* mice but not in the *Pxr-/-* mice [42]. The authors concluded that PXR contributes to the development of vascular adaptations to pregnancy. Thus, PXR agonists reduced vasodilatation in aorta but enhanced vascular relaxation in mesenteric arteries [42,44]. Pulakazhi Venu et al. [44] speculated that these contrasting findings could be explained by different modes of vascular tone regulation; endothelium-produced endothelial nitric oxide (NO) synthase in the aorta and endothelium-derived hyperpolarizing factors in mesenteric arteries. PXR activation is known to reduce NO release, although the model used was not linked to vascular regulation (intestinal Caco-2 cell line) [45]. It is also interesting that laminar shear stress, the atheroprotective blood flow, activates PXR in bovine aortic and human umbilical vein endothelial cells, whereas atherogenic oscillatory shear stress suppresses PXR [43]. It should also be noted that in our ambulatory BP study, the heart rate and renin activity were elevated in addition to systolic and diastolic BP [14]. All of these effects are also seen when the sympathetic nervous system is activated [46,47]. However, to the best of our knowledge, the effect of PXR activation on the sympathetic nervous system is yet to be explored.

In addition to direct PXR action on vasculature, 4β-hydroxycholesterol (4βHC), a cholesterol metabolite produced by CYP3A enzymes in the liver [48] and a liver X receptor (LXR) agonist [49], may also be linked with BP regulation. Both LXRα and LXRβ are activated by 4βHC [50]. We showed in our ambulatory BP study [14] that plasma 4βHC concentration strongly negatively correlated with 24-hour systolic BP. This negative correlation was present in both rifampicin and placebo arms (rifampicin, r = −0.69, $p < 0.001$; placebo, r = −0.70, $p < 0.001$), although rifampicin dosing elevated 4βHC concentration more than 3-fold, and 24 h BP was increased as detailed above. This could be interpreted to indicate that 4βHC is a negative regulator of BP acting to reverse PXR-mediated hypertension.

The activation of LXRα by synthetic LXR agonists T0901317 and GW3965 reduces the experimentally stimulated RAAS and/or BP [44,51,52]. However, in experimental models without prior hypertension-inducing procedures or treatments, both T0901317 and 22(R)-hydroxycholesterol treatment elevated BP in mice [53]. Both LXRα and LXRβ activate transcriptionally the expression of renin in vitro and in vivo in acute experiments [54]. In our in vitro experiments [14], 4βHC was able to activate renin expression via LXRα in human Calu-6 cells but only modestly with unphysiologically high 4βHC concentrations arguing against a direct role of 4βHC in human renin regulation. Thus, LXR activation seems to induce renin expression in rodent kidneys and a human cell model, while the experimentally stimulated RAAS activity and elevated BP are perhaps blunted by LXR activation. It is known that LXR activation induces endothelial NO synthase [55], which could possibly explain the negative association of plasma 4βHC with lower BP (circulating 4βHC–endothelial LXR activation–endothelial NO production).

In addition to CYP3A4, the polymorphic CYP3A5 enzyme synthesizes 4βHC [48]. The concentration of 4βHC increases with the number of functional *CYP3A5*1* alleles [48]. A relationship between *CYP3A5* gene polymorphisms and hypertension has been suggested, but studies have yielded conflicting results [56]. There are many confounding factors such as ethnicity, the modulating effect of salt intake, and concomitant hypertension medications, some of which are CYP3A5 substrates [56]. In a meta-analysis, there was no overall effect of CYP3A5 expressor status on BP or hypertension [57]. However, in white populations, the carriers of *CYP3A5*1* allele had lower systolic BP compared with noncarriers. Since the *CYP3A5*1* carriers have higher circulating 4βHC concentration and higher 4βHC is associated with lower 24-hour BP [14], the increased 4βHC production could offer a mechanistic explanation for the influence of the genotype. However, more studies are still needed in this field.

To conclude, PXR activation elevates BP and heart rate in humans, while plasma 4βHC is associated with lower BP. The exact mechanisms behind these phenomena are uncertain, but direct vascular PXR action and endothelial LXR activation by 4βHC may be involved.

5. HDL Cholesterol Metabolism and the PXR—4βHC Axis

Low HDL-C (<1.3 mmol/L in women and <1.0 mmol/L in men) is one of the metabolic syndrome criteria. The ability of HDL to accept cholesterol from peripheral macrophages appears to be the crucial functional aspect of HDL-C metabolism and a key step in the beneficial reverse cholesterol transport (RCT) from the periphery to the liver and intestine for excretion [58,59]. Although there is no direct evidence that PXR regulates HDL-C metabolism, there are certain links between CYP3A activity and HDL-C. The treatment with PXR agonists such as carbamazepine, phenobarbital, and phenytoin is associated with increased HDL-C, while total cholesterol remains constant [60,61]. It has also been shown that CYP content of liver biopsy samples correlates with HDL-C in patients with epilepsy [62]. In psychiatric patients, CYP3A activity measured with midazolam phenotyping correlated strongly with HDL-C [63]. Phenytoin increased HDL-C and especially HDL2 but not HDL3, total cholesterol, or LDL in a placebo-controlled parallel trial in patients with low HDL-C [64]. In addition, occupational exposure to pesticide lindane, a potent PXR agonist [65], associates with remarkably high HDL-C concentrations [66].

We have recently demonstrated that 4βHC, through its LXR agonism, could be a link between PXR activation and HDL-C metabolism as it regulates the expression of cholesterol transporters in macrophages [67]. The expression and function of efflux transporter ATP-binding cassette transporter A1 (ABCA1) and ABCG1 were induced by 4βHC in vitro. Both *ABCA1* and *ABCG1* are known transcriptional targets of LXR [58]. The efflux, facilitated by ApoAI as an acceptor for cholesterol, was augmented by 4βHC more than the efflux to HDL2 [67]. Furthermore, 4βHC incubation repressed the expression and function of influx transporter lectin-like oxidized LDL receptor-1 (LOX-1). Thus, we could show that 4βHC is able to stimulate cholesterol efflux in the macrophages, the starting point of the beneficial RCT pathway. We also showed in humans and rats that dosing with prototypical PXR agonists rifampicin and PCN was able to induce plasma/serum 4βHC significantly (>2-fold in humans and >8-fold in rats). Crucially, the expression of ABCA1 mRNA in mononuclear cells of healthy volunteers in vivo was induced by rifampicin dosing. In rats, PCN induced the expression of ABCA1 and ABCG1, especially in the heart in vivo. Thus, the evidence suggests the existence of a novel hepatic PXR–circulating 4βHC–peripheral LXR pathway that links the hepatic xenobiotic exposure and the regulation of cholesterol transport in peripheral tissues [27] (Figure 2). It may be incidental, but hepatic CYP3A4 levels, plasma 4βHC and HDL-C levels are all higher in women than men [68].

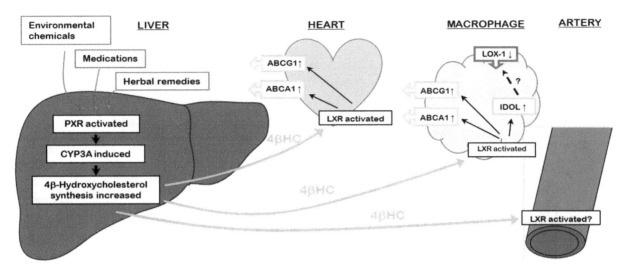

Figure 2. PXR–4β-hydroxycholesterol–LXR pathway as a regulator of cholesterol transporters and its putative role in vascular tone regulation. PXR activation by xenobiotics elevates circulating 4βHC, leading to the induction of cholesterol efflux transporters ABCA1 and ABCG1 and the repression of cholesterol influx transporter LOX-1. In addition to ABCA1 and ABCG1, inducible degrader of the LDL receptor (IDOL), another LXR target, is induced by 4βHC. The exact mechanism of LOX-1 repression is currently not known. The effects of 4βHC in vascular tone regulation are yet to be explored.

The results reviewed above indicate that PXR activation and especially elevated 4βHC levels could be beneficial factors in the regulation of HDL metabolism. This contrasts with the mostly harmful effects of PXR action on the other components MetS (obesity, hypertension, glucose metabolism). However, as obesity is a major driver of the MetS and both CYP3A4 activity and circulating 4βHC are known to be repressed by obesity and MetS [69,70], the repression of hepatic CYP3A4–circulating 4βHC–peripheral LXR pathway could link obesity and disrupted HDL-C metabolism in the obese patients with MetS.

6. PXR and Hypertriglyceridemia

Elevated triglyceride level is one of the diagnostic criteria for MetS. However, unlike the other components of the MetS, PXR activation appears to have little effect on the plasma triglyceride level. Efavirenz and quetiapine both induced plasma cholesterol through mechanisms dependent on PXR; however, they did not affect plasma triglyceride level [71,72]. Furthermore, the *Pxr* KO did not affect plasma triglyceride levels under HFD [17,18]. In contrast, PXR activation has been observed in many studies to promote liver steatosis. Although non-alcoholic fatty liver disease (NAFLD) is now often considered a hepatic manifestation of MetS, it does not belong to the current official criteria and will not be further discussed here, but the reader is advised to see recent reviews on the topic [13,73,74].

7. Conclusions

The current evidence indicates that apart from plasma triglyceride level, PXR activation can modulate all the components of the MetS (Table 2). In particular, there is robust evidence in humans that glucose tolerance is impaired and that blood pressure is elevated by PXR activation. As a major xenosensor, PXR is activated by various EDCs and PXR could mediate their metabolism-disrupting effect. Thus, PXR activation may contribute to the incidence of MetS. Emerging evidence in humans also indicates that circulating 4βHC regulates reverse cholesterol transport and blood pressure in beneficial ways. There is not yet any direct human evidence that PXR activation is a causative factor of obesity, hypertension, or type 2 diabetes. This may putatively be related to the fact that PXR activation and the effects of 4βHC may in certain aspects counteract each other.

Table 2. Components of the metabolic syndrome and the suggested role of PXR and the PXR–4βHC axis in mice and humans.

Components of MetS	PXR and/or 4βHC Implicated		Suggested Mechanism		Ref.
	Mouse	Human	Mouse	Human	
Abdominal obesity	+ (or −)		Effect on energy expenditure		[17,18,20]
Elevated triglycerides	± (plasma) + (liver steatosis)		Increased lipogenesis		[71,72,74]
Low HDL cholesterol		+		Obesity-repressed 4βHC	[67]
Hypertension	+	+	Vascular vasoconstrictive effects	Vascular vasoconstrictive effects?	[14,44]
Hyperglycemia	+	+	Reduced hepatic glucose uptake	Increased gluconeogenesis, reduced hepatic glucose uptake	[22,25]

+, increasing effect; −, decreasing effect; ±, no effect.

Author Contributions: J.H. (Janne Hukkanen) and J.H. (Jukka Hakkola) contributed equally to the writing and editing. All authors have read and agreed to the published version of the manuscript.

References

1. Mottillo, S.; Filion, K.B.; Genest, J.; Joseph, L.; Pilote, L.; Poirier, P.; Rinfret, S.; Schiffrin, E.L.; Eisenberg, M.J. The metabolic syndrome and cardiovascular risk a systematic review and meta-analysis. *J. Am. Coll. Cardiol.* **2010**, *56*, 1113–1132. [CrossRef] [PubMed]
2. Ford, E.S.; Li, C.; Sattar, N. Metabolic Syndrome and Incident Diabetes: Current state of the evidence. *Diabetes Care* **2008**, *31*, 1898–1904. [CrossRef] [PubMed]
3. Moore, J.X.; Chaudhary, N.; Akinyemiju, T. Metabolic Syndrome Prevalence by Race/Ethnicity and Sex in the United States, National Health and Nutrition Examination Survey, 1988–2012. *Prev. Chronic Dis.* **2017**, *14*, E24. [CrossRef] [PubMed]
4. Grundy, S.M. Metabolic syndrome pandemic. *Arterioscler. Thromb. Vasc. Biol.* **2008**, *28*, 629–636. [CrossRef]
5. Alberti, K.G.; Eckel, R.H.; Grundy, S.M.; Zimmet, P.Z.; Cleeman, J.I.; Donato, K.A.; Fruchart, J.C.; James, W.P.; Loria, C.M.; Smith, S.C. Harmonizing the metabolic syndrome: A joint interim statement of the International Diabetes Federation Task Force on Epidemiology and Prevention; National Heart, Lung, and Blood Institute; American Heart Association; World Heart Federation; International Atherosclerosis Society; and International Association for the Study of Obesity. *Circulation* **2009**, *120*, 1640–1645.
6. Heindel, J.J.; Blumberg, B.; Cave, M.; Machtinger, R.; Mantovani, A.; Mendez, M.A.; Nadal, A.; Palanza, P.; Panzica, G.; Sargis, R.; et al. Metabolism disrupting chemicals and metabolic disorders. *Reprod. Toxicol.* **2017**, *68*, 3–33. [CrossRef] [PubMed]
7. Lind, L.; Lind, P.M. Can persistent organic pollutants and plastic-associated chemicals cause cardiovascular disease? *J. Intern. Med.* **2012**, *271*, 537–553. [CrossRef]
8. Neel, B.A.; Sargis, R.M. The Paradox of Progress: Environmental Disruption of Metabolism and the Diabetes Epidemic. *Diabetes* **2011**, *60*, 1838–1848. [CrossRef]
9. Hukkanen, J.; Hakkola, J.; Rysa, J. Pregnane X receptor (PXR) - a contributor to the diabetes epidemic? *Drug Metabol. Drug Interact.* **2014**, *29*, 3–15. [CrossRef] [PubMed]
10. Baillie-Hamilton, P.F. Chemical Toxins: A Hypothesis to Explain the Global Obesity Epidemic. *J. Altern. Complement. Med.* **2002**, *8*, 185–192. [CrossRef]

11. Grün, F.; Blumberg, B. Endocrine disrupters as obesogens. *Mol. Cell. Endocrinol.* **2009**, *304*, 19–29. [CrossRef]

12. Papalou, O.; Kandaraki, E.A.; Papadakis, G.; Diamanti-Kandarakis, E. Endocrine Disrupting Chemicals: An Occult Mediator of Metabolic Disease. *Front. Endocrinol.* **2019**, *10*, 112. [CrossRef] [PubMed]

13. Hakkola, J.; Rysä, J.; Hukkanen, J. Regulation of hepatic energy metabolism by the nuclear receptor PXR. *Biochim. Biophys. Acta Bioenerg.* **2016**, *1859*, 1072–1082. [CrossRef]

14. Hassani-Nezhad-Gashti, F.; Salonurmi, T.; Hautajärvi, H.; Rysä, J.; Hakkola, J.; Hukkanen, J. Pregnane X Receptor Activator Rifampin Increases Blood Pressure and Stimulates Plasma Renin Activity. *Clin. Pharmacol. Ther.* **2020**, *108*, 856–865. [CrossRef]

15. Heindel, J.J.; Newbold, R.; Schug, T.T. Endocrine disruptors and obesity. *Nat. Rev. Endocrinol.* **2015**, *11*, 653–661. [CrossRef]

16. Casals-Casas, C.; Desvergne, B. Endocrine Disruptors: From Endocrine to Metabolic Disruption. *Annu. Rev. Physiol.* **2011**, *73*, 135–162. [CrossRef]

17. Spruiell, K.; Richardson, R.M.; Cullen, J.M.; Awumey, E.M.; Gonzalez, F.J.; Gyamfi, M.A. Role of Pregnane X Receptor in Obesity and Glucose Homeostasis in Male Mice. *J. Biol. Chem.* **2013**, *289*, 3244–3261. [CrossRef]

18. He, J.; Gao, J.; Xu, M.; Ren, S.; Stefanovic-Racic, M.; O'Doherty, R.M.; Xie, W. PXR Ablation Alleviates Diet-Induced and Genetic Obesity and Insulin Resistance in Mice. *Diabetes* **2013**, *62*, 1876–1887. [CrossRef]

19. Zhao, L.-Y.; Xu, J.-Y.; Shi, Z.; Englert, N.A.; Zhang, S.-Y. Pregnane X receptor (PXR) deficiency improves high fat diet-induced obesity via induction of fibroblast growth factor 15 (FGF15) expression. *Biochem. Pharmacol.* **2017**, *142*, 194–203. [CrossRef]

20. Ma, Y.; Liu, D. Activation of Pregnane X Receptor by Pregnenolone 16 α-carbonitrile Prevents High-Fat Diet-Induced Obesity in AKR/J Mice. *PLoS ONE* **2012**, *7*, e38734. [CrossRef]

21. Spruiell, K.; Jones, D.Z.; Cullen, J.M.; Awumey, E.M.; Gonzalez, F.J.; Gyamfi, M.A. Role of human pregnane X receptor in high fat diet-induced obesity in pre-menopausal female mice. *Biochem. Pharmacol.* **2014**, *89*, 399–412. [CrossRef]

22. Rysä, J.; Buler, M.; Savolainen, M.J.; Ruskoaho, H.; Hakkola, J.; Hukkanen, J. Pregnane X Receptor Agonists Impair Postprandial Glucose Tolerance. *Clin. Pharmacol. Ther.* **2013**, *93*, 556–563. [CrossRef]

23. Stage, T.B.; Damkier, P.; Christensen, M.M.H.; Nielsen, L.B.-K.; Højlund, K.; Nielsen, F. Impaired Glucose Tolerance in Healthy Men Treated with St. John's Wort. *Basic Clin. Pharmacol. Toxicol.* **2015**, *118*, 219–224. [CrossRef]

24. Ling, Z.; Shu, N.; Xu, P.; Wang, F.; Zhong, Z.; Sun, B.; Li, F.; Zhang, M.; Zhao, K.; Tang, X.; et al. Involvement of pregnane X receptor in the impaired glucose utilization induced by atorvastatin in hepatocytes. *Biochem. Pharmacol.* **2016**, *100*, 98–111. [CrossRef] [PubMed]

25. Hassani-Nezhad-Gashti, F.; Rysä, J.; Kummu, O.; Näpänkangas, J.; Buler, M.; Karpale, M.; Hukkanen, J.; Hakkola, J. Activation of nuclear receptor PXR impairs glucose tolerance and dysregulates GLUT2 expression and subcellular localization in liver. *Biochem. Pharmacol.* **2018**, *148*, 253–264. [CrossRef]

26. Hukkanen, J.; Rysa, J.; A Makela, K.; Herzig, K.-H.; Hakkola, J.; Savolainen, M.J. The effect of pregnane X receptor agonists on postprandial incretin hormone secretion in rats and humans. *J. Physiol. Pharmacol. Off. J. Pol. Physiol. Soc.* **2015**, *66*, 831–839.

27. Postic, C.; Shiota, M.; Niswender, K.D.; Jetton, T.L.; Chen, Y.; Moates, J.M.; Shelton, K.D.; Lindner, J.; Cherrington, A.D.; Magnuson, M.A. Dual roles for glucokinase in glucose homeostasis as determined by liver and pancreatic beta cell-specific gene knock-outs using Cre recombinase. *J. Biol. Chem.* **1999**, *274*, 305–315. [CrossRef]

28. Burcelin, R.; Muñoz, M.D.C.; Guillam, M.T.; Thorens, B. Liver hyperplasia and paradoxical regulation of glycogen metabolism and glucose-sensitive gene expression in GLUT2-null hepatocytes. Further evidence for the existence of a membrane-based glucose release pathway. *J. Biol. Chem.* **2000**, *275*, 10930–10936. [CrossRef]

29. Bhalla, S.; Ozalp, C.; Fang, S.; Xiang, L.; Kemper, J.K. Ligand-activated Pregnane X Receptor Interferes with HNF-4 Signaling by Targeting a Common Coactivator PGC-1α. *J. Biol. Chem.* **2004**, *279*, 45139–45147. [CrossRef]

30. Kodama, S.; Moore, R.; Yamamoto, Y.; Negishi, M. Human nuclear pregnane X receptor cross-talk with CREB to repress cAMP activation of the glucose-6-phosphatase gene. *Biochem. J.* **2007**, *407*, 373–381. [CrossRef]

31. Kodama, S.; Koike, C.; Negishi, M.; Yamamoto, Y. Nuclear Receptors CAR and PXR Cross Talk with FOXO1 To Regulate Genes That Encode Drug-Metabolizing and Gluconeogenic Enzymes. *Mol. Cell. Biol.* **2004**, *24*, 7931–7940. [CrossRef] [PubMed]

32. Staudinger, J.L.; Goodwin, B.; Jones, S.A.; Hawkins-Brown, D.; MacKenzie, K.I.; Latour, A.; Liui, Y.; Klaasseni, C.D.; Brown, K.K.; Reinhard, J.; et al. The nuclear receptor PXR is a lithocholic acid sensor that protects against liver toxicity. *Proc. Natl. Acad. Sci. USA* **2001**, *98*, 3369–3374. [CrossRef] [PubMed]

33. Xie, W.; Barwick, J.L.; Downes, M.; Blumberg, B.; Simon, C.M.; Nelson, M.C.; Neuschwander-Tetri, B.A.; Brunt, E.M.; Guzelian, P.S.; Evans, R.M. Humanized xenobiotic response in mice expressing nuclear receptor SXR. *Nat. Cell Biol.* **2000**, *406*, 435–439. [CrossRef]

34. Gotoh, S.; Negishi, M. Serum- and glucocorticoid-regulated kinase 2 determines drug-activated pregnane X receptor to induce gluconeogenesis in human liver cells. *J. Pharmacol. Exp. Ther.* **2013**, *348*, 131–140. [CrossRef]

35. Gotoh, S.; Negishi, M. Statin-activated nuclear receptor PXR promotes SGK2 dephosphorylation by scaffolding PP2C to induce hepatic gluconeogenesis. *Sci. Rep.* **2015**, *5*, 14076. [CrossRef]

36. Gotoh, S.; Miyauchi, Y.; Moore, R.; Negishi, M. Glucose elicits serine/threonine kinase VRK1 to phosphorylate nuclear pregnane X receptor as a novel hepatic gluconeogenic signal. *Cell. Signal.* **2017**, *40*, 200–209. [CrossRef]

37. Oladimeji, P.; Lin, W.; Brewer, C.T.; Chen, T. Glucose-dependent regulation of pregnane X receptor is modulated by AMP-activated protein kinase. *Sci. Rep.* **2017**, *7*, 46751. [CrossRef] [PubMed]

38. Hassani-Nezhad-Gashti, F.; Kummu, O.; Karpale, M.; Rysä, J.; Hakkola, J. Nutritional status modifies pregnane X receptor regulated transcriptome. *Sci. Rep.* **2019**, *9*, 16728. [CrossRef]

39. Zhai, Y.; Pai, H.V.; Zhou, J.; Amico, J.; Vollmer, R.R.; Xie, W. Activation of Pregnane X Receptor Disrupts Glucocorticoid and Mineralocorticoid Homeostasis. *Mol. Endocrinol.* **2007**, *21*, 138–147. [CrossRef]

40. Watlington, C.O.; Kramer, L.B.; Schuetz, E.G.; Zilai, J.; Grogan, W.M.; Guzelian, P.; Gizek, F.; Schoolwerth, A.C. Corticosterone 6 beta-hydroxylation correlates with blood pressure in spontaneously hypertensive rats. *Am. J. Physiol. Physiol.* **1992**, *262*, F927–F931. [CrossRef]

41. Swales, K.E.; Moore, R.; Truss, N.J.; Tucker, A.; Warner, T.D.; Negishi, M.; Bishop-Bailey, D. Pregnane X receptor regulates drug metabolism and transport in the vasculature and protects from oxidative stress. *Cardiovasc. Res.* **2011**, *93*, 674–681. [CrossRef]

42. Hagedorn, K.A.; Cooke, C.-L.; Falck, J.R.; Mitchell, B.F.; Davidge, S.T. Regulation of Vascular Tone During Pregnancy. *Hypertension* **2007**, *49*, 328–333. [CrossRef]

43. Wang, X.; Fang, X.; Zhou, J.; Chen, Z.; Zhao, B.; Xiao, L.; Liu, A.; Li, Y.-S.J.; Shyy, J.Y.-J.; Guan, Y.; et al. Shear stress activation of nuclear receptor PXR in endothelial detoxification. *Proc. Natl. Acad. Sci. USA* **2013**, *110*, 13174–13179. [CrossRef] [PubMed]

44. Pulakazhi Venu, V.K.; Saifeddine, M.; Mihara, K.; Tsai, Y.C.; Nieves, K.; Alston, L.; Mani, S.; McCoy, K.D.; Hollenberg, M.D.; Hirota, S.A. PMC6732469; The pregnane X receptor and its microbiota-derived ligand indole 3-propionic acid regulate endothelium-dependent vasodilation. *Am. J. Physiol Endocrinol Metab* **2019**, *317*, E350–E361. [CrossRef] [PubMed]

45. Esposito, G.; Gigli, S.; Seguella, L.; Nobile, N.; D'Alessandro, A.; Pesce, M.; Capoccia, E.; Steardo, L.; Cirillo, C.; Cuomo, R.; et al. Rifaximin, a non-absorbable antibiotic, inhibits the release of pro-angiogenic mediators in colon cancer cells through a pregnane X receptor-dependent pathway. *Int. J. Oncol.* **2016**, *49*, 639–645. [CrossRef]

46. Fisher, J.P.; Paton, J.F.R. The sympathetic nervous system and blood pressure in humans: Implications for hypertension. *J. Hum. Hypertens.* **2011**, *26*, 463–475. [CrossRef]

47. Schweda, F.; Kurtz, A. Regulation of Renin Release by Local and Systemic Factors. *Rev. Physiol. Biochem. Pharmacol.* **2009**, *161*, 1–44. [CrossRef]

48. Diczfalusy, U.; Nylen, H.; Elander, P.; Bertilsson, L. 4beta-Hydroxycholesterol, an endogenous marker of CYP3A4/5 activity in humans. *Br. J. Clin. Pharmacol.* **2011**, *71*, 183–189. [CrossRef]

49. Janowski, B.A.; Willy, P.J.; Devi, T.R.; Falck, J.R.; Mangelsdorf, D.J. An oxysterol signalling pathway mediated by the nuclear receptor LXRα. *Nat. Cell Biol.* **1996**, *383*, 728–731. [CrossRef]

50. Nury, T.; Samadi, M.; Varin, A.; Lopez, T.; Zarrouk, A.; Boumhras, M.; Riedinger, J.-M.; Masson, D.; Vejux, A.; Lizard, G. Biological activities of the LXRα and β agonist, 4β-hydroxycholesterol, and of its isomer, 4α-hydroxycholesterol, on oligodendrocytes: Effects on cell growth and viability, oxidative and inflammatory status. *Biochimie* **2013**, *95*, 518–530. [CrossRef] [PubMed]

51. Kuipers, I.; Van Der Harst, P.; Kuipers, F.; Van Genne, L.; Goris, M.; Lehtonen, J.Y.; Van Veldhuisen, D.J.; Van Gilst, W.H.; A De Boer, R. Activation of liver X receptor-α reduces activation of the renal and cardiac renin–angiotensin–aldosterone system. *Lab. Investig.* **2010**, *90*, 630–636. [CrossRef]

52. Mitro, N.; Vargas, L.; Romeo, R.; Koder, A.; Saez, E. T0901317 is a potent PXR ligand: Implications for the biology ascribed to LXR. *FEBS Lett.* **2007**, *581*, 1721–1726. [CrossRef]

53. Valbuena-Diez, A.C.; Blanco, F.J.; Oujo, B.; Langa, C.; Gonzalez-Nuñez, M.; Llano, E.; Pendas, A.M.; Díaz, M.; Castrillo, A.; Lopez-Novoa, J.M.; et al. Oxysterol-Induced Soluble Endoglin Release and Its Involvement in Hypertension. *Circulation* **2012**, *126*, 2612–2624. [CrossRef]

54. Morello, F.; De Boer, R.A.; Steffensen, K.R.; Gnecchi, M.; Chisholm, J.W.; Boomsma, F.; Anderson, L.M.; Lawn, R.M.; Gustafsson, J.A.; Lopez-Ilasaca, M.; et al. Liver X receptors alpha and beta regulate renin expression in vivo. *J. Clin Invest.* **2005**, *115*, 1913–1922. [CrossRef]

55. Hayashi, T.; Kotani, H.; Yamaguchi, T.; Taguchi, K.; Iida, M.; Ina, K.; Maeda, M.; Kuzuya, M.; Hattori, Y.; Ignarro, L.J. Endothelial cellular senescence is inhibited by liver X receptor activation with an additional mechanism for its atheroprotection in diabetes. *Proc. Natl. Acad. Sci. USA* **2014**, *111*, 1168–1173. [CrossRef]

56. Bochud, M.; Bovet, P.; Burnier, M.; Eap, C.B. CYP3A5andABCB1genes and hypertension. *Pharmacogenomics* **2009**, *10*, 477–487. [CrossRef]

57. Xi, B.; Wang, C.; Liu, L.; Zeng, T.; Liang, Y.; Li, J.; Mi, J. Association of the CYP3A5 polymorphism (6986G>A) with blood pressure and hypertension. *Hypertens. Res.* **2011**, *34*, 1216–1220. [CrossRef]

58. Lee, S.D.; Tontonoz, P. Liver X receptors at the intersection of lipid metabolism and atherogenesis. *Atherosclerosis* **2015**, *242*, 29–36. [CrossRef]

59. Temel, R.E.; Brown, J.M. A new model of reverse cholesterol transport: EnTICEing strategies to stimulate intestinal cholesterol excretion. *Trends Pharmacol. Sci.* **2015**, *36*, 440–451. [CrossRef] [PubMed]

60. A Nikkila, E.; Kaste, M.; Ehnholm, C.; Viikari, J. Increase of serum high-density lipoprotein in phenytoin users. *BMJ* **1978**, *2*, 99. [CrossRef] [PubMed]

61. O'Neill, B.; Callaghan, N.; Stapleton, M.; Molloy, W. Serum elevation of high density lipoprotein (HDL) cholesterol in epileptic patients taking carbamazepine or phenytoin. *Acta Neurol. Scand.* **2009**, *65*, 104–109. [CrossRef] [PubMed]

62. Luoma, P.V.; Sotaniemi, E.A.; Pelkonen, R.O.; Myllyla, V.V. Plasma high-density lipoprotein cholesterol and hepatic cytochrome P-450 concentrations in epileptics undergoing anticonvulsant treatment. *Scand. J. Clin. Lab. Investig.* **1980**, *40*, 163–167. [CrossRef] [PubMed]

63. Choong, E.; Polari, A.; Kamdem, R.H.; Gervasoni, N.; Spisla, C.; Sirot, E.J.; Bickel, G.G.; Bondolfi, G.; Conus, P.; Eap, C.B. Pharmacogenetic Study on Risperidone Long-Acting Injection. *J. Clin. Psychopharmacol.* **2013**, *33*, 289–298. [CrossRef]

64. Miller, M.; Burgan, R.G.; Osterlund, L.; Segrest, J.P.; Garber, D.W. A Prospective, Randomized Trial of Phenytoin in Nonepileptic Subjects With Reduced HDL Cholesterol. *Arter. Thromb. Vasc. Biol.* **1995**, *15*, 2151–2156. [CrossRef] [PubMed]

65. Kojima, H.; Sata, F.; Takeuchi, S.; Sueyoshi, T.; Nagai, T. Comparative study of human and mouse pregnane X receptor agonistic activity in 200 pesticides using in vitro reporter gene assays. *Toxicology* **2011**, *280*, 77–87. [CrossRef]

66. Carlson, L.A.; Kolmodin-Hedman, B. HYPER-α-LIPOPROTEINEMIA IN MEN EXPOSED TO CHLORINATED HYDROCARBON PESTICIDES. *Acta Medica Scand.* **2009**, *192*, 29–32. [CrossRef]

67. Salonurmi, T.; Nabil, H.; Ronkainen, J.; Hyotylainen, T.; Hautajarvi, H.; Savolainen, M.J.; Tolonen, A.; Oresic, M.; Kansakoski, P.; Rysa, J.; et al. 4beta-Hydroxycholesterol Signals From the Liver to Regulate Peripheral Cholesterol Transporters. *Front. Pharmacol.* **2020**, *11*, 361. [CrossRef]

68. Zanger, U.M.; Schwab, M. Cytochrome P450 enzymes in drug metabolism: Regulation of gene expression, enzyme activities, and impact of genetic variation. *Pharmacol. Ther.* **2013**, *138*, 103–141. [CrossRef]

69. Tremblay-Franco, M.; Zerbinati, C.; Pacelli, A.; Palmaccio, G.; Lubrano, C.; Ducheix, S.; Guillou, H.; Iuliano, L. Effect of obesity and metabolic syndrome on plasma oxysterols and fatty acids in human. *Steroids* **2015**, *99*, 287–292. [CrossRef]

70. Rodríguez-Morató, J.; Goday, A.; Langohr, K.; Pujadas, M.; Civit, E.; Pérez-Mañá, C.; Papaseit, E.; Ramon, J.M.; Benaiges, D.; Castañer, O.; et al. Short- and medium-term impact of bariatric surgery on the activities of CYP2D6, CYP3A4, CYP2C9, and CYP1A2 in morbid obesity. *Sci. Rep.* **2019**, *9*, 20405–20409. [CrossRef]

71. Gwag, T.; Meng, Z.; Sui, Y.; Helsley, R.N.; Park, S.-H.; Wang, S.; Greenberg, R.N.; Zhou, C. Non-nucleoside reverse transcriptase inhibitor efavirenz activates PXR to induce hypercholesterolemia and hepatic steatosis. *J. Hepatol.* **2019**, *70*, 930–940. [CrossRef]

72. Meng, Z.; Gwag, T.; Sui, Y.; Park, S.-H.; Zhou, X.; Zhou, C. The atypical antipsychotic quetiapine induces hyperlipidemia by activating intestinal PXR signaling. *JCI Insight* **2019**, *4*, 4. [CrossRef]

73. Staudinger, J.L. Clinical applications of small molecule inhibitors of Pregnane X receptor. *Mol. Cell. Endocrinol.* **2019**, *485*, 61–71. [CrossRef] [PubMed]

74. Cave, M.C.; Clair, H.B.; Hardesty, J.E.; Falkner, K.C.; Feng, W.; Clark, B.J.; Sidey, J.; Shi, H.; Aqel, B.A.; McClain, C.J.; et al. Nuclear receptors and nonalcoholic fatty liver disease. *Biochim. Biophys. Acta Bioenerg.* **2016**, *1859*, 1083–1099. [CrossRef]

4

Sleep Apnea and Sleep Habits: Relationships with Metabolic Syndrome

Anne-Laure Borel [1,2]

[1]   Department of Endocrinology, Diabetes and Nutrition, Grenoble Alpes University Hospital, 38043 Grenoble, France; alborel@chu-grenoble.fr

[2]   "Hypoxia, Pathophysiology" (HP2) Laboratory INSERM U1042, Grenoble Alpes University, 38043 Grenoble, France

Abstract: Excess visceral adiposity is a primary cause of metabolic syndrome and often results from excess caloric intake and a lack of physical activity. Beyond these well-known etiologic factors, however, sleep habits and sleep apnea also seem to contribute to abdominal obesity and metabolic syndrome: Evidence suggests that sleep deprivation and behaviors linked to evening chronotype and social jetlag affect eating behaviors like meal preferences and eating times. When circadian rest and activity rhythms are disrupted, hormonal and metabolic regulations also become desynchronized, and this is known to contribute to the development of metabolic syndrome. The metabolic consequences of obstructive sleep apnea syndrome (OSAS) also contribute to incident metabolic syndrome. These observations, along with the first sleep intervention studies, have demonstrated that sleep is a relevant lifestyle factor that needs to be addressed along with diet and physical activity. Personalized lifestyle interventions should be tested in subjects with metabolic syndrome, based on their specific diet and physical activity habits, but also according to their circadian preference. The present review therefore focuses (i) on the role of sleep habits in the development of metabolic syndrome, (ii) on the reciprocal relationship between sleep apnea and metabolic syndrome, and (iii) on the results of sleep intervention studies.

Keywords: metabolic syndrome; sleep; sleep apnea; sleep habit; sleep duration; chronotype; social jetlag

1. Introduction

Metabolic syndrome defines a group of risk factors underlying cardiovascular and metabolic diseases: abdominal obesity, atherogenic dyslipidemia, elevated blood pressure, and fasting plasma glucose [1]. The combined criteria used to define this syndrome identify a phenotype which is related to a greatest risk of developing cardiovascular and metabolic diseases than the simple addition of risks associated with each criterion [2].

Excess visceral adipose tissue is believed to be a primary driver of the cardiometabolic complications of metabolic syndrome [3]. An increase in visceral adiposity is thought to reflect the relative inability of the subcutaneous adipose tissue depot to sufficiently metabolize and store excess calories [2]. The specific characteristics of visceral adiposity, as opposed to subcutaneous adiposity elsewhere in the body, drive altered glucose homeostasis, proinflammatory adipocytokine release, and endothelial dysfunction that are the primary causes of metabolic syndrome [3].

Excess visceral fat is a modifiable risk factor that is usually associated with both excess caloric intake and a lack of physical activity [4]. Beyond these well-known, lifestyle-related etiologies, it also seems reasonable to assume that sleep habits could also contribute to abdominal obesity and, thus, metabolic syndrome. In addition, sleep apnea has been shown to increase the risk of cardiometabolic disease, and patients with metabolic syndrome are prone to develop sleep apnea [5].

The present narrative review focuses (i) on the role of sleep habits in the development of metabolic syndrome and (ii) on the reciprocal relationship between sleep apnea and metabolic syndrome. Finally, emerging evidence is reviewed regarding sleep intervention studies and how targeting of one specific lifestyle habits may impact other behaviors.

2. Sleep Habits and Metabolic Syndrome

2.1. Definitions

Metabolic syndrome: In 1998, the World Health Organization (WHO) became the first organization to introduce the term metabolic syndrome, with a primary focus on insulin resistance and hyperglycemia [3]. In 2001, the National Cholesterol Education Program's Adult Treatment Panel III (NCEP-ATP III) released its own definition, adding abdominal adiposity, specifically an increased waist circumference, as a major component of the syndrome [4]. Several definitions followed, issued from different societies, which mainly diverged on the clinical evaluation of abdominal adiposity. In 2009, the International Diabetes Federation Task Force on Epidemiology and Prevention; the National Heart, Lung, and Blood Institute; the American Heart Association; the World Heart Federation; and the International Atherosclerosis Society joined to release a statement harmonizing the criteria for defining the metabolic syndrome. This is the definition that is in use today, and it takes into account population-specific cutoffs for waist circumference [5]. Metabolic syndrome is defined by three of five criteria, with dyslipidemia being two criteria among: Fasting glucose $\geq$ 100 mg/dL or antidiabetic therapy, increased waist circumference, TG $\geq$ 150 mg/dl, and/or HDL-C $<$ 40/50 in men/women or antilipidic therapy, $\geq$130/85 mmHg or therapy.

Sleep characteristics: Recent research has indicated that people's sleep habits are changing. In this paper, we use the following definitions for terms commonly used in this field [6,7]:

'Sleep duration' is the time between falling asleep and waking up.

'Sleep debt' is a value calculated as the weekend sleep duration (i.e., Friday and Saturday nights) minus the sleep duration during the rest of the week.

'Chronotype' defines an individual's circadian preference: 'early' or 'morning' people tend to go to bed and wake up early, whereas 'late' or 'evening' people go to bed and wake up late [8,9]. The chronotype is calculated as follows [10]:

$$\text{Chronotype} = \text{Mid-sleep time on free days (MSF)} - 0.5 \times \text{sleep debt}$$

MSF represents the 'mid sleep time' that is calculated as the mid-point between sleep onset and wake time on free days, i.e., days when people do not have to get up for work.

Whether people are a 'night owl' or an 'early bird' can also be assessed using the Morningness–Eveningness Questionnaire, a 19-item scale validated by Horne and Östberg that addresses the timing preference for different daily activities [11].

'Social jetlag' refers to a misalignment of sleep timing between work and free days. Work, school, and other schedules often interfere with an individual's sleep preferences. Evening people, for example, are more likely to accumulate a sleep debt during the workdays which will be recovered during work-free days. This is calculated as the absolute difference between mid-sleep time on free days (MSF) and week days (MSW) i.e., social jetlag = |MSF − MSW| [12].

2.2. Epidemiological Evidence Related to Metabolic Syndrome

A normal amount of sleep is considered to be 7 to 8 h per night. Fewer than 6 h per night is classed as sleep deprivation and more than 9 h per night is considered as oversleeping. Sleep duration has decreased over the last 50 years in industrialized countries: In the USA, the percentage of those who self-reported that they did not sleep enough increased during this period from about 15% to 30% [13]. In France, it is estimated that average sleep duration has shown a 1 h 30 min reduction in the last 50 years (https://www.inserm.fr/en/health-information/health-and-research-from-z/sleep). In a 2017 telephone survey to investigate public health in France called the "Baromètre de Santé publique France 2017" (Public health barometer France 2017), 12,637 men and women aged between 18 and 75 years answered questions about their sleeping habits; 36% reported sleeping fewer than 6 h per night.

Several epidemiological studies and their meta-analysis have revealed sleep restriction to be associated with an increased prevalence of obesity [14]. Children seem particularly vulnerable: Reviews of child and adolescent data demonstrated an increased incidence of obesity in groups sleeping less than the time recommended for their age group [15]; this association was not so clearly marked in adults [16].

Regarding the specific association between sleep deprivation and metabolic syndrome, numerous studies have reported an association between a short sleep duration and an increased prevalence of metabolic syndrome. Some, but not all, research has also reported a similar association with long sleep duration. Eighteen such cross-sectional studies were included in a recent meta-analysis into (sleep) dose–(metabolic) response association [16]. A total of 75,657 adults were included, 51% of whom were men, and the age range was 18–96 years. Most studies reported odds ratios (OR) adjusted for age, sex, smoking, and alcohol intake. Short sleep was associated with metabolic syndrome, with a pooled estimate of the OR of 1.23 (95% CI, 1.11–1.37; $p < 0.001$; I^2, 71%). Thus, there was a significantly higher proportion of metabolic syndrome in those who had short sleep durations, with low heterogeneity between studies. In addition, a dose–response relationship was found for durations of sleep <5 h, 5–6 h, and 6–7 h: Pooled ORs for having metabolic syndrome for these sleep groups were 1.51 (95% CI, 1.10–2.08; $p = 0.01$; I^2, 88%), 1.28 (95% CI, 1.11–1.48; $p < 0.001$; I^2, 67%), and 1.16 (95% CI, 1.02–1.31; $p = 0.02$; I^2, 81%), respectively. There was no significant association with long sleep durations (pooled OR of 15 studies = 1.13, 95% CI, 0.97–1.32; $p = 0.10$; I^2, 89%). These results were consistent with a previous meta-analysis [17].

In children, sleep deprivation has also been associated with an increase in cardiometabolic risk. This pattern has been seen in cross-sectional analyses based on both self-reported sleeping habits [18] and objective, actimetry-measured sleep patterns [19].

Although these relationships found in cross-sectional studies appear to be robust, there is less evidence for longitudinal associations. A large-scale prospective study into the risk of developing metabolic syndrome used data collected from 162,121 adults aged 20–80 years (men 47.4%) who had participated in a medical screening program in Taiwan [20]. At the start of the screening, no participant was either obese or had any characteristic of metabolic syndrome. Follow-up data were available annually from 98% of participants, and the number of visits made by each participant ranged from 2 to 19. Of these, 18.6% of people were short sleepers (<6 h/day), 72.8% were regular sleepers (6–8 h/day, control values) and 8.6% were long sleepers (>8 h/day). More than half of the participants (57.6%) reported that they had insomnia symptoms. Compared to regular sleep data, short sleep duration was associated with a 12% (adjusted HR 1.12 [1.07–1.17]) increase in risk of becoming centrally obese during the follow-up period. Short sleepers were also more likely to develop metabolic syndrome (adjusted HR 1.09 [1.05–1.13]) compared to regular sleepers ($p < 001$). By contrast, long sleep was associated with a decreased risk of metabolic syndrome (adjusted HR 0.93 [0.88–0.99]). Similar results were found in two other longitudinal studies [21,22].

It is also interesting to note that in 1344 participants of the Penn State Adult Cohort, the cardiovascular mortality associated with metabolic syndrome showed an interaction with sleep duration as measured in a single polysomnography. In this sample, the mean age was 48.8 (14.2) years, and 57.8% were women and 9.5% black. The initial prevalence of metabolic syndrome was 39.2%. Overall, those with metabolic syndrome had a higher crude mortality rate than those without (32.7% versus 15.1%); $p < 0.01$ after 16.6 (4.2) years of follow-up. The mean sleep duration for the entire sample was 5.9 (1.3) h. There was a significant interaction between metabolic syndrome and objective sleep duration for mortality risk. The risk of cardiovascular mortality associated with metabolic syndrome as a function of objective short sleep duration was 1.49 (95% CI = 0.75–2.97) for subjects who slept ≥6 h/night and 2.10 (95% CI = 1.39–3.16) for those who slept <6 h per night [23].

The impact of work on sleep quality has been shown as a major contributor on occupational health disparities. For instance, the 2011–2012 US National Health and Nutrition Examination Survey (NHANES) compared the metabolic health of 260 long-haul truck drivers from North Carolina with the general population. The results showed that more years of driving and poorer quality sleep were statistically significant predictors for the higher cardiometabolic risk that was observed in the drivers [24]. In 39,182 male employees in Japan that were followed up for up to seven years, it was also found that short sleep duration and shift work were independently associated with the development of metabolic syndrome [25].

Numerous studies have also found that subjects with late chronotypes tend to have poorer metabolic health as compared with those with early chronotypes: They present more often with obesity [26–28], central repartition of adiposity [29,30], and with metabolic syndrome [19,30,31]. Indeed, in the Obesity, Nutrigenetics, Timing, and Mediterranean (ONTIME) study of 404 men and 1722 women, all of whom were overweight or obese, those with late chronotypes had higher BMI scores, higher triglycerides, lower HDL-cholesterol, higher levels of homeostasis model assessment for insulin resistance (HOMA-IR), and higher total metabolic syndrome scores [31].

In 1620 subjects derived from the Ansan cohort of the Korean Genome Epidemiology Study (KoGES), metabolic characteristics, body composition assessed by Dual-energy X-ray absorptiometry (DEXA), and visceral adiposity measured by computed tomography were collected and compared according to "morningness/eveningness" preference (Horne-Ostberg Morningness-Eveningness Questionnaire). In men, eveningness was associated with higher triglycerides levels but surprisingly lower systolic blood pressure. Anthropometrics measurements found less muscle mass in men with evening preference. In women, eveningness was associated with lower HDL-cholesterol and higher triglycerides and C-reactive protein (CRP) levels. Anthropometrics showed more visceral fat in women with evening preference [30].

Social jetlag, which is of greater amplitude in subjects with late chronotype, has also been independently linked with obesity [12,29] and metabolic disturbances [7]. However, few studies did not find such an association [32,33]. For instance, chronotype and social jetlag, objectively measured by wrist actimetry in 390 healthy young adults (21–35 years old), did not show any association with excess body weight, nor with elevated blood pressure [32].

2.3. Mechanisms of Action

Environmental cues, or "natural zeitgebers", like the alternation between day and night or cycles in external temperatures, usually synchronize circadian rhythms including patterns of rest and activity, food intake, and daily variations in metabolic fluxes and levels of hormones [34]. The timing of such patterns also varies with a normal distribution according to individuals' circadian preferences or chronotype. This normal distribution is in part dependent on genetic variations. In a twin study that measured circadian variations by wrist temperature, the results showed that between 46% and 70% of the observed circadian variance in temperatures could be attributed to genetic factors [35]. Three genome wide association studies (GWAS) performed in participants of European descent using data from the UK Biobank and the US genetics company 23andMe have also reported several single-nucleotide polymorphisms (SNPs) that are associated with chronotype [36–38]. Variations in other sleep characteristics, including sleep duration, have also been linked with polymorphisms at other loci [39].

However, sleep timing is also dependent upon extrinsic or "social zeitgebers" which may be related to work or leisure activities whose schedules conflict with intrinsic factors. A typical example of this conflict is found in shift workers: The work activities, food intake, and exposure to artificial lights at night cause a loss of internal synchrony and, in consequence, adverse effects on body weight and metabolism [40].

It has been shown that subjects with late chronotype have a tendency to eat less in the morning, while in the evening, they have higher global energy intakes and also higher intakes in sucrose, fat, and saturated fatty acids than subjects with morning chronotypes [41]. A daily caloric distribution with larger evening meals has been associated with a higher risk of obesity, particularly in those with evening chronotypes [42]. In patients with type 2 diabetes, late chronotypes have been associated with higher levels of glycated hemoglobin compared to early chronotypes and also with behaviors such as more frequently skipping breakfast [43]. Furthermore, food addiction, defined as an addictive behavior towards palatable foods, seems to be more frequent in subjects with late chronotype and is reported to be mediated by a higher frequency of insomnia and impulsivity [44]. Multiple studies have shown that an evening chronotype is associated with unhealthier diets and behaviors, such as smoking or drinking more alcohol [45–47]. People who are evening chronotypes are also more likely to be less physically active and to have more sedentary activities [45,47–49].

The role of gene variants that are associated with a latter chronotype to explain higher BMI and unfavorable metabolic traits has been evaluated in the GWAS based on UK-biobank data [37]. A reciprocal Mendelian randomization analysis, using a genetic risk score based on the 13 known variants of chronotype-linked genes, found no consistent evidence that early or late chronotypes led to higher BMI. This contrasts with another study that showed that a genetic risk score (GRS) for longer sleep duration was negatively associated with obesity [50].

The ONTIME study, reported by Vera et al. [31], addressed the question of the respective role gene versus behaviors to explain the deleterious metabolic profile of subjects with late chonotype. Firstly, the study showed that the GRS related to late chronotype, derived from GWAS studies, provided a reliable indication of subjects' circadian preferences. Second, the study identified that people with late chronotype had a higher metabolic risk score than people with an early chronotype. The analyses then showed that lifestyle factors, not chronotype GRS, underlay the relationship between evening chronotypes and metabolic alterations. Late chronotypes ate all three main meals later in the day, were more likely to have larger portion sizes, second helpings, to choose energy-dense foods, and to have a higher emotional eating score. However, evening types did not have a higher caloric intake, but they were less physically active and spent longer sitting down each day. These data therefore suggest that while the GRS can capture late chronotype, it does not associate with their metabolic risks. Metabolic alterations in people with late chronotype seem linked to unhealthy behaviors rather than to genetic predisposition.

Therefore, based on current knowledge, it seems that extrinsic factors linked to circadian preference, rather than intrinsic factors, are implicated in the cardiometabolic risk profile of an individual (Figure 1).

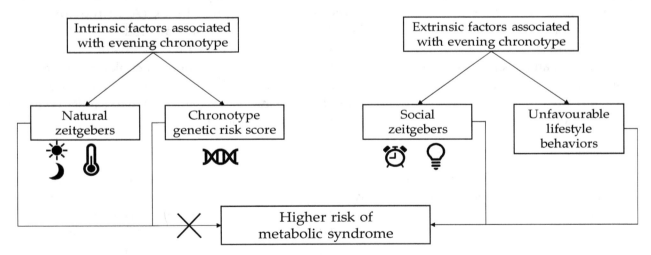

Figure 1. Schema showing the roles of intrinsic and extrinsic factors associated with evening chronotype in the risk of developing metabolic syndrome.

However, there are several data that suggest a gene–environment interaction between genetic traits that underlie our sleep characteristics and the risk of developing metabolic diseases under exposition to unhealthy food or physical inactivity. For instance, in the PREVIMED study, a significant association between the CLOCK-rs4580704 SNP and the risk of developing type 2 diabetes was observed after 4.8 years of follow-up. A gene–diet effect was found since only patients in the intervention group had a protective effect of the G variant for type 2 diabetes incidence and not the control group [51].

Dashti et al. [52] performed cross-sectional meta-analyses of population-based cohorts using data from the CHARGE (Cohorts for Heart and Aging Research in Genomic Epidemiology) Consortium. They studied whether dietary intake and sleep duration modified associations between five common circadian-related gene variants (CLOCK-rs1801260, CRY2-rs11605924, MTNR1B-rs1387153, MTNR1Brs10830963, and NR1D1-rs2314339) and glycemic traits, anthropometrics, and HDL-c levels. They found that higher intakes of carbohydrates and lower intakes of fat were linked to lower fasting glucose and HOMA-IR levels. Both short and long sleep durations were associated with higher fasting glucose levels, increased BMI, and greater waist circumference. Accordingly, known associations of selected SNPs on cardiometabolic traits were essentially replicated, but no diet–gene or sleep–gene interactions were found at the prespecified Bonferroni-corrected significance level of $p < 0.003$.

Thus, some evidence argues for a gene–environment interaction with circadian-related genes. It suggests a different metabolic answer to unhealthy behaviors as well as a different benefit from lifestyle interventions according to circadian genetic traits. If confirmed in further studies, such interactions will allow personalized risk prediction and personalized lifestyle intervention.

3. Obstructive Sleep Apnea and Metabolic Syndrome

3.1. Definition

Obstructive sleep apnea syndrome (OSAS) is caused by the complete or partial collapse of the pharynx repeatedly during sleep. These repeated collapses have four main consequences: desaturation–reoxygenation sequences, transitory episodes of hypercapnia, increased respiratory effort, and repeated micro-awakenings that end the respiratory event. Central obesity predisposes individuals to OSAS due to an infiltration of fat in the neck that causes upper airway collapse and increases abdominal pressure, leading to a reduction in lung volume. It has also been suggested that adipose tissue accumulation alters the neuromechanical control of the upper airway via the effects of leptin on central respiratory drive [5,53].

OSAS is defined as the presence of apnea (a 10-second interruption in airflow) and/or hypopnea (a ≤30% decrease in respiratory airflow with an associated oxygen desaturation >3% and/or micro-arousals). It is considered as mild if the Apnea–Hypopnea Index (AHI: the sum of the number of apnea and hypopnea events per hour) is between 5 and 14.9, as moderate if the score is between 15 and 29.9, and severe if the score is >30 events per hour. Clinical signs of OSAS include daytime fatigue and sleepiness, severe and daily snoring, reported sensations of choking or suffocation during sleep, nycturia, and morning headaches. The associated daytime loss of vigilance can be dangerous due to the risk of falling asleep while driving or at work [54,55]. It also causes cognitive disorders as a result of loss of attention, memory, and concentration [56].

3.2. Epidemiological Evidence Relating OSAS to Metabolic Syndrome

Metabolic syndrome and OSAS share a common risk factor, abdominal obesity, and 50%–60% of people with metabolic syndrome also have OSAS [57,58]. However, studies have also shown an association, independent of obesity, between OSAS and cardiometabolic risk factors, including hypertension [59], insulin resistance [60], and type 2 diabetes [61]. OSAS has been found to be associated with metabolic syndrome in several case-control and cross-sectional studies: A meta-analysis of 13 studies ($n = 7934$ subjects) reported an increased risk of metabolic syndrome in patients with OSAS with a pooled odds ratio (OR) of 1.72 (95% CI: 1.31–2.26, $p < 0.001$) and with a BMI-adjusted pooled OR of 1.97 (95% CI: 1.34–2.88, $p < 0.001$) [62].

A recent cohort study evaluated the influence of OSAS on the incidence of metabolic syndrome in a multiethnic sample of 1853 people from two population-based samples (Episono in Brazil and HypnoLaus in Switzerland) [63]. Participants included in the analysis were mainly female (56%) and Caucasian (88%), with an average age of 51.9 (±13.1) years and a BMI of 24.9 (±3.7) kg/m^2. The mean follow-up duration was 5.9 (±1.3) years, and 17.2% developed a metabolic syndrome during this time. The OR for developing metabolic syndrome when having moderate-to-severe OSAS was 2.245 (95%CI: 1.214 - 4.149), $p = 0.010$) after adjustments for cohort, age, BMI, and the number of metabolic syndrome components present at baseline. Of note, to assess whether the relationship between OSAS and metabolic syndrome could be bidirectional, a subset analysis was performed on 547 participants free of OSAS at baseline from the Episono cohort. After adjustment for sex, age, and baseline AHI and BMI, metabolic syndrome was not found a significant predictor of incident OSAS.

3.3. Mechanism of Action

The immediate consequences of OSAS-related respiratory events are intermittent hypoxia and fragmented sleep. These intermittent hypoxic respiratory events lead to the development of chronic adaptative mechanisms.

Studies in animals and humans have shown that intermittent exposure to hypoxia leads to sympathetic hyperactivity [64,65], to systemic and vascular inflammation via NFkB [66–69], to oxidative stress [70], and to pro-inflammatory stimulation of the adipose tissue via hypoxia and hypoxia inducible factor 1 (HIF-1) [71,72]. Sleep fragmentation also disrupts the nychthemeral cycle of cortisol secretion and the somatotropic axis, leading to an increase in nocturnal cortisol and a decrease in IGF-1 [73–76].

These mechanisms are involved in the development of insulin resistance, endothelial dysfunction, and vascular remodeling that is characterized by increased arterial rigidity. OSAS also alters the nictemeral cycle of arterial pressure: Patients lose the normal nocturnal reduction in arterial pressure of 10%–20% in comparison to daytime pressure, and this is responsible for the so-called 'non-dipper' or 'reverse dipper' blood pressure profile [49–51] which can evolve toward permanent, 24 h hypertension [54–56].

The above mechanisms may, at least in part, explain the development of cardiometabolic abnormalities in patients with OSAS. Nevertheless, the relationship between the two disorders is bidirectional (Figure 2): Visceral adiposity is strongly associated with development of OSAS. Central obesity, as described above, is associated with an increase in neck fat infiltration that reduces upper airway volume. Excess intraabdominal fat accumulation increases abdominal pressure, leading to lung volume reduction [5]. In addition to these mechanical effects, visceral adiposity generates low-grade inflammation [77]. Visceral fat adipocytes secrete low levels of TNF-alpha, which then stimulates preadipocytes and surrounding endothelial cells to produce monocyte chemoattract protein-1 (MCP-1). MCP-1, in turn, promotes macrophage recruitment and adhesion to endothelial cells [78] where they secrete proinflammatory cytokines like TNF-alpha, IL-6, and IL-1b, which results in increased plasma C-reactive protein (CRP).

It has been shown that anti-inflammatory therapy can modestly reduce OSAS severity in the absence of other treatments: A placebo-controlled, double-blind study of eight men with obesity and severe OSAS found that a three-week trial of the TNF-alpha antagonist etanercept significantly reduced AHI, IL-6 levels, and objectively measured daytime sleepiness [79]. These data therefore suggest systemic inflammation plays a role in the pathogenesis of OSAS.

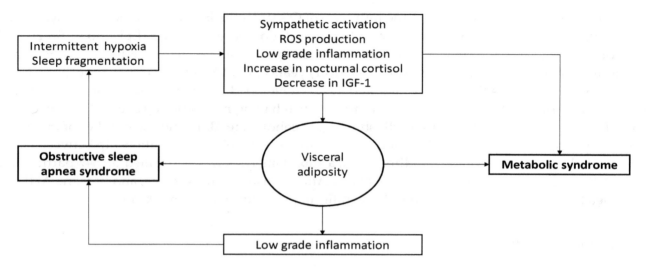

Figure 2. Bidirectional relationship between obstructive sleep apnea syndrome and metabolic syndrome. ROS, reactive oxygen species; IGF-1, insulin-like growth factor 1.

4. Sleep as a Component of a Comprehensive Lifestyle Intervention

4.1. First Steps of Chronotherapy as a Lifestyle Intervention

With regard to the timing of food intake, people with an evening chronotype have a later intake of all three main meals. The timing and daily distribution of this energy intake has been linked to a deleterious cardiometabolic risk profile, as described above. Thus, emerging evidence suggests that meal timing (when) is a dimension of dietary intake that matters, in addition to meal composition (what) and eating behaviors (how) [31,80].

Few works have studied the role of food intake timing. One study that included 32 young, normal weight women in a randomized, crossover protocol compared two different lunch-eating conditions: early lunch eating at 13:00 and late lunch eating at 16:30 [81]. Breakfast, lunch, and dinner composition were standardized. Those who ate lunch later had a lower pre-meal resting energy expenditure and glucose tolerance. Early eating, by contrast, was associated with improved circadian cortisol and temperature profiles.

A second study recruited eight overweight individuals who had an average eating duration (time range between the first and last daily food intake) >14 h [82]. The study consisted in a 16-week pilot intervention where participants were asked to restrict their eating duration to a self-selected window of 10–12 h and then to maintain this pattern during both weekdays and weekends to minimize metabolic jetlag. After 16 weeks, the participants had successfully reduced their eating time range and had lost a mean of 3.3 kg (95% CI: 0.9–5.6). Unexpectedly, they also reported greater sleep satisfaction. These results were maintained one year after the intervention. Thus, it appeared that changing the timing of meals not only may affect body weight, resting energy expenditure, and metabolic health but that it may also improve sleep quality.

Fewer studies have investigated the cardiometabolic effect of interventions aiming at improving sleep. A recent review [83] found only seven studies using a variety of interventions to extend sleep that also described the effects of this sleep extension on at least one cardiometabolic risk factor. The research was conducted in both subjects who were healthy and those who were hypertensive. Most had short sleep, although in one study, the subjects had normal sleep ($n = 14$). The interventions were short-term, lasting from 3 days to 6 weeks. These interventions were successful to increase sleep duration from 21 to 177 min. In intervention arms, subjects reported a reduction in their overall appetite, a decreased desire for sweet and salty foods, a lowered daily intake of free sugar, and less caloric intake from protein. Metabolically, insulin sensitivity improved in two studies [84,85].

An additional cross-over study, published since that review, included 21 nondiabetic subjects that usually slept <6 h per night. In the intention-to-treat analysis, the sleep extension group had their sleep extended by 36.0 (45.2) min. There was no improvement in plasma glucose/insulin homeostasis (as measured by oral glucose tolerance tests), but per-protocol analysis of the eight subjects who achieved a sleep duration >6 h during the sleep extension phase showed that sleep extension was associated with improved insulin sensitivity and insulin secretion [86].

Finally, physical activity has also been proven to have a positive impact on both sleep quality and sleep latency, the time in bed before falling asleep, without changing sleep duration [87]. It appears that the timing of physical activity is also important with regard to the cardiometabolic benefit: For instance, postprandial glucose increases were lower if patients with type 2 diabetes carried out physical activity after meals rather than before [88,89]. Thus, the introduction of chronotherapy in either diet or physical activity interventions could improve the cardiometabolic benefits. These interventions do not only change the targeted behavior but also have a positive impact on other behaviors: Changing food timing and increasing physical activity improve sleep quality and promoting sleep extension positively impacts food choices.

4.2. Effect of OSAS Treatment

Continuous positive airway pressure (CPAP) is currently the main treatment for moderate-to-severe OSAS. CPAP provides a pneumatic splint to prevent pharyngeal collapse, and it must be applied to the upper airways via a nasal or oronasal mask for ≥4 h per night in order to achieve its therapeutic goals [90]. The beneficial effects of CPAP on daily sleepiness and quality of life have been clearly demonstrated in patients with moderate-to-severe forms of OSAS [91].

Whereas the severity of OSAS is clearly parallel to the severity of excess weight [92], CPAP treatment in itself does not allow body weight reduction and was even associated with a small increase in body weight in a meta-analysis of randomized controlled trials (RCTs) [93]. Accordingly, CPAP did not impact visceral adiposity accumulation or body composition in a three-month RCT [94].

Regarding the cardiometabolic impact of CPAP treatment, the most robust evidence is related to blood pressure. Regular CPAP therapy results in modest reductions in blood pressure [95]. This is supported by a recent meta-analysis that pooled the results of 24 h recordings from five randomized trials and found a reduction in systolic and diastolic blood pressure of 4.78 mmHg (IC95%: −7.95 to −1.61) and 2.95 mmHg (IC 95%: −5.37 to −0.53), respectively, in patients with resistant hypertension who had been treated with CPAP [96]. CPAP also modestly improves insulin sensitivity. This was shown in a meta-analysis that included 12 observational studies: CPAP significantly improved the HOMA-IR index [97]. A modest, but significant, effect on insulin sensitivity was also found in a meta-analysis that included 244 patients without diabetes in five RCTs that compared the effects of CPAP and a placebo treatment applied between 6 weeks and 6 months [94,98–100]. In patients with type 2 diabetes, CPAP did not improve HbA1c in RCTs, although there was some evidence to suggest that CPAP decreased nocturnal glucose levels and insulin sensitivity [61].

The hypothesis that CPAP might reduce the rate of cardiovascular events was tested in four RCTs. The results all showed that CPAP did not impact the rate of cardiovascular events. This finding was further confirmed by a meta-analysis of 10 RCTs which involved comparison of CPAP to placebo treatments in studies with various main objectives, not only those related to cardiovascular events [101].

Despite the neutral or slightly negative effect of CPAP on body weight per se, it has been suggested that CPAP treatment could be a useful adjunct to improve the overall success of a lifestyle intervention. For example, a diet and physical activity intervention aimed at viscerally obese men (an ancillary study of the SYNERGY trial) found that those who did not have sleep apnea had all-round better results following the intervention than men who had presented with untreated apnea. Despite a similar level of adherence to the diet and physical activity recommendations, the men with apnea showed smaller reductions in BMI, waist circumference, and plasma triglycerides as well as smaller increases in HDL cholesterol and adiponectin [102].

Chirinos et al. [103] have treated people having OSAS by CPAP, weight loss intervention or both combined. When both interventions were cumulated, an incremental reduction in insulin resistance and serum triglyceride levels was obtained compared to weight loss intervention alone. In addition, providing a good adherence to a regimen of weight loss and CPAP resulted in incremental reductions in blood pressure as compared to either intervention alone.

5. Conclusions

This review provides evidence that sleep matters in terms of cardiometabolic health, and more specifically, metabolic syndrome. Sleep deprivation, behaviors linked to an evening chronotype, and social jetlag impact food timing, food preference, and food behavior. In addition, when an individual does not respect their own intrinsic circadian rhythm of rest and activity, dysregulation of hormonal and metabolic regulations occurs, and this strongly contributes to the development of metabolic syndrome.

In addition to sleep habits, the metabolic consequences of OSAS also contribute to metabolic syndrome: Both conditions are linked by a bidirectional autoaggravating relationship through the excess of visceral fat. Central obesity promotes sleep apnea through mechanical action and low-grade inflammation, while OSAS promotes metabolic syndrome through sympathetic nervous overactivity, reactive oxygen production, low-grade inflammation, and alterations in cortisol and IGF-1 circadian fluctuations.

From these observations, sleep has emerged as a relevant lifestyle factor that needs to be addressed along with diet and physical activity as part of a holistic treatment plan for those with metabolic syndrome. Recent intervention studies have demonstrated that improving one behavior, be it diet, physical activity or sleep, may positively impact the others. Early research on the first interventions targeting sleep extension or food timing seem promising. Further interventional studies should address comprehensive interventions, including chronotherapy through sleep, food, and physical activity timing. Personalized behavioral interventions should be tested in subjects with metabolic syndrome, based on their specific diet and physical activity habits, but also according to their circadian preference.

Acknowledgments: I thank J.R. and J.D.P. for English revision.

References

1. Alberti, K.G.; Eckel, R.H.; Grundy, S.M.; Zimmet, P.Z.; Cleeman, J.I.; Donato, K.A.; Fruchart, J.C.; James, W.P.; Loria, C.M.; Smith, S.C., Jr. Harmonizing the Metabolic Syndrome: A Joint Interim Statement of the International Diabetes Federation Task Force on Epidemiology and Prevention; National Heart, Lung, and Blood Institute; American Heart Association; World Heart Federation; International Atherosclerosis Society; and International Association for the Study of Obesity. *Circulation* **2009**, *120*, 1640–1645.
2. Sperling, L.S.; Mechanick, J.I.; Neeland, I.J.; Herrick, C.J.; Despres, J.P.; Ndumele, C.E.; Vijayaraghavan, K.; Handelsman, Y.; Puckrein, G.A.; Araneta, M.R.; et al. The CardioMetabolic Health Alliance: Working Toward a New Care Model for the Metabolic Syndrome. *J. Am. Coll. Cardiol.* **2015**, *66*, 1050–1067. [CrossRef] [PubMed]
3. Despres, J.P.; Lemieux, I. Abdominal Obesity and Metabolic Syndrome. *Nature* **2006**, *444*, 881–887. [CrossRef] [PubMed]
4. Neeland, I.J.; Poirier, P.; Despres, J.P. Cardiovascular and Metabolic Heterogeneity of Obesity: Clinical Challenges and Implications for Management. *Circulation* **2018**, *137*, 1391–1406. [CrossRef] [PubMed]
5. Levy, P.; Kohler, M.; McNicholas, W.T.; Barb, F.; Mcevoy, R.D.; Somers, V.K.; Lavie, L.; Pepin, J.L. Obstructive Sleep Apnoea Syndrome. *Nat. Rev. Dis. Primers* **2015**, *1*, 15015. [CrossRef] [PubMed]
6. Larcher, S.; Benhamou, P.Y.; Pepin, J.L.; Borel, A.L. Sleep Habits and Diabetes. *Diabetes Metab.* **2015**, *41*, 263–271. [CrossRef]
7. Larcher, S.; Gauchez, A.S.; Lablanche, S.; Pepin, J.L.; Benhamou, P.Y.; Borel, A.L. Impact of Sleep Behavior on Glycemic Control in Type 1 Diabetes: The Role of Social Jetlag. *Eur. J. Endocrinol.* **2016**, *175*, 411–419. [CrossRef]

8. Baehr, E.K.; Revelle, W.; Eastman, C.I. Individual Differences in the Phase and Amplitude of the Human Circadian Temperature Rhythm: With an Emphasis on Morningness-Eveningness. *J. Sleep Res.* **2000**, *9*, 117–127. [CrossRef]

9. Roenneberg, T.; Kuehnle, T.; Juda, M.; Kantermann, T.; Allebrandt, K.; Gordijn, M.; Merrow, M. Epidemiology of the Human Circadian Clock. *Sleep Med. Rev.* **2007**, *11*, 429–438. [CrossRef]

10. Roenneberg, T.; Wirz-Justice, A.; Merrow, M. Life between Clocks: Daily Temporal Patterns of Human Chronotypes. *J. Biol. Rhythm.* **2003**, *18*, 80–90. [CrossRef]

11. Horne, J.A.; Ostberg, O. A Self-Assessment Questionnaire to Determine Morningness-Eveningness in Human Circadian Rhythms. *Int. J. Chronobiol.* **1976**, *4*, 97–110. [PubMed]

12. Roenneberg, T.; Allebrandt, K.V.; Merrow, M.; Vetter, C. Social Jetlag and Obesity. *Curr. Biol.* **2012**, *22*, 939–943. [CrossRef] [PubMed]

13. Knutson, K.L.; Van Cauter, E.; Rathouz, P.J.; DeLeire, T.; Lauderdale, D.S. Trends in the Prevalence of Short Sleepers in the USA: 1975–2006. *Sleep* **2010**, *33*, 37–45. [CrossRef] [PubMed]

14. Cappuccio, F.P.; Taggart, F.M.; Kandala, N.B.; Currie, A.; Peile, E.; Stranges, S.; Miller, M.A. Meta-Analysis of Short Sleep Duration and Obesity in Children and Adults. *Sleep* **2008**, *31*, 619–626. [CrossRef]

15. Miller, M.A.; Kruisbrink, M.; Wallace, J.; Ji, C.; Cappuccio, F.P. Sleep Duration and Incidence of Obesity in Infants, Children, and Adolescents: A Systematic Review and Meta-Analysis of Prospective Studies. *Sleep* **2018**, *41*. [CrossRef]

16. Magee, L.; Hale, L. Longitudinal Associations between Sleep Duration and Subsequent Weight Gain: A Systematic Review. *Sleep Med. Rev.* **2012**, *16*, 231–241. [CrossRef]

17. Xi, B.; He, D.; Zhang, M.; Xue, J.; Zhou, D. Short Sleep Duration Predicts Risk of Metabolic Syndrome: A Systematic Review and Meta-Analysis. *Sleep Med. Rev.* **2014**, *18*, 293–297. [CrossRef]

18. Pulido-Arjona, L.; Correa-Bautista, J.E.; Agostinis-Sobrinho, C.; Mota, J.; Santos, R.; Correa-Rodriguez, M.; Garcia-Hermoso, A.; Ramirez-Velez, R. Role of Sleep Duration and Sleep-Related Problems in the Metabolic Syndrome Among Children and Adolescents. *Ital. J. Pediatr.* **2018**, *44*, 9. [CrossRef]

19. Lucas-De La Cruz, L.; Martin-Espinosa, N.; Cavero-Redondo, I.; Gonzalez-Garcia, A.; Diez-Fernandez, A.; Martinez-Vizcaino, V.; Notario-Pacheco, B. Sleep Patterns and Cardiometabolic Risk in Schoolchildren from Cuenca, Spain. *PLoS ONE* **2018**, *13*, e0191637. [CrossRef]

20. Deng, H.B.; Tam, T.; Zee, B.C.; Chung, R.Y.; Su, X.; Jin, L.; Chan, T.C.; Chang, L.Y.; Yeoh, E.K.; Lao, X.Q. Short Sleep Duration Increases Metabolic Impact in Healthy Adults: A Population-Based Cohort Study. *Sleep* **2017**, *40*. [CrossRef]

21. Kim, J.Y.; Yadav, D.; Ahn, S.V.; Koh, S.B.; Park, J.T.; Yoon, J.; Yoo, B.S.; Lee, S.H. A Prospective Study of Total Sleep Duration and Incident Metabolic Syndrome: The ARIRANG Study. *Sleep Med.* **2015**, *16*, 1511–1515. [CrossRef] [PubMed]

22. Song, Q.; Liu, X.; Zhou, W.; Wang, X.; Wu, S. Changes in sleep Duration and Risk of Metabolic Syndrome: The Kailuan Prospective Study. *Sci. Rep.* **2016**, *6*, 36861. [CrossRef] [PubMed]

23. Fernandez-Mendoza, J.; He, F.; LaGrotte, C.; Vgontzas, A.N.; Liao, D.; Bixler, E.O. Impact of the Metabolic Syndrome on Mortality is Modified by Objective Short Sleep Duration. *J. Am. Heart Assoc.* **2017**, *6*. [CrossRef] [PubMed]

24. Hege, A.; Lemke, M.K.; Apostolopoulos, Y.; Sonmez, S. Occupational Health Disparities among U.S. long-Haul Truck Drivers: The Influence of Work Organization and Sleep on Cardiovascular and Metabolic Disease Risk. *PLoS ONE* **2018**, *13*, e0207322. [CrossRef] [PubMed]

25. Itani, O.; Kaneita, Y.; Tokiya, M.; Jike, M.; Murata, A.; Nakagome, S.; Otsuka, Y.; Ohida, T. Short Sleep Duration, Shift Work, and Actual Days Taken off Work are Predictive Life-Style Risk Factors for New-Onset Metabolic Syndrome: A Seven-Year Cohort Study of 40,000 Male Workers. *Sleep Med.* **2017**, *39*, 87–94. [CrossRef] [PubMed]

26. Maukonen, M.; Kanerva, N.; Partonen, T.; Mannisto, S. Chronotype and Energy Intake Timing in Relation to Changes in Anthropometrics: A 7-Year Follow-Up Study in Adults. *Chronobiol. Int.* **2019**, *36*, 27–41. [CrossRef]

27. Zhang, Y.; Xiong, Y.; Dong, J.; Guo, T.; Tang, X.; Zhao, Y. Caffeinated Drinks Intake, Late Chronotype, and Increased Body Mass Index among Medical Students in Chongqing, China: A Multiple Mediation Model. *Int. J. Environ. Res. Public Health* **2018**, *15*, 1721. [CrossRef]

28. Ruiz-Lozano, T.; Vidal, J.; De Hollanda, A.; Canteras, M.; Garaulet, M.; Izquierdo-Pulido, M. Evening Chronotype Associates with Obesity in Severely Obese Subjects: Interaction with CLOCK 3111T/C. *Int. J. Obes.* **2016**, *40*, 1550–1557. [CrossRef]

29. Malone, S.K.; Zemel, B.; Compher, C.; Souders, M.; Chittams, J.; Thompson, A.L.; Pack, A.; Lipman, T.H. Social Jet Lag, Chronotype and Body Mass Index in 14–17-Year-Old Adolescents. *Chronobiol. Int.* **2016**, *33*, 1255–1266. [CrossRef]

30. Yu, J.H.; Yun, C.H.; Ahn, J.H.; Suh, S.; Cho, H.J.; Lee, S.K.; Yoo, H.J.; Seo, J.A.; Kim, S.G.; Choi, K.M.; et al. Evening Chronotype is Associated with Metabolic Disorders and Body Composition in Middle-Aged Adults. *J. Clin. Endocrinol. Metab.* **2015**, *100*, 1494–1502. [CrossRef]

31. Vera, B.; Dashti, H.S.; Gomez-Abellan, P.; Hernandez-Martinez, A.M.; Esteban, A.; Scheer, F.; Saxena, R.; Garaulet, M. Modifiable Lifestyle Behaviors, but not a Genetic Risk Score, Associate with Metabolic Syndrome in Evening Chronotypes. *Sci. Rep.* **2018**, *8*, 945. [CrossRef] [PubMed]

32. McMahon, D.M.; Burch, J.B.; Youngstedt, S.D.; Wirth, M.D.; Hardin, J.W.; Hurley, T.G.; Blair, S.N.; Hand, G.A.; Shook, R.P.; Drenowatz, C.; et al. Relationships between Chronotype, Social Jetlag, Sleep, Obesity and Blood Pressure in Healthy Young Adults. *Chronobiol. Int.* **2019**, *36*, 493–509. [CrossRef] [PubMed]

33. Marinac, C.R.; Quante, M.; Mariani, S.; Weng, J.; Redline, S.; Cespedes Feliciano, E.M.; Hipp, J.A.; Wang, D.; Kaplan, E.R.; James, P.; et al. Associations between Timing of Meals, Physical Activity, Light Exposure, and Sleep With Body Mass Index in Free-Living Adults. *J. Phys. Act. Health* **2019**, *16*, 214–221. [CrossRef] [PubMed]

34. Yetish, G.; Kaplan, H.; Gurven, M.; Wood, B.; Pontzer, H.; Manger, P.R.; Wilson, C.; McGregor, R.; Siegel, J.M. Natural Sleep and its Seasonal Variations in Three Pre-Industrial Societies. *Curr. Biol.* **2015**, *25*, 2862–2868. [CrossRef]

35. Lopez-Minguez, J.; Ordonana, J.R.; Sanchez-Romera, J.F.; Madrid, J.A.; Garaulet, M. Circadian System Heritability as Assessed by Wrist Temperature: A Twin Study. *Chronobiol. Int.* **2015**, *32*, 71–80. [CrossRef]

36. Lane, J.M.; Vlasac, I.; Anderson, S.G.; Kyle, S.D.; Dixon, W.G.; Bechtold, D.A.; Gill, S.; Little, M.A.; Luik, A.; Loudon, A.; et al. Genome-Wide Association Analysis Identifies Novel Loci for Chronotype in 100,420 Individuals from the UK Biobank. *Nat. Commun.* **2016**, *7*, 10889. [CrossRef]

37. Jones, S.E.; Tyrrell, J.; Wood, A.R.; Beaumont, R.N.; Ruth, K.S.; Tuke, M.A.; Yaghootkar, H.; Hu, Y.; Teder-Laving, M.; Hayward, C.; et al. Genome-Wide Association Analyses in 128,266 Individuals Identifies New Morningness and Sleep Duration Loci. *PLoS Genet.* **2016**, *12*, e1006125. [CrossRef]

38. Hu, Y.; Shmygelska, A.; Tran, D.; Eriksson, N.; Tung, J.Y.; Hinds, D.A. GWAS of 89,283 Individuals Identifies Genetic Variants Associated with Self-Reporting of being a Morning Person. *Nat. Commun.* **2016**, *7*, 10448. [CrossRef]

39. Goel, N. Genetic Markers of Sleep and Sleepiness. *Sleep Med. Clin.* **2017**, *12*, 289–299. [CrossRef]

40. Guerrero-Vargas, N.N.; Espitia-Bautista, E.; Buijs, R.M.; Escobar, C. Shift-Work: Is Time of Eating Determining Metabolic Health? Evidence from Animal Models. *Proc. Nutr. Soc.* **2018**, *77*, 199–215. [CrossRef]

41. Maukonen, M.; Kanerva, N.; Partonen, T.; Kronholm, E.; Tapanainen, H.; Kontto, J.; Mannisto, S. Chronotype Differences in Timing of Energy and Macronutrient Intakes: A Population-Based Study in Adults. *Obesity* **2017**, *25*, 608–615. [CrossRef] [PubMed]

42. Xiao, Q.; Garaulet, M.; Scheer, F. Meal Timing and Obesity: Interactions with Macronutrient Intake and Chronotype. *Int. J. Obes.* **2019**, *43*, 1701–1711. [CrossRef] [PubMed]

43. Reutrakul, S.; Hood, M.M.; Crowley, S.J.; Morgan, M.K.; Teodori, M.; Knutson, K.L. The Relationship between Breakfast Skipping, Chronotype, and Glycemic Control in Type 2 Diabetes. *Chronobiol. Int.* **2014**, *31*, 64–71. [CrossRef] [PubMed]

44. Kandeger, A.; Selvi, Y.; Tanyer, D.K. The Effects of Individual Circadian Rhythm Differences on Insomnia, Impulsivity, and Food Addiction. *Eat. Weight Disord.* **2019**, *24*, 47–55. [CrossRef]

45. Maukonen, M.; Kanerva, N.; Partonen, T.; Kronholm, E.; Konttinen, H.; Wennman, H.; Mannisto, S. The Associations between Chronotype, a Healthy Diet and Obesity. *Chronobiol. Int.* **2016**, *33*, 972–981. [CrossRef] [PubMed]

46. Mota, M.C.; Waterhouse, J.; De-Souza, D.A.; Rossato, L.T.; Silva, C.M.; Araujo, M.B.; Tufik, S.; De Mello, M.T.; Crispim, C.A. Association between Chronotype, Food Intake and Physical Activity in Medical Residents. *Chronobiol. Int.* **2016**, *33*, 730–739. [CrossRef] [PubMed]

47. Patterson, F.; Malone, S.K.; Lozano, A.; Grandner, M.A.; Hanlon, A.L. Smoking, Screen-Based Sedentary Behavior, and Diet Associated with Habitual Sleep Duration and Chronotype: Data from the UK Biobank. *Ann. Behav. Med.* **2016**, *50*, 715–726. [CrossRef]

48. Wennman, H.; Kronholm, E.; Partonen, T.; Peltonen, M.; Vasankari, T.; Borodulin, K. Evening Typology and Morning Tiredness Associates with Low Leisure Time Physical Activity and High Sitting. *Chronobiol. Int.* **2015**, *32*, 1090–1100. [CrossRef]

49. Olds, T.S.; Maher, C.A.; Matricciani, L. Sleep Duration or Bedtime? Exploring the Relationship between Sleep Habits and Weight Status and Activity Patterns. *Sleep* **2011**, *34*, 1299–1307. [CrossRef]

50. Dashti, H.S.; Redline, S.; Saxena, R. Polygenic Risk Score Identifies Associations between Sleep Duration and Diseases Determined from an Electronic Medical Record Biobank. *Sleep* **2019**, *42*. [CrossRef]

51. Corella, D.; Asensio, E.M.; Coltell, O.; Sorli, J.V.; Estruch, R.; Martinez-Gonzalez, M.A.; Salas-Salvado, J.; Castaner, O.; Aros, F.; Lapetra, J.; et al. CLOCK Gene Variation is Associated with Incidence of Type-2 Diabetes and Cardiovascular Diseases in Type-2 Diabetic Subjects: Dietary Modulation in the PREDIMED Randomized Trial. *Cardiovasc. Diabetol.* **2016**, *15*, 4. [CrossRef] [PubMed]

52. Dashti, H.S.; Follis, J.L.; Smith, C.E.; Tanaka, T.; Garaulet, M.; Gottlieb, D.J.; Hruby, A.; Jacques, P.F.; Kiefte-De Jong, J.C.; Lamon-Fava, S.; et al. Gene-Environment Interactions of Circadian-Related Genes for Cardiometabolic Traits. *Diabetes Care* **2015**, *38*, 1456–1466. [CrossRef] [PubMed]

53. Balachandran, J.S.; Patel, S.R. In the Clinic. Obstructive Sleep Apnea. *Ann. Intern. Med.* **2014**, *161*. [CrossRef] [PubMed]

54. Tregear, S.; Reston, J.; Schoelles, K.; Phillips, B. Obstructive Sleep Apnea and Risk of Motor Vehicle Crash: Systematic Review and Meta-Analysis. *J. Clin. Sleep Med.* **2009**, *5*, 573–581. [PubMed]

55. Mulgrew, A.T.; Nasvadi, G.; Butt, A.; Cheema, R.; Fox, N.; Fleetham, J.A.; Ryan, C.F.; Cooper, P.; Ayas, N.T. Risk and Severity of Motor Vehicle Crashes in Patients with Obstructive Sleep Apnoea/Hypopnoea. *Thorax* **2008**, *63*, 536–541. [CrossRef] [PubMed]

56. Mazza, S.; Pepin, J.L.; Naegele, B.; Rauch, E.; Deschaux, C.; Ficheux, P.; Levy, P. Driving Ability in Sleep Apnoea Patients before and after CPAP Treatment: Evaluation on a Road Safety Platform. *Eur. Respir. J.* **2006**, *28*, 1020–1028. [CrossRef]

57. Drager, L.F.; Togeiro, S.M.; Polotsky, V.Y.; Lorenzi-Filho, G. Obstructive Sleep Apnea: A Cardiometabolic Risk in Obesity and the Metabolic Syndrome. *J. Am. Coll. Cardiol.* **2013**, *62*, 569–576. [CrossRef]

58. Resta, O.; Foschino-Barbaro, M.P.; Legari, G.; Talamo, S.; Bonfitto, P.; Palumbo, A.; Minenna, A.; Giorgino, R.; De Pergola, G. Sleep-Related Breathing Disorders, Loud Snoring and Excessive Daytime Sleepiness in Obese Subjects. *Int. J. Obes. Relat. Metab. Disord.* **2001**, *25*, 669–675. [CrossRef]

59. Pepin, J.L.; Borel, A.L.; Tamisier, R.; Baguet, J.P.; Levy, P.; Dauvilliers, Y. Hypertension and Sleep: Overview of a Tight Relationship. *Sleep Med. Rev.* **2014**, *18*, 509–599. [CrossRef]

60. Borel, A.L.; Monneret, D.; Tamisier, R.; Baguet, J.P.; Faure, P.; Levy, P.; Halimi, S.; Pepin, J.L. The Severity of Nocturnal Hypoxia but not Abdominal Adiposity is Associated with Insulin Resistance in non-Obese Men with Sleep Apnea. *PLoS ONE* **2013**, *8*, e71000. [CrossRef]

61. Borel, A.L.; Tamisier, R.; Bohme, P.; Priou, P.; Avignon, A.; Benhamou, P.Y.; Hanaire, H.; Pepin, J.L.; Kessler, L.; Valensi, P.; et al. Obstructive Sleep Apnoea Syndrome in Patients Living with Diabetes: Which Patients should be Screened? *Diabetes Metab.* **2018**. [CrossRef] [PubMed]

62. Qian, Y.; Xu, H.; Wang, Y.; Yi, H.; Guan, J.; Yin, S. Obstructive Sleep Apnea Predicts Risk of Metabolic Syndrome Independently of Obesity: A Meta-Analysis. *Arch. Med. Sci.* **2016**, *12*, 1077–1087. [CrossRef] [PubMed]

63. Hirotsu, C.; Haba-Rubio, J.; Togeiro, S.M.; Marques-Vidal, P.; Drager, L.F.; Vollenweider, P.; Waeber, G.; Bittencourt, L.; Tufik, S.; Heinzer, R. Obstructive Sleep Apnoea as a Risk Factor for Incident Metabolic Syndrome: A Joined Episono and HypnoLaus Prospective Cohorts Study. *Eur. Respir. J.* **2018**, *52*. [CrossRef] [PubMed]

64. Fletcher, E.C. Sympathetic over Activity in the Etiology of Hypertension of Obstructive Sleep Apnea. *Sleep* **2003**, *26*, 15–19. [CrossRef]

65. Somers, V.K.; Dyken, M.E.; Clary, M.P.; Abboud, F.M. Sympathetic Neural Mechanisms in Obstructive Sleep Apnea. *J. Clin. Investig.* **1995**, *96*, 1897–1904. [CrossRef]

66. Ryan, S.; Mc Nicholas, W.T. Intermittent Hypoxia and Activation of Inflammatory Molecular Pathways in OSAS. *Arch. Physiol. Biochem.* **2008**, *114*, 261–266. [CrossRef]

67. Ryan, S.; Taylor, C.T.; Mc Nicholas, W.T. Selective Activation of Inflammatory Pathways by Intermittent Hypoxia in Obstructive Sleep Apnea Syndrome. *Circulation* **2005**, *112*, 2660–2667. [CrossRef]

68. Ryan, S.; Taylor, C.T.; Mc Nicholas, W.T. Systemic Inflammation: A Key Factor in the Pathogenesis of Cardiovascular Complications in Obstructive Sleep Apnoea Syndrome? *Thorax* **2009**, *64*, 631–636. [CrossRef]

69. Arnaud, C.; Beguin, P.C.; Lantuejoul, S.; Pepin, J.L.; Guillermet, C.; Pelli, G.; Burger, F.; Buatois, V.; Ribuot, C.; Baguet, J.P.; et al. The Inflammatory Preatherosclerotic Remodeling Induced by Intermittent Hypoxia is Attenuated by RANTES/CCL5 inhibition. *Am. J. Respir. Crit. Care. Med.* **2011**, *184*, 724–731. [CrossRef]

70. Jelic, S.; Padeletti, M.; Kawut, S.M.; Higgins, C.; Canfield, S.M.; Onat, D.; Colombo, P.C.; Basner, R.C.; Factor, P.; LeJemtel, T.H. Inflammation, Oxidative Stress, and Repair Capacity of the Vascular Endothelium in Obstructive Sleep Apnea. *Circulation* **2008**, *117*, 2270–2278. [CrossRef]

71. Lee, Y.S.; Kim, J.W.; Osborne, O.; Oh, D.Y.; Sasik, R.; Schenk, S.; Chen, A.; Chung, H.; Murphy, A.; Watkins, S.M.; et al. Increased Adipocyte O_2 Consumption Triggers HIF-1alpha, Causing Inflammation and Insulin Resistance in Obesity. *Cell* **2014**, *157*, 1339–1352. [CrossRef] [PubMed]

72. Poulain, L.; Thomas, A.; Rieusset, J.; Casteilla, L.; Levy, P.; Arnaud, C.; Dematteis, M. Visceral white Fat Remodelling Contributes to Intermittent Hypoxia-Induced Atherogenesis. *Eur. Respir. J.* **2014**, *43*, 513–522. [CrossRef] [PubMed]

73. Leproult, R.; Copinschi, G.; Buxton, O.; Van Cauter, E. Sleep Loss Results in an Elevation of Cortisol Levels the next Evening. *Sleep* **1997**, *20*, 865–870.

74. Vgontzas, A.N.; Pejovic, S.; Zoumakis, E.; Lin, H.M.; Bentley, C.M.; Bixler, E.O.; Sarrigiannidis, A.; Basta, M.; Chrousos, G.P. Hypothalamic-Pituitary-Adrenal Axis Activity in Obese Men with and without Sleep Apnea: Effects of Continuous Positive Airway Pressure Therapy. *J. Clin. Endocrinol. Metab.* **2007**, *92*, 4199–4207. [CrossRef] [PubMed]

75. Bratel, T.; Wennlund, A.; Carlstrom, K. Pituitary Reactivity, Androgens and Catecholamines in Obstructive Sleep Apnoea. Effects of Continuous Positive Airway Pressure Treatment (CPAP). *Respir. Med.* **1999**, *93*, 1–7. [CrossRef]

76. Leproult, R.; Van Cauter, E. Role of Sleep and Sleep Loss in Hormonal Release and Metabolism. *Endocr. Dev.* **2010**, *17*, 11–21. [PubMed]

77. Hotamisligil, G.S. Inflammation and Metabolic Disorders. *Nature* **2006**, *444*, 860–867. [CrossRef] [PubMed]

78. Xu, H.; Barnes, G.T.; Yang, Q.; Tan, G.; Yang, D.; Chou, C.J.; Sole, J.; Nichols, A.; Ross, J.S.; Tartaglia, L.A.; et al. Chronic Inflammation in Fat Plays a Crucial Role in the Development of Obesity-Related Insulin Resistance. *J. Clin. Investig.* **2003**, *112*, 1821–1830. [CrossRef]

79. Vgontzas, A.N.; Zoumakis, E.; Lin, H.M.; Bixler, E.O.; Trakada, G.; Chrousos, G.P. Marked Decrease in Sleepiness in Patients with Sleep Apnea by Etanercept, a Tumor Necrosis Factor-Alpha Antagonist. *J. Clin. Endocrinol. Metab.* **2004**, *89*, 4409–4413. [CrossRef]

80. Jiang, P.; Turek, F.W. Timing of Meals: When is as Critical as what and how much. *Am. J. Physiol. Endocrinol. Metab.* **2017**, *312*, E369–E380. [CrossRef]

81. Bandin, C.; Scheer, F.A.; Luque, A.J.; Avila-Gandia, V.; Zamora, S.; Madrid, J.A.; Gomez-Abellan, P.; Garaulet, M. Meal Timing Affects Glucose Tolerance, Substrate Oxidation and Circadian-Related Variables: A Randomized, Crossover Trial. *Int. J. Obes.* **2015**, *39*, 828–833. [CrossRef] [PubMed]

82. Gill, S.; Panda, S. A Smartphone App Reveals Erratic Diurnal Eating Patterns in Humans that Can Be Modulated for Health Benefits. *Cell Metab.* **2015**, *22*, 789–798. [CrossRef] [PubMed]

83. Henst, R.H.P.; Pienaar, P.R.; Roden, L.C.; Rae, D.E. The Effects of Sleep Extension on Cardiometabolic Risk Factors: A Systematic Review. *J. Sleep Res.* **2019**, e12865. [CrossRef] [PubMed]

84. Al Khatib, H.K.; Hall, W.L.; Creedon, A.; Ooi, E.; Masri, T.; McGowan, L.; Harding, S.V.; Darzi, J.; Pot, G.K. Sleep Extension is a Feasible Lifestyle Intervention in Free-Living Adults who are Habitually Short Sleepers: A Potential Strategy for Decreasing Intake of Free Sugars? A Randomized Controlled Pilot Study. *Am. J. Clin. Nutr.* **2018**, *107*, 43–53. [CrossRef] [PubMed]

85. Tasali, E.; Chapotot, F.; Wroblewski, K.; Schoeller, D. The Effects of Extended Bedtimes on Sleep Duration and Food Desire in Overweight Young Adults: A Home-Based Intervention. *Appetite* **2014**, *80*, 220–224. [CrossRef]

86. So-Ngern, A.; Chirakalwasan, N.; Saetung, S.; Chanprasertyothin, S.; Thakkinstian, A.; Reutrakul, S. Effects of Two-Week Sleep Extension on Glucose Metabolism in Chronically Sleep-Deprived Individuals. *J. Clin. Sleep Med.* **2019**, *15*, 711–718. [CrossRef]

87.   Yang, P.Y.; Ho, K.H.; Chen, H.C.; Chien, M.Y. Exercise Training Improves Sleep Quality in Middle-Aged and Older Adults with Sleep Problems: A Systematic Review. *J. Physiother.* **2012**, *58*, 157–163. [CrossRef]

88.   Reynolds, A.N.; Mann, J.I.; Williams, S.; Venn, B.J. Advice to Walk after Meals is more Effective for Lowering Postprandial Glycaemia in Type 2 Diabetes Mellitus than Advice that does not Specify Timing: A Randomised Crossover Study. *Diabetologia* **2016**, *59*, 2572–2578. [CrossRef]

89.   Borror, A.; Zieff, G.; Battaglini, C.; Stoner, L. The Effects of Postprandial Exercise on Glucose Control in Individuals with Type 2 Diabetes: A Systematic Review. *Sports Med.* **2018**, *48*, 1479–1491. [CrossRef]

90.   Sullivan, C.E.; Issa, F.G.; Berthon-Jones, M.; Eves, L. Reversal of Obstructive Sleep Apnoea by Continuous Positive Airway Pressure Applied Through the Nares. *Lancet* **1981**, *1*, 862–865. [CrossRef]

91.   McDaid, C.; Griffin, S.; Weatherly, H.; Duree, K.; Van Der Burgt, M.; Van Hout, S.; Akers, J.; Davies, R.J.; Sculpher, M.; Westwood, M. Continuous Positive Airway Pressure Devices for the Treatment of Obstructive Sleep Apnoea-Hypopnoea Syndrome: A Systematic Review and Economic Analysis. *Health Technol. Assess.* **2009**, *13*, iii–iv, xi–xiv, 1–119, 143–274. [CrossRef] [PubMed]

92.   Peppard, P.E.; Young, T.; Palta, M.; Dempsey, J.; Skatrud, J. Longitudinal Study of Moderate Weight Change and Sleep-Disordered Breathing. *JAMA* **2000**, *284*, 3015–3021. [CrossRef] [PubMed]

93.   Drager, L.F.; Brunoni, A.R.; Jenner, R.; Lorenzi-Filho, G.; Bensenor, I.M.; Lotufom, P.A. Effects of CPAP on Body Weight in Patients with Obstructive Sleep Apnoea: A Meta-Analysis of Randomised Trials. *Thorax* **2015**, *70*, 258–264. [CrossRef] [PubMed]

94.   Hoyos, C.M.; Killick, R.; Yee, B.J.; Phillips, C.L.; Grunstein, R.R.; Liu, P.Y. Cardiometabolic Changes after Continuous Positive Airway Pressure for Obstructive Sleep Apnoea: A Randomised Sham-Controlled Study. *Thorax* **2012**, *67*, 1081–1089. [CrossRef]

95.   Furlan, S.F.; Braz, C.V.; Lorenzi-Filho, G.; Drager, L.F. Management of Hypertension in Obstructive Sleep Apnea. *Curr. Cardiol. Rep.* **2015**, *17*, 108. [CrossRef]

96.   Liu, L.; Cao, Q.; Guo, Z.; Dai, Q. Continuous Positive Airway Pressure in Patients With Obstructive Sleep Apnea and Resistant Hypertension: A Meta-Analysis of Randomized Controlled Trials. *J. Clin. Hypertens.* **2016**, *18*, 153–158. [CrossRef]

97.   Yang, D.; Liu, Z.; Yang, H.; Luo, Q. Effects of Continuous Positive Airway Pressure on Glycemic Control and Insulin Resistance in Patients with Obstructive Sleep Apnea: A Meta-Analysis. *Sleep Breath.* **2013**, *17*, 33–38. [CrossRef]

98.   Weinstock, T.G.; Wang, X.; Rueschman, M.; Ismail-Beigi, F.; Aylor, J.; Babineau, D.C.; Mehra, R.; Redline, S. A Controlled Trial of CPAP Therapy on Metabolic Control in Individuals with Impaired Glucose Tolerance and Sleep Apnea. *Sleep* **2012**, *35*, 617–625B. [CrossRef]

99.   Coughlin, S.R.; Mawdsley, L.; Mugarza, J.A.; Wilding, J.P.; Calverley, P.M. Cardiovascular and Metabolic Effects of CPAP in Obese Males with OSA. *Eur. Respir. J.* **2007**, *29*, 720–727. [CrossRef]

100. Craig, S.E.; Kohler, M.; Nicoll, D.; Bratton, D.J.; Nunn, A.; Davies, R.; Stradling, J. Continuous Positive Airway Pressure Improves Sleepiness but not Calculated Vascular Risk in Patients with Minimally Symptomatic Obstructive Sleep Apnoea: The MOSAIC Randomised Controlled Trial. *Thorax* **2012**, *67*, 1090–1096. [CrossRef]

101. Yu, J.; Zhou, Z.; McEvoy, R.D.; Anderson, C.S.; Rodgers, A.; Perkovic, V.; Neal, B. Association of Positive Airway Pressure with Cardiovascular Events and Death in Adults With Sleep Apnea: A Systematic Review and Meta-analysis. *JAMA* **2017**, *318*, 156–166. [CrossRef] [PubMed]

102. Borel, A.L.; Leblanc, X.; Almeras, N.; Tremblay, A.; Bergeron, J.; Poirier, P.; Despres, J.P.; Series, F. Sleep Apnoea Attenuates the Effects of a Lifestyle Intervention Programme in Men with Visceral Obesity. *Thorax* **2012**, *67*, 735–741. [CrossRef] [PubMed]

103. Chirinos, J.A.; Gurubhagavatula, I.; Teff, K.; Rader, D.J.; Wadden, T.A.; Townsend, R.; Foster, G.D.; Maislin, G.; Saif, H.; Broderick, P.; et al. CPAP, Weight Loss, or Both for Obstructive Sleep Apnea. *N. Engl. J. Med.* **2014**, *370*, 2265–2275. [CrossRef] [PubMed]

5

Eating Habits and Lifestyle during COVID-19 Lockdown in the United Arab Emirates

Leila Cheikh Ismail [1,2,3,*], Tareq M. Osaili [1,3,4], Maysm N. Mohamad [5], Amina Al Marzouqi [6], Amjad H. Jarrar [5], Dima O. Abu Jamous [3], Emmanuella Magriplis [7], Habiba I. Ali [5], Haleama Al Sabbah [8], Hayder Hasan [1,3], Latifa M. R. AlMarzooqi [9], Lily Stojanovska [5,10], Mona Hashim [1,3], Reyad R. Shaker Obaid [1,3], Sheima T. Saleh [1] and Ayesha S. Al Dhaheri [5]

[1] Department of Clinical Nutrition and Dietetics, College of Health Sciences, University of Sharjah, Sharjah 27272, UAE; tosaili@sharjah.ac.ae (T.M.O.); haidarah@sharjah.ac.ae (H.H.); mhashim@sharjah.ac.ae (M.H.); robaid@sharjah.ac.ae (R.R.S.O.); U14120207@sharjah.ac.ae (S.T.S.)

[2] Nuffield Department of Women's & Reproductive Health, University of Oxford, Oxford OX1 2JD, UK

[3] Research Institute of Medical and Health Sciences (RIMHS), University of Sharjah, Sharjah 27272, UAE; d_abujamous@yahoo.com

[4] Department of Nutrition and Food Technology, Faculty of Agriculture, Jordan University of Science and Technology, Irbid 22110, Jordan

[5] Department of Nutrition and Health, College of Medicine and Health Sciences, United Arab Emirates University, Al Ain 15551, UAE; drmaysm@gmail.com (M.N.M.); amjadj@uaeu.ac.ae (A.H.J.); habAli@uaeu.ac.ae (H.I.A.); lily.stojanovska@uaeu.ac.ae (L.S.); ayesha_aldhaheri@uaeu.ac.ae (A.S.A.D.)

[6] Department of Health Services Administration, College of Health Sciences, University of Sharjah, Sharjah 27272, UAE; amalmarzouqi@sharjah.ac.ae

[7] Department of Food Science and Human Nutrition, Agricultural University of Athens, Iera Odos 75, 11855 Athens, Greece; emagriplis@aua.gr

[8] College of Natural and Health Sciences, Zayed University, Dubai 19282, UAE; haleemah.alsabah@zu.ac.ae

[9] Nutrition Section, Ministry of Health and Prevention, Dubai 1853, UAE; latefa.rashed@moh.gov.ae

[10] Institute for Health and Sport, Victoria University, Melbourne 14428, Australia

* Correspondence: lcheikhismail@sharjah.ac.ae

Abstract: The coronavirus disease is still spreading in the United Arab Emirates (UAE) with subsequent lockdowns and social distancing measures being enforced by the government. The purpose of this study was to assess the effect of the lockdown on eating habits and lifestyle behaviors among residents of the UAE. A cross-sectional study among adults in the UAE was conducted using an online questionnaire between April and May 2020. A total of 1012 subjects participated in the study. During the pandemic, 31% reported weight gain and 72.2% had less than eight cups of water per day. Furthermore, the dietary habits of the participants were distanced from the Mediterranean diet principles and closer to "unhealthy" dietary patterns. Moreover, 38.5% did not engage in physical activity and 36.2% spent over five hours per day on screens for entertainment. A significantly higher percentage of participants reported physical exhaustion, emotional exhaustion, irritability, and tension "all the time" during the pandemic compared to before the pandemic ($p < 0.001$). Sleep disturbances were prevalent among 60.8% of the participants during the pandemic. Although lockdowns are an important safety measure to protect public health, results indicate that they might cause a variety of lifestyle changes, physical inactivity, and psychological problems among adults in the UAE.

Keywords: United Arab Emirates; COVID-19; eating habits; lifestyle behaviors

1. Introduction

The novel coronavirus disease (COVID-19) pandemic has added various challenges and changes to human life worldwide, causing an unprecedented impact on human health, lifestyle, and social life, and has affected the local and international economy [1]. Following its first emergence in December 2019, in the city of Wuhan in China and its subsequent outbreak throughout the world in the following months it was characterized as a global pandemic by the World Health Organization (WHO) on 11 March 2020 [2]. On 28 September 2020, over 32.7 million confirmed cases of novel coronavirus and around 991,000 deaths worldwide were reported by the WHO [3]. In the United Arab Emirates (UAE) a total of 90,618 confirmed cases were reported in the same period [3]. In response to the rapid spread of the disease governments all around the world had to implement strict measures such as complete or partial lockdowns, isolation, quarantine and social distancing [4,5].

In the UAE, as a response to this outbreak, the government had to act quickly to contain the spread of the virus. Parallel with measures taken by most countries worldwide, complete and partial lockdowns were implemented, non-essential public places were closed, telework and distance learning was initiated, delivery services like delivering drugs to chronically ill patients were provided and sanitizing cities during night as part of the National Disinfection Program was implemented [6]. According to the World Bank, the total population of the UAE in 2019 was about 9.8 million [7]. However, nearly 75% of the population is concentrated in Abu Dhabi and Dubai as they have more than 3 million residents each. Moreover, the UAE is a multicultural country with expatriates and immigrants accounting for about 88% of the population [8]. Thus, this study provides unique opportunities to examine the impact of COVID-19 on lifestyle behaviors in the UAE.

There is no doubt that during times of confinement, food accessibility and availability may be affected, which in turn affects diet quality [9]. The imposed possibility of reduced income, job losses and anxiety about an uncertain future might lead the population to cut down expenditure including their expenses for food, making them go for more palatable, affordable and possibly unhealthy options [10]. Diet can affect many areas, but most importantly it can affect immune status [11] in the short term, a time during which heightened activity should be at its best. Available literature, however, has shown trends toward unfavorable dietary behaviors during the lockdown such as increased caloric intake, more frequent snacking, reduced consumption of fresh fruits and vegetable, and weight gain [10,12]. Traditionally, the diet in the UAE consists of fruits (such as dates), vegetables and fish and it is characterized by a high-fiber content and low fat and cholesterol content [13]; foods that characterize the Mediterranean diet and that are rich in vitamins A, D, C, folate, E and B-complex, required for an optimal immune response. Moreover, a large portion of UAE residents are from Arab countries in which fruits, vegetables and olive oils constitute key components of their diets. Therefore, it would be of interest to assess any shift in dietary habits during the COVID-19 situation.

Levels of physical activity were also negatively affected during quarantine [10,14,15]. Factors like complete lockdowns, closure of sport facilities and parks, and overall movement restrictions have reduced the ability to engage in physical activity. This was accompanied with an increase in sedentary behaviors related to quarantine, including distance learning and telework [16]. A meta-analysis on physical activity prior to COVID-19 pandemic revealed that a quarter of the population residing in the UAE had a sedentary lifestyle and were not engaged in any type of physical activity [17].

The emergence of infectious diseases reaching pandemic levels induces a huge psychological impact and distressed mental health symptoms in the population with anxiety being the most common as was shown following the Middle East respiratory syndrome coronavirus (MERS-CoV), severe acute respiratory syndrome coronavirus (SARS-CoV), and severe acute respiratory syndrome coronavirus 2 (SARS-CoV-2) [18,19]. Anxiety and uncertainty along with food insecurity and restricted healthcare access might also impact individuals with eating disorders and obesity [20,21]. Multiple factors influence the extent of psychological impact of outbreaks including unknown means of virus transmission, future unpredictability, media misinformation, and quarantine [19,22]. Consequently, such stressful events strongly aggravate disturbed sleep patterns and insomnia, poor eating habits along with decreased levels of physical activity and increased sedentary behaviors [23,24].

This study aimed to investigate the effect of quarantine on eating habits, physical activity, stress and sleep behaviors among adult UAE residents using a formulated online survey. A comparison of lifestyle and dietary behaviors before and during the lockdown was also conducted to allow better understanding of the effects of Covid-19-induced confinement policies on lifestyle changes among the UAE residents. Dietary intake was examined during the lockdown to evaluate potential risks of nutritional inadequacies.

2. Materials and Methods

2.1. Study Design and Participants

To assess the effect of the coronavirus pandemic and the effect of lockdown on eating habits and lifestyle of residents of the UAE, a population-based (cross-sectional) study was conducted in the UAE between April and May 2020. Although cross-sectional studies are rarely used to compare before and after, since there is no temporal sequence, it is the best design to use when previous information is not available, in order to draw inferences. Considering the sudden outbreak of COVID-19, this study aimed to evaluate the effect of the pandemic by examining highly modifiable factors including lifestyle and dietary.

The target population included all adults ≥18 years and from all seven emirates, residing in UAE. These were invited to participate in an online survey using snowball sampling methods in order to guarantee a large-scale distribution and recruitment of participants. A total of 1012 participants (24.1% males) were included in this study.

A web link was retrieved for the survey and was distributed using e-mail invitations and social media platforms, e.g., LinkedIn™ (Mountain View, CA, USA), Facebook™ (Cambridge, MA, USA), and WhatsApp™ (Menlo Park, CA, USA). The first page of the survey included an information sheet and consent form indicating the participants' right to withdraw at any time. Consenting participants then chose their desired language and proceeded to complete and submit their responses. All data were collected anonymously with no indication of any personal information and participants were not rewarded. The study protocol was approved by the Research Ethics Committee at the University of Sharjah (REC-20-04-25-02) and the Social Sciences Research Ethics Committee at United Arab of Emirates University (ERS_2020_6106).

2.2. Survey Questionnaire

A multicomponent, self-administered online survey was designed using Google document forms in English, Arabic, and French. This survey contained questions on dietary and lifestyle habits prior to and during the COVID-19 confinement. A researcher from the College of Health Sciences at the University of Sharjah (UAE) and a researcher from the College of Food and Agriculture at United Arab Emirates University (UAE) developed the draft of the survey in English. Questions were developed based on a previous national nutrition survey [25], the International Physical Activity Questionnaire Short Form (IPAQ-SF) [26] and the Copenhagen Psychosocial Questionnaire (COPSOQ-II) [27]. It was then translated and culturally adapted following an internationally accepted methodology [28,29]. The survey was later reviewed by the research team and was pilot tested with 25 people from the UAE. Following the pilot-testing, slight modifications were made to the survey. The online survey included 37 questions and was divided into seven sections: (1) socio-demographic background (10 questions): gender, age, marital status, number of children the participant has, education level, employment status, whether they were working or studying from home during the lockdown, weight change, perceived health status, and emirate of residence; (2) sources of information (2 questions): where do they obtain health and nutrition related information; (3) eating habits (8 questions): meal type, meal frequency, eating breakfast, skipping meals, reasons for skipping meals, water intake, and food frequency of specific foods; (4) shopping habits (5 questions): preparing a grocery list, stocking up on foods, using online shopping, reading food labels, and cleaning/sanitizing groceries; (5) physical activity (4 questions): exercising frequency, household chores frequency, computer time for work or study, and screen time for entertainment; (6) stress and irritability (4 questions): physical exhaustion, emotional exhaustion, irritability, and tension; (7) sleep (4 questions) sleep duration, sleep quality, sleep disturbances, and energy level. The full version of the questionnaire is available as a Supplementary File.

Questions on eating habits, physical activity, stress and irritability, and sleep were asked twice, once regarding the period before the pandemic (pre-COVID-19) and the other regarding the period during lockdown (during COVID-19).

2.2.1. Dietary Assessment

A total of 10 specific dietary questions were included in the questionnaire to assess frequency of specific food groups only during COVID-19 pandemic [30]. Food groups were included based on usual intakes of the population residing in the United Arab Emirates [31,32]. These characterize the basic Mediterranean type diet but also include food high in sugar and fat, observed to be recently trending in the UAE [25]. Specifically, the questionnaire included the following food groups: fruit, vegetables, milk and milk products, meat and meat products (red meat, chicken and fish), grains (bread, rice pasta), sweets, sugar sweetened beverages (ssbs), coffee and tea, and energy drinks. Response options included never; 1–4 times per week; once a day; 2–3 times a day; 4 or more times a day. Internal consistency of the food added in the food frequency questionnaire was evaluated using Cronbach's alpha for this section of the questionnaire specifically, to decrease false high internal consistency, since this test is affected by the length of the test [33]. A value of 0.81 was derived showing strong inter-relatedness of the food items, ensuring validity (Cronbach's alpha = 0.81, from a scale of 0 to 1.0; small cohort error variance of 0.34).

2.2.2. Physical Activity Assessment

A modified version of the International Physical Activity Questionnaire Short Form (IPAQ-SF) was used to assess frequency of physical activity pre-COVID-19 and during COVID-19 among surveyed participants [26]. Participants were asked to indicate "how many days per week did they engage in moderate to vigorous physical activity", and "how many days per week did they engage in household chores". They were also asked to indicate "how many hours per day did they spend on the computer for work or study", and "how many hours per day did they spend on screens for fun and entertainment".

2.2.3. Stress, Irritability and Sleep Assessment

Questions on stress and sleep were adopted from the second version of the Copenhagen Psychosocial Questionnaire (COPSOQ-II) with modifications [27]. Regarding stress and irritability, participants were asked to provide the frequency of experiencing physical exhaustion; emotional exhaustion; irritability; and tension. The same questions were asked once regarding the period before the pandemic (pre-COVID-19) and once during the pandemic. The response options included all the time; a small part of the time; part of the time; a large part of the time; all the time.

With regard to sleep, participants were asked if they experienced sleep disturbances including sleeping badly and restlessly; having difficulty to go to sleep; waking up too early and not being able to get back to sleep; waking up several times and found it difficult to get back to sleep; or none of the options. The questionnaire also included the following questions: "number of sleeping hours per night", "rating sleep quality", and "describing energy level during the day". The repose options for rating sleep quality were very good; good; poor. The repose options for describing energy level were energized; neutral; lazy. Questions were repeated twice, once about the period pre-COVID-19 and the second regarding the period during COVID-19.

2.3. Statistical Analysis

Categorical variables are presented as counts and percentages. The chi square test was used to determine the association between categorical variables, and the McNemar test was used to investigate the difference between categorical variables before and during the COVID-19 pandemic. A sub-analysis was also performed for weight and specific behavioral variables' differences between groups. Specifically, data were stratified (i) by sex, (ii) by age group (18–35 and ≥36 years), and (iii) level of education. Principal component analysis (PCA) was used to group related dietary practice into components [34]. The correlation of each food group with the underlying component was calculated with component loadings. In this analysis, values >0.3 were considered as having an effect in the component construction. Each participant was given a score based on the sum of the component loadings of each food group. The identified components were rotated (varimax rotation) to retrieve orthogonal, uncorrelated factors, decreasing variance errors. The Kaiser–Meyer–Olkin (KMO) measure of sample adequacy was used to assess PCA adequacy. Results were significant for p value < 0.05. Statistical analysis was performed using Statistical Package for the Social Sciences (SPSS) version 26.0 (IBM, Chicago, IL, USA).

3. Results

3.1. Demographic Characteristics

The survey was completed by 1012 participants. The sample distribution from different emirates was representative of the population distribution in the UAE. With the highest number of participants residing in Abu Dhabi and Dubai. More specifically, local coverage spreads over all regions in the UAE: 33.9% of participants live in the capital Abu Dhabi, 32.5% in Dubai, and 33.6% in Sharjah and northern Emirates. The majority of the participants completed the survey in Arabic (60.4%), followed by English (39.3%), and only 0.3% chose the French language. Comprehensive information relating to demographic characteristics of the study population is presented in Table 1. The majority of participants were females (75.9%), aged 26–35 years (29.1%), were married (56.4%), had no children (50%), completed a bachelor's degree (54.1%), worked full-time (53.3%), and were working or studying from home during quarantine (61.6%). Almost one third of the participants reported weight gain since the start of the lockdown (31%). However, 20.9% reported weight loss, 40.1% maintained their weight, and 7.9% did not know if there was a change in their weight. The majority of participants described their health status during the outbreak as very good (39.7%) and only 0.7% indicated poor health status.

Table 1. Demographic characteristics of study participants (n = 1012).

Characteristics	n	%
Gender		
Male	244	24.1
Female	768	75.9
Age (years)		
18–25	280	27.7
26–35	294	29.1
36–45	240	23.7
46–55	154	15.2
>55	44	4.3
Marital status		
Married	571	56.4
Single	403	39.8
Divorced	30	3.0
Widowed	8	0.8

Table 1. *Cont.*

Characteristics	*n*	%
Number of children		
None	506	50.0
1–2	230	22.7
≥ 3	276	27.3
Education level		
Less than high school	8	0.8
High school	111	11.0
College/Diploma	102	10.1
Bachelor's degree	547	54.1
Higher than bachelor's degree	244	24.1
Employment status		
Full-time	539	53.3
Part-time	44	4.3
Self-employed	31	3.1
Student	156	15.4
Unemployed	230	22.7
Retired	12	1.2
Working/studying from home		
Yes	623	61.6
No	309	30.5
Not applicable	80	7.9
Weight change during pandemic		
Lost weight	212	20.9
Gained weight	314	31.0
Maintained weight	406	40.1
Do not know	80	7.9
Perceived health state during pandemic		
Excellent	217	21.4
Very good	402	39.7
Good	284	28.1
Fair	102	10.1
Poor	7	0.7
Emirate of residence		
Abu Dhabi	343	33.9
Dubai	329	32.5
Sharjah	244	24.1
Ajman	52	5.1
Ras al Khaimah	20	2.0
Fujairah	16	1.6
Umm al Quwain	8	0.8

3.2. Source of Information

When asked about the most common source of information for health and nutrition updates, 69.1% and 67.8% of participants reported relying on social media applications, respectively (Table 2). Local and international health authorities were selected as the second source of information for both health and nutrition updates (65.4% and 48.7%, respectively).

Table 2. Source of health and nutrition information during COVID-19 pandemic ($n = 1012$).

Source of Information *	Health-Related Information, n (%)	Nutrition-Related Information, n (%)
Local and international health authorities	662 (65.4)	493 (48.7)
Social media	699 (69.1)	686 (67.8)
Healthcare professionals	409 (40.4)	462 (45.7)
Television	231 (22.8)	172 (17.0)
Newspapers	75 (7.4)	51 (5.0)
Friends and family	339 (33.5)	386 (38.1)

* As multiple responses were allowed, the total number of responses is greater than the number of surveyed participants and the percent of cases is displayed.

3.3. Eating Habits

Table 3 presents the eating habits of the study participants pre- and during the COVID-19 pandemic. Results showed a significant increase in the percentage of participants consuming mostly homemade meals during the pandemic and a significant reduction in those mainly consuming fast-food ($p < 0.001$). Moreover, the percentage of participants consuming five or more meals per day increased from 2.1% before the pandemic to 7% during the pandemic ($p < 0.001$). Also, the percentage of participants consuming breakfast increased from 66% to 74.2%, and the percentage of those skipping meals decreased from 64.5% to 46.2% during the pandemic ($p < 0.001$). Participants reported skipping meals mainly due to lack of time before the pandemic (62.3%), however, the main reason behind that was lack of appetite (36%). With regards to water intake, only 24.1% of participants consumed eight or more cups per day before the pandemic, and the percentage increased to 27.8% during the pandemic ($p = 0.003$).

Table 3. Eating habits pre- and during COVID-19 pandemic ($n = 1012$).

Variables	Pre-COVID-19 n (%)	During COVID-19 n (%)	p-Value (2-Sided)
Most consumed meals during the week *			
Homemade	838 (82.8)	974 (96.2)	<0.001
Frozen ready-to-eat meals	119 (11.8)	97 (9.6)	0.032
Fast food	270 (26.7)	80 (7.9)	<0.001
Restaurants [1]	289 (28.6)	58 (5.7)	<0.001
Healthy restaurants [2]	98 (9.7)	46 (4.5)	<0.001
Number of meals per day			
1–2 meals	470 (46.4)	369 (36.5)	<0.001
3–4 meals	521 (51.5)	572 (56.5)	0.009
≥5 meals	21 (2.1)	71 (7.0)	<0.001
Eating breakfast on most days			
Yes	668 (66.0)	751 (74.2)	<0.001
No	344 (34.0)	261 (25.8)	
Skipping meals			
Yes	663 (65.5)	468 (46.2)	<0.001
No	349 (34.5)	544 (53.8)	
Reasons for skipping meals (If the answer was yes) *			
To reduce food intake	143 (21.7)	136 (29.1)	0.011
Lack of time	410 (62.3)	143 (30.6)	<0.001
To lose weight	122 (18.5)	110 (23.6)	0.001
Lack of appetite	182 (27.7)	168 (36.0)	0.016
Fasting	68 (10.3)	120 (25.7)	<0.001

Table 3. *Cont.*

Variables	Pre-COVID-19 n (%)	During COVID-19 n (%)	p-Value (2-Sided)
Amount of water consumed per day			
1–4 cups	410 (40.5)	337 (33.3)	<0.001
5–7 cups	358 (35.4)	394 (38.9)	0.036
≥8 cups	244 (24.1)	281 (27.8)	0.003

* As multiple responses were allowed, the total number of responses is greater than the number of surveyed participants and the percent of cases is displayed. [1] Restaurants: included all ethnic restaurants (Asian, Middle Eastern, International, etc.), casual dining and family style restaurants; [2] healthy restaurants: included food outlets with the "Weqaya logo", restaurants categorized as "healthy" on food mobile apps (such as Zomato, Talabat, and Uber Eats) or catering services providing meal plan services based on nutritional needs (such as Kcal, right bite, Eat Clean ME, etc.).

The frequency of consumption for particular food products during the COVID-19 pandemic among residents of the UAE are presented in Table 4. Over half of the participants (51.2%) did not consume fruits daily, 37% did not consume vegetables daily, and 46.2% did not consume milk and dairy products on daily basis. However, 46.1% of the participants consumed sweets and desserts at least once per day, and 37.1% reported consuming salty snacks (chips, crackers, and nuts) every day.

Table 4. The frequency of consumption of particular foods during COVID-19 pandemic (*n* = 1012).

Food Items	≥4 Times/Day	2–3 Times/Day	Once/Day	1–4 Times/Week	Never
			n (%)		
Fruits	20 (2.0)	133 (13.1)	341 (33.7)	462 (45.7)	56 (5.5)
Vegetables	32 (3.2)	244 (24.1)	362 (35.8)	356 (35.2)	18 (1.8)
Milk and milk products	17 (1.7)	167 (16.5)	361 (35.7)	374 (37.0)	93 (9.2)
Meat/fish/chicken	32 (3.2)	133 (13.1)	440 (43.5)	383 (37.8)	24 (2.4)
Bread/rice/pasta	43 (4.2)	263 (26.0)	350 (34.6)	311 (30.7)	45 (4.4)
Sweets/desserts	29 (2.9)	106 (10.5)	331 (32.7)	437 (43.2)	109 (10.8)
Salty snacks	14 (1.4)	85 (8.4)	276 (27.3)	500 (49.4)	137 (13.5)
Coffee/tea	80 (7.9)	321 (31.7)	300 (29.6)	222 (21.9)	89 (8.8)
Sweetened drinks	18 (1.8)	51 (5.0)	156 (15.4)	340 (33.6)	447 (44.2)
Energy drinks	4 (0.4)	11 (1.1)	35 (3.5)	87 (8.6)	875 (86.5)

Additionally, 69.2% had tea or coffee at least once per day. Sweet drinks such as fruit juices and beverages were less popular among the study participants, as 44.2% reported never consuming them and an even higher percentage (86.5%) reported never consuming energy drinks during the pandemic.

A total of two components from the PCA output were derived, based on eigenvalue (at least 1) and scree plots obtained (Table 5). These two components explained 47% of the variance in eating behavior and were named based on the interpretation of the component loadings. The first pattern explained 31% of eating variation and was named "Western-type diet" since it was characterized by significantly positive loadings in dairy, meat, sweets, salted foods and vegetables. The second pattern explained 16% of the variance and loaded positively with ssbs and energy drinks and negatively on fruits and vegetables. Therefore, it was named "Free Sugars diet". A KMO of 0.78 was obtained, which is considered substantial.

Table 5. Component loading for the two major dietary patterns of the participants during COVID-19.

Food Groups	Western	Free Sugars
Fruits	0.2839	**−0.3807**
Vegetable	**0.3302**	**−0.4219**
Milk	**0.3247**	−0.1932
Meat	**0.3599**	−0.0732
Carbs	**0.3975**	−0.0764
Sweets	**0.3845**	0.2917
Salted Foods	**0.3356**	0.2776
Coffee/Tea	0.2457	−0.1641
Sweet Drinks	0.2678	**0.4929**
Energy Drinks	0.1575	**0.4433**
KMO	**0.78**	

KMO: Kaiser–Meyer–Olkin (KMO) test. The unique characteristics of each component (dietary pattern) are presented in bold. Marginally unique dietary characteristic for each component. Loadings ≥0.30 and ≤−0.30.

3.4. Shopping

The results revealed that the majority of participants prepared a shopping list beforehand (80.3%), started stocking up on foods during the pandemic (43.9%), did not order their groceries online (58.0%), read the food label before purchasing products (52.4%), and sanitized or cleaned groceries before storing them (71.9%) (Table 6).

Table 6. Shopping practices during COVID-19 pandemic ($n = 1012$).

Variables	n	%
Prepare shopping list		
Yes	813	80.3
No	199	19.7
Start stocking up on foods		
Yes	444	43.9
No	412	40.7
Already stocking up	156	15.4
Online grocery shopping		
Yes	425	42.0
No	587	58.0
Reading food labels		
Yes	530	52.4
No	113	11.2
Sometimes	369	36.5
Sanitizing/cleaning groceries		
Yes	728	71.9
No	113	11.2
Sometimes	171	16.9

3.5. Physical Activity

Figure 1a shows that 32.1% of the participants reported not engaging in any physical activity before the coronavirus pandemic, and the percentage increased to 38.5% during the pandemic ($p < 0.001$). Moreover, Figure 1b shows that there was a significant association between the frequency of performing physical activity during the pandemic and the reported change in weight among participants ($p < 0.001$). Of those who reported performing physical activity more than three times per week, 29.9% lost weight and 49.5% maintained their weight ($p < 0.001$). Furthermore, 40.3% of people who did not perform physical activity reported weight gain.

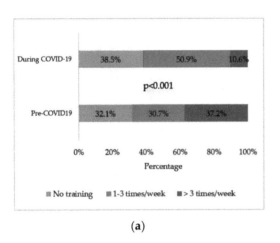

(a)

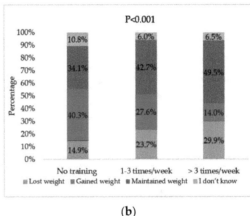

(b)

Figure 1. Physical activity pre- and during COVID-19 pandemic (**a**) Frequency; (**b**) Change in weight. The p values indicate the statistical significance of McNemar test. The p values indicate the statistical significance of chi-square test.

A significantly higher percentage of participants spent more than five hours per day on the computer for study or work purposes during the pandemic (47.6%) compared to before the pandemic (32%) ($p < 0.001$). Similarly, the percentage of participants spending more than five hours per day on screens for fun increased from 12.9% before the lockdown to 36.2% during the lockdown ($p < 0.001$) (Table 7).

Table 7. Daily activities pre- and during COVID-19 pandemic ($n = 1012$).

Variables	Pre-COVID-19 n (%)	During COVID-19 n (%)	p-Value (2-Sided)
Doing household chores			
Never	302 (29.8)	207 (20.5)	<0.001
1–3 times/week	404 (39.8)	333 (32.9)	<0.001
4–5 times/week	62 (6.1)	114 (11.3)	<0.001
Everyday	244 (24.1)	358 (35.4)	<0.001
Screen time for study or work			
None	188 (18.6)	160 (15.8)	0.004
1–2 h/day	282 (27.9)	136 (13.4)	<0.001
3–5 h/day	218 (21.5)	234 (23.1)	0.375
>5 h/day	324 (32.0)	482 (47.6)	<0.001
Screen time for entertainment			
Less than 30 min/day	113 (11.2)	62 (6.1)	<0.001
1–2 h/day	456 (45.1)	231 (22.8)	<0.001
3–5 h/day	312 (30.8)	353 (34.9)	0.053
>5 h/day	131 (12.9)	366 (36.2)	<0.001

3.6. Stress

Participants were asked to indicate the frequency of experiencing physical exhaustion; emotional exhaustion; irritability; and tension before and during the pandemic. Figure 2 presented the response distribution in percentages for each of the four stress parameters.

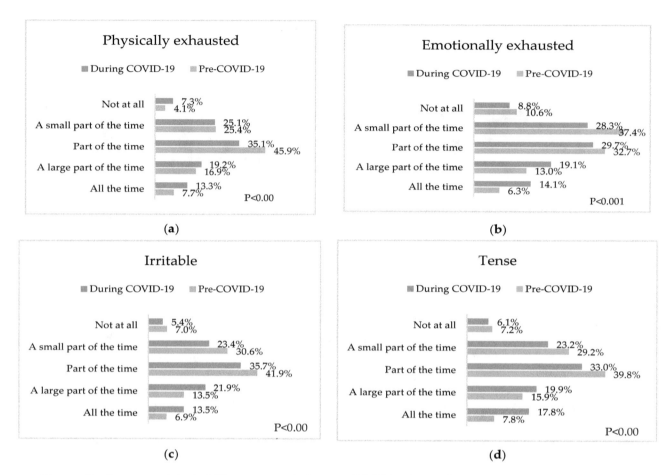

Figure 2. Stress and irritability pre- and during COVID-19 pandemic (**a**) Physical exhaustion; (**b**) Emotional exhaustion; (**c**) Irritability; (**d**) Tension. The *p* values indicate the statistical significance of McNemar test.

The results indicate a significant increase in the percentage of participants reporting all four stress parameters "all the time" during the coronavirus pandemic compared to before the pandemic (13.3% vs. 7.7% for physical exhaustion; 14.1% vs. 6.3% for emotional exhaustion; 13.5% vs. 6.9% for irritability; and 17.8% vs. 6.3% for tension) (all $p < 0.001$).

3.7. Sleep

Results showed a significant decrease in the percentage of participants who reported sleeping less than seven hours per night from 51.7% before the pandemic to 39% during the pandemic ($p < 0.001$) (Table 8). However, a higher percentage of participants reported poor sleep quality during the pandemic (28.1%) compared to before the pandemic (17.3) ($p < 0.001$), and sleep disturbances were also more common during the pandemic (60.8%) compared to before (52.9%). Consequently, 30.9% of the surveyed participants reported feeling lazy and less energized during the pandemic, compared to only 4.7% before the pandemic ($p < 0.001$) (Table 8).

An analysis of weight and behavioral factors by sex and age groups is depicted in Table 9. Significantly more males reported decreased engagement in physical activity (50% vs. 39.3%; $p = 0.013$) and increased screen time (54.5% vs. 51%; $p = 0.002$). Sleep disturbances increase was, however, significantly higher in females ($p = 0.011$). Moreover, those aged over 36 years reported a higher weight gain as well as an increase in the number of meals consumed per day ($p = 0.042$ and $p = 0.024$, respectively). Sleep duration and quality was most affected among participants aged 18–35 ($p < 0.001$). There was no significant association between different education levels and lifestyle changes (Table 9).

Table 8. Sleep pre- and during COVID-19 pandemic ($n = 1012$).

Variables	Pre-COVID-19 n (%)	During COVID-19 n (%)	p-Value (2-Sided)
Hours of sleep per night			
<7 h	523 (51.7)	395 (39.0)	<0.001
7–9 h	459 (45.4)	499 (49.3)	0.057
>9 h	30 (3.0)	118 (11.7)	<0.001
How would you rate your sleep quality			
Very good	308 (30.4)	282 (27.9)	0.134
Good	529 (52.3)	446 (44.1)	<0.001
Poor	175 (17.3)	284 (28.1)	<0.001
Did you experience any of the following *			
Slept badly and restlessly	251 (24.8)	285 (28.2)	0.057
Hard to go to sleep	199 (19.7)	358 (35.4)	<0.001
Woken up too early and not been able to get back to sleep	232 (22.9)	147 (14.5)	<0.001
Woken up several times and found it difficult to get back to sleep	187 (18.5)	334 (33.0)	<0.001
None	477 (47.1)	397 (39.2)	<0.001
Describe your energy level			
Energized	369 (36.5)	189 (18.7)	<0.001
Neutral	596 (58.9)	510 (50.4)	<0.001
Lazy	47 (4.7)	313 (30.9)	<0.001

* As multiple responses were allowed, the total number of responses is greater than the number of surveyed participants and the percent of cases is displayed.

Table 9. Lifestyle changes during COVID-19 pandemic by demographic factors ($n = 1012$).

Variables	All $n = 1012$	Gender			Age Group (Year)			Education Level		
		Female $n = 768$	Male $n = 244$	p Value	18–35 $n = 574$	≥36 $n = 438$	p Value	High School $n = 119$	Higher Degree $n = 893$	p Value
Weight, n, (%)										
Decreased	212 (20.9)	166 (21.6)	46 (18.9)	0.143	131 (22.8)	81 (18.5)	0.042	19 (16.0)	193 (21.6)	0.350
Same as before	486 (48.0)	376 (49.0)	110 (45.1)		273 (47.6)	213 (48.6)		62 (52.1)	424 (47.5)	
Increased	314 (31.0)	226 (29.4)	88 (36.1)		170 (29.6)	144 (32.9)		38 (31.9)	276 (30.9)	
Meals per day, n (%)										
Decreased	124 (12.3)	96 (12.5)	28 (11.5)	0.140	84 (14.6)	40 (9.1)	0.024	13 (10.9)	111 (12.4)	0.352
Same as before	628 (62.1)	464 (60.4)	164 (67.2)		342 (59.6)	272 (61.9)		69 (58.0)	559 (62.6)	
Increased	260 (25.7)	208 (27.1)	52 (21.3)		148 (25.8)	127 (29.0)		37 (31.1)	223 (25.0)	
Physical activity, n (%)										
Decreased	424 (41.9)	302 (39.3)	122 (50.0)	0.013	226 (39.4)	198 (45.2)	0.171	42 (35.3)	382 (42.8)	0.169
Same as before	438 (43.3)	346 (45.1)	92 (37.7)		258 (44.9)	180 (41.1)		61 (51.3)	377 (42.2)	
Increased	150 (14.8)	120 (15.6)	30 (12.3)		90 (15.7)	60 (13.7)		16 (13.4)	134 (15.0)	

Table 9. *Cont.*

Variables	All n = 1012	Gender			Age Group (Year)			Education Level		
		Female n = 768	Male n = 244	p Value	18–35 n = 574	≥36 n = 438	p Value	High School n = 119	Higher Degree n = 893	p Value
Screen time (entertainment), n (%)										
Decreased	72 (7.1)	67 (8.7)	5 (2.0)	0.002	46 (8.0)	26 (5.9)	0.150	8 (6.7)	64 (7.2)	0.984
Same as before	415 (41.0)	309 (40.2)	106 (43.4)		222 (38.7)	193 (44.1)		49 (41.2)	366 (41.0)	
Increased	525 (51.9)	392 (51.0)	133 (54.5)		306 (53.3)	219 (50.0)		62 (52.1)	463 (51.8)	
Sleep (h), n (%)										
Decreased	148 (14.6)	124 (16.1)	24 (9.8)	0.051	100 (17.4)	48 (11.0)	<0.001	23 (19.3)	125 (14.0)	0.302
Same as before	534 (52.8)	397 (51.7)	137 (56.1)		270 (47.0)	264 (60.3)		59 (49.6)	475 (53.2)	
Increased	330 (32.6)	247 (32.2)	83 (34.0)		204 (35.5)	126 (28.8)		37 (31.1)	293 (32.8)	
Sleep disturbances, n (%)										
Decreased	157 (15.5)	119 (15.5)	38 (15.6)	0.011	90 (15.7)	67 (15.3)	<0.001	16 (13.4)	141 (15.8)	0.135
Same as before	552 (54.5)	401 (52.2)	151 (61.9)		285 (49.7)	267 (61.0)		58 (48.7)	494 (55.3)	
Increased	303 (29.9)	248 (32.3)	55 (22.5)		199 (34.7)	104 (23.7)		45 (37.8)	258 (28.9)	

p value was based on chi-square test at 5% level.

4. Discussion

This population-based, cross-sectional study assessed eating habits and lifestyle behaviors among residences of the UAE, via an online survey during the COVID-19 pandemic between April and May 2020. The results indicate that the COVID-19 pandemic and the subsequent lockdown resulted in weight gain in about one-third of the respondents with changes in important and highly modifiable dietary and lifestyle behaviors that are considered essential for optimal somatic and psychological health. Specifically, participants also reported an increase in the number of meals consumed per day and a reduction in the percentage of skipping meals particularly breakfast during the pandemic. The present study also indicated that dietary habits were distanced from the Mediterranean diet principles and closer to "unhealthy" dietary patterns, characterized as high in energy but with low nutrient density; viewed as a detrimental combination for immune status. Although more homemade meals were prepared, a factor associated with healthy weight status, at the same time more non-nutritious foods were chosen, as well as being more frequently consumed (since an increase was also seen among frequency of meals per day). These data, therefore, are informative on the potential alterations of food prepared and consumed although at home.

In agreement with our study, the results from Kuwait, United States, Italy and France revealed an increase in caloric intake and indicated weight gain during the current COVID-19 home confinement [10,35–37]. Data from Kuwait, a close Gulf country to UAE, showed a significant increase in weight of respondents during the quarantine and the weight gain was 4.5 times higher among those consuming unhealthy diets [38]. The actual weight increase was not assessed in this study considering the short time interval of COVID-19 lockdown, however, the large percentage of the population that reported an increase in weight can be used as a proxy pertaining to changes in eating behavior and activity level. It has been suggested that the negative alterations in eating behaviors could be due to anxiety or boredom [39], lack of motivation to maintain healthy habits [40], or reduced availability of goods and limited access to food due to restricted store opening hours [41]. The prevalence of overweight and obesity in the UAE even before COVID-19 was high and has increased over time [42]. It is estimated that over one third of the population in the UAE is living with obesity with higher rates among females [43]. Thus, extra efforts are needed to reduce the burden of obesity and its risk factors especially during the COVID-19 pandemic.

Over half of the surveyed participants in this study did not consume fruits daily and about one third did not consume vegetables and dairy products on daily basis. Instead, almost half of the same population reported consuming sweets and desserts at least once per day and over one third consumed salty snacks daily. This transition towards a Westernized diet in the UAE was reported in 1998, where the consumption of fresh fruit and vegetables and of milk and dairy products was found low [32]. Moreover, in 2003, 77.5% of males and 75.7% of females in the UAE had less than five servings of fruit and vegetables per day [44]. Likewise, a recent study among Emirati adolescents revealed that only 28% of them met the recommended daily fruit and vegetable intake [45]. This is concerning especially as fruits and vegetables are an important source of fiber, vitamins, minerals, and antioxidants. Diets rich in antioxidants (such as the Mediterranean diet and Dietary Approaches to Stop Hypertension (DASH) diet) are vascular protective. The Mediterranean diet is recognized as an anti-inflammatory dietary pattern, focusing on high consumption of plant foods, low red meat and dairy and moderate consumption of monounsaturated fat sources such as olive oil [46]. Evidence suggests that the Mediterranean diet is associated with better health status, lower risk of chronic disease and inflammation as well as increased immunity [47–49]. The Mediterranean diet is not only a healthy dietary pattern, but is also a sustainable diet that has a lower environmental impact than the typical Western diet [50]. Moreover, mounting evidence indicates that the Mediterranean diet has a favorable effect on diseases related to chronic inflammation, including visceral obesity, type 2 diabetes mellitus and the metabolic syndrome [51–55]. Knowing that the prevalence of cardiovascular disease incidence is high in the UAE (40%) [56] and rates of dyslipidemia are strikingly elevated (72.5%) [57] makes it imperative that diets such as the Mediterranean diet should be encouraged to prevent the potentially negative effect of quarantine on dietary habits and overall health [41].

Due to the increase in obesogenic behaviors related to the COVID-19 pandemic, two dietary patterns were revealed among the studied population, named the "Western-type diet" and the "Free Sugars diet". These patterns indicate unhealthy eating behaviors during the period of the pandemic. This is in agreement with previous studies reporting a transformation of the diet in Eastern Mediterranean countries from a traditional Mediterranean diet to a more Westernized diet which is high in energy, saturated fat, cholesterol, salt, and refined carbohydrates, and low in fruits, vegetables, fiber, and polyunsaturated fats [25,58–60]. Therefore, current dietary behaviors in the UAE may not be effective against the COVID-19 virus since it can adversely affect the immune system response among other health factors. Furthermore, it is unclear whether these dietary patterns were due to the lockdown that followed the COVID-19 outbreak; however, the implications can be detrimental considering an adequate supply of macro- and micro-nutrients are essential for optimal immune function and response [11,61].

Amidst these passive changes in food behavior, some beneficial aspects emerged from this study, such as a significant increase in home-made food preparations, regular breakfast consumption and lower intakes of fast foods. Similarly, a consumer online based survey conducted by Ipsos across the Middle East and North Africa (MENA) region revealed that 57% out of the 5000 consumers who took part in the survey were preparing their own meals, and 79% were eating less often at restaurants [62].

Among the surveyed participants, more than one third reported a non-engagement in any physical activity during coronavirus pandemic lockdown. This was mostly observed among males in this study, with a simultaneously greater likelihood of increased sedentary time, compared to females. The findings of this questionnaire are in accordance with other studies indicating that the current COVID-19 pandemic had a dramatic impact on lifestyle behaviors globally, including diminished engagement in sports and physical activity in general [63–65]. Moreover, the "Effects of home Confinement on multiple Lifestyle Behaviours during the COVID-19 outbreak (ECLB-COVID-19)" international survey revealed that the COVID-19 pandemic had a negative effect on all levels of physical activity (vigorous, moderate, walking and overall) and increased daily sedentary time by more than 28% [14]. Similarly, in the current study the proportion of participants who spent more than five hours per day on screens for entertainment increased by 23.3%. Together with the unhealthy diet, the reduction of physical activity would not only contribute to weight gain, but also to an increase in cardiovascular risk during quarantine. Thus, awareness about the importance of regular physical activity and its benefits on overall health is necessary during such times [66,67]. It is also important to identify groups at a higher risk of unhealthy lifestyle behaviors during the COVID-19 pandemic to design interventions targeted towards these groups.

During the COVID-19 pandemic higher levels of anxiety, stress and depression have been observed among individuals [68–70]. In this study, the percentage of participants experiencing exhaustion, irritability, and tension more often during the coronavirus pandemic increased significantly. Sleep was mostly affected in females and needs to be further evaluated since it is linked with multiple endocrine functions, as well risk for obesity and depression. The risk of obesity is underlined by the significant increase in daily meal frequency among participants over 36 years with the majority being female. Also, despite WHO recommendations to minimize listening to unreliable news that could cause anxiety or distress and to seek information only from trusted sources [71], over two thirds of participants in this survey used social media as a main source for health updates. Studies have shown the negative and harmful effect of misinformation overload "infodemic" on the mental health of individuals [72,73]. Moreover, stress and anxiety could disrupt sleep quality during the night and energy levels during the day. Results of the current survey indicated a 10.8% increase in participants reporting poor sleep quality and 26.2% increase in those feeling lazy during the pandemic. Xiao and his co-workers found a significant negative correlation between anxiety levels and sleep quality and suggested the use of telepsychiatry consultation as an important therapeutic strategy [74]. The use of telehealth has been shown to be useful in providing support to patients and is appropriate for the delivery of mental health services [75]. Additionally, the Mediterranean diet does not only have a protective effect on the risk of cardiovascular diseases and certain types of cancer [54,76], but also an increased compliance with it could be associated with lesser mental distress, better sleep quality, and higher scoring for self-perceived health status [77–79].

It is acknowledged that this study has limitations related to the use of self-reported questionnaire, snowball sampling method and the cross-sectional study design. The study information was acquired after lockdown, and although comparisons are critical to be made in order to draw inferences, no conclusive remarks can be drawn. Results stratified by sex should be interpreted with caution, since the majority of the participants were females. Furthermore, in order to minimize selection bias that may arise with snowball sampling (including interrelated-similar individuals), each individual could refer a maximum of three people who were not family members, and only one individual per age group (young adults, older adults, elderly) was enrolled from a household. Moreover, the change in dietary pattern was not assessed in this study, since data on food frequency were only obtained during COVID-19 pandemic, although these can be used as a reference for further studies performed, in these uncertain times. This was done to reduce the probability of including recall bias, since the participants had to respond to multiple questions on food frequency and quantity during COVID-19 lockdown and for a prolonged period prior to that. Also, the presence of obesity and eating disorders were not determined in the study, nor was information on infection with COVID-19 reported. Such analysis would require a longer questionnaire, hence may have decreased the compliance and response rate, but also would have required a larger sample size based on the prevalence of all factors to acquire adequate study power. Another potential limitation of the study was that respondents were mostly females. Although this is usual in online questionnaires [80], it should be considered when generalizing the results. However, using an online survey facilitated data collection during COVID-19 pandemic from all seven emirates. It also guaranteed the anonymity of the participants, thus reducing the social desirability bias. The strengths of this research include data collection timing one month after lockdown which minimizes memory failure for previous habits. In addition, the survey provided was in multiple languages in a multilingual environment like UAE.

The results of the study indicate that individuals in the UAE experienced negative lifestyle changes, unbalanced food choices, a reduction in physical activity, and psychological problems during the COVID-19 pandemic. Although quarantine is an essential measure to protect public health and control the transmission of the virus, these findings should be taken into consideration for future regulations in the UAE.

Author Contributions: Conceptualization, L.C.I., T.M.O. and A.S.A.D.; methodology, L.C.I., T.M.O., A.S.A.D., M.N.M., M.H., and S.T.S.; validation, L.C.I., T.M.O., A.S.A.D., M.N.M. and E.M.; formal analysis, L.C.I., M.N.M., S.T.S., E.M. and H.H.; investigation, L.C.I., T.M.O., M.N.M., A.S.A.D., A.A.M., A.H.J., D.O.A.J., H.I.A., H.A.S., H.H., L.M.R.A., L.S., M.H., R.R.S.O., and S.T.S.; writing—original draft preparation, L.C.I., M.N.M., A.S.A.D. and S.T.S.; writing—review and editing, L.C.I., T.M.O., M.N.M., A.S.A.D., A.A.M., A.H.J., D.O.A.J., E.M.,H.I.A., H.A.S., H.H., L.M.R.A., L.S., M.H., R.R.S.O., and S.T.S. All authors have read and agreed to the published version of the manuscript.

References

1. Barro, R.J.; Ursúa, J.F.; Weng, J. *The Coronavirus and the Great Influenza Pandemic: Lessons from the "Spanish flu" for the Coronavirus's Potential Effects on Mortality and Economic Activity*; 0898-2937; National Bureau of Economic Research: Cambridge, MA, USA, 2020.
2. WHO. WHO Director-General's Opening Remarks at the Media Briefing on COVID-19—11 March 2020. Available online: https://www.who.int/dg/speeches/detail/who-director-general-s-opening-remarks-at-the-media-briefing-on-covid-19---11-march-2020 (accessed on 16 August 2020).
3. WHO. Coronavirus Disease (COVID-19) Weekly Epidemiological and Operational Updates September 2020. Available online: https://www.who.int/docs/default-source/coronaviruse/situation-reports/20200928-weekly-epi-update.pdf?sfvrsn=9e354665_6 (accessed on 29 September 2020).
4. Wilder-Smith, A.; Freedman, D. Isolation, quarantine, social distancing and community containment: Pivotal role for old-style public health measures in the novel coronavirus (2019-nCoV) outbreak. *J. Travel Med.* **2020**, *27*, taaa020. [CrossRef] [PubMed]
5. Koh, D. COVID-19 lockdowns throughout the world. *Occup. Med.* **2020**. [CrossRef]
6. Bloukh, S.H.; Shaikh, A.; Pathan, H.M.; Edis, Z. Prevalence of COVID-19: A Look behind the Scenes from the UAE and India. *Preprints* **2020**. [CrossRef]
7. Bank, T.W. United Arab Emirates: Data Source: United Nations World Population Prospects. Available online: https://data.worldbank.org/country/AE (accessed on 16 August 2020).
8. De Bel-Air, F. *Demography, Migration, and the Labour Market in the UAE*; Migration Policy Center, Gulf Labour Markets and Migration (GLMM): Firenze, Italy, 2015.
9. Scarmozzino, F.; Visioli, F. Covid-19 and the Subsequent Lockdown Modified Dietary Habits of Almost Half the Population in an Italian Sample. *Foods* **2020**, *9*, 675. [CrossRef] [PubMed]
10. Deschasaux-Tanguy, M.; Druesne-Pecollo, N.; Esseddik, Y.; Szabo de Edelenyi, F.; Alles, B.; Andreeva, V.A.; Baudry, J.; Charreire, H.; Deschamps, V.; Egnell, M.; et al. Diet and physical activity during the COVID-19 lockdown period (March-May 2020): Results from the French NutriNet-Sante cohort study. *medRxiv* **2020**. [CrossRef]
11. Calder, P.C. Nutrition, immunity and COVID-19. *BMJ Nutr. Prev. Health* **2020**, *3*, 74. [CrossRef]
12. Zachary, Z.; Brianna, F.; Brianna, L.; Garrett, P.; Jade, W.; Alyssa, D.; Mikayla, K. Self-quarantine and Weight Gain Related Risk Factors During the COVID-19 Pandemic. *Obes. Res. Clin. Pract.* **2020**. [CrossRef]
13. Musaiger, A.O. Diet and Prevention of Coronary Heart Disease in the Arab Middle East Countries. *Med. Princ. Pract.* **2002**, *11*, 9–16. [CrossRef]
14. Ammar, A.; Brach, M.; Trabelsi, K.; Chtourou, H.; Boukhris, O.; Masmoudi, L.; Bouaziz, B.; Bentlage, E.; How, D.; Ahmed, M. Effects of COVID-19 Home Confinement on Eating Behaviour and Physical Activity: Results of the ECLB-COVID19 International Online Survey. *Nutrients* **2020**, *12*, 1583. [CrossRef]
15. Lippi, G.; Henry, B.M.; Sanchis-Gomar, F. Physical inactivity and cardiovascular disease at the time of coronavirus disease 2019 (COVID-19). *Eur. J. Prev. Cardiol.* **2020**. [CrossRef]

16.   Hall, G.; Laddu, D.R.; Phillips, S.A.; Lavie, C.J.; Arena, R. A tale of two pandemics: How will COVID-19 and global trends in physical inactivity and sedentary behavior affect one another? *Prog. Cardiovasc. Dis.* **2020**. [CrossRef] [PubMed]

17.   Yammine, K. The prevalence of physical activity among the young population of UAE: A meta-analysis. *Perspect. Public Health* **2017**, *137*, 275–280. [CrossRef] [PubMed]

18.   Wu, P.; Fang, Y.; Guan, Z.; Fan, B.; Kong, J.; Yao, Z.; Liu, X.; Fuller, C.J.; Susser, E.; Lu, J. The psychological impact of the SARS epidemic on hospital employees in China: Exposure, risk perception, and altruistic acceptance of risk. *Can. J. Psychiatry* **2009**, *54*, 302–311. [CrossRef]

19.   Pfefferbaum, B.; North, C.S. Mental health and the Covid-19 pandemic. *N. Engl. J. Med.* **2020**. [CrossRef] [PubMed]

20.   Todisco, P.; Donini, L.M. Eating disorders and obesity (ED&O) in the COVID-19 storm. *Eat. Weight Disord.* **2020**, *1*. [CrossRef]

21.   Touyz, S.; Lacey, H.; Hay, P. Eating disorders in the time of COVID-19. *J. Eat. Disord.* **2020**, *8*, 19. [CrossRef] [PubMed]

22.   Rajkumar, R.P. COVID-19 and mental health: A review of the existing literature. *Asian J. Psychiatry* **2020**, *52*, 102066. [CrossRef]

23.   Holmes, E.A.; O'Connor, R.C.; Perry, V.H.; Tracey, I.; Wessely, S.; Arseneault, L.; Ballard, C.; Christensen, H.; Silver, R.C.; Everall, I. Multidisciplinary research priorities for the COVID-19 pandemic: A call for action for mental health science. *Lancet Psychiatry* **2020**. [CrossRef]

24.   Torales, J.; O'Higgins, M.; Castaldelli-Maia, J.M.; Ventriglio, A. The outbreak of COVID-19 coronavirus and its impact on global mental health. *Int. J. Soc. Psychiatry* **2020**. [CrossRef]

25.   Ng, S.W.; Zaghloul, S.; Ali, H.; Harrison, G.; Yeatts, K.; El Sadig, M.; Popkin, B.M. Nutrition transition in the United Arab Emirates. *Eur. J. Clin. Nutr.* **2011**, *65*, 1328–1337. [CrossRef]

26.   Lee, P.H.; Macfarlane, D.J.; Lam, T.H.; Stewart, S.M. Validity of the international physical activity questionnaire short form (IPAQ-SF): A systematic review. *Int. J. Behav. Nutr. Phys. Act.* **2011**, *8*, 115. [CrossRef] [PubMed]

27.   Pejtersen, J.H.; Kristensen, T.S.; Borg, V.; Bjorner, J.B. The second version of the Copenhagen Psychosocial Questionnaire. *Scand. J. Public Health* **2010**, *38*, 8–24. [CrossRef]

28.   Wild, D.; Grove, A.; Martin, M.; Eremenco, S.; McElroy, S.; Verjee-Lorenz, A.; Erikson, P. Principles of good practice for the translation and cultural adaptation process for patient-reported outcomes (PRO) measures: Report of the ISPOR task force for translation and cultural adaptation. *Value Health* **2005**, *8*, 94–104. [CrossRef] [PubMed]

29.   Beaton, D.E.; Bombardier, C.; Guillemin, F.; Ferraz, M.B. Guidelines for the process of cross-cultural adaptation of self-report measures. *Spine* **2000**, *25*, 3186–3191. [CrossRef]

30.   Osler, M.; Heitmann, B.L. The Validity of a Short Food Frequency Questionnaire and its Ability to Measure Changes in Food Intake: A Longitudinal Study. *Int. J. Epidemiol.* **1996**, *25*, 1023–1029. [CrossRef] [PubMed]

31.   Cooper, R.; Al-Alami, U. Food consumption patterns of female undergraduate students in the United Arab Emirates. *West Afr. J. Med.* **2011**, *30*, 42–46. [CrossRef] [PubMed]

32.   Musaiger, A.O.; Abuirmeileh, N.M. Food consumption patterns of adults in the United Arab Emirates. *J. R. Soc. Promot. Health* **1998**, *118*, 146–150. [CrossRef]

33.   Streiner, D.L. Starting at the Beginning: An Introduction to Coefficient Alpha and Internal Consistency. *J. Personal. Assess.* **2003**, *80*, 99–103. [CrossRef]

34.   Panagiotakos, D.B.; Pitsavos, C.; Stefanadis, C. Dietary patterns: A Mediterranean diet score and its relation to clinical and biological markers of cardiovascular disease risk. *Nutr. Metab. Cardiovasc. Dis.* **2006**, *16*, 559–568. [CrossRef]

35.   Bhutani, S.; Cooper, J.A. COVID-19 related home confinement in adults: Weight gain risks and opportunities. *Obesity* **2020**. [CrossRef]

36.   Di Renzo, L.; Gualtieri, P.; Pivari, F.; Soldati, L.; Attinà, A.; Cinelli, G.; Leggeri, C.; Caparello, G.; Barrea, L.; Scerbo, F.; et al. Eating habits and lifestyle changes during COVID-19 lockdown: An Italian survey. *J. Transl. Med.* **2020**, *18*, 229. [CrossRef] [PubMed]

37.   Husain, W.; Ashkanani, F. Does COVID-19 Change Dietary Habits and Lifestyle Behaviours in Kuwait? *Environ. Health Prev. Med.* **2020**. [CrossRef] [PubMed]

38. ALMughamis, N.S.; AlAsfour, S.; Mehmood, S. Poor Eating Habits and Predictors of Weight Gain During the COVID-19 Quarantine Measures in Kuwait: A Cross Sectional Study. *Res. Sq.* **2020**. [CrossRef]

39. Moynihan, A.B.; Van Tilburg, W.A.; Igou, E.R.; Wisman, A.; Donnelly, A.E.; Mulcaire, J.B. Eaten up by boredom: Consuming food to escape awareness of the bored self. *Front. Psychol.* **2015**, *6*, 369. [CrossRef] [PubMed]

40. Gardner, B.; Rebar, A.L. Habit Formation and Behavior Change. In *Oxford Research Encyclopedia of Psychology*; Oxford University Press: Oxford, UK, 2019.

41. Mattioli, A.V.; Puviani, M.B.; Nasi, M.; Farinetti, A. COVID-19 pandemic: The effects of quarantine on cardiovascular risk. *Eur. J. Clin. Nutr.* **2020**. [CrossRef]

42. Sulaiman, N.; Elbadawi, S.; Hussein, A.; Abusnana, S.; Madani, A.; Mairghani, M.; Alawadi, F.; Sulaiman, A.; Zimmet, P.; Huse, O. Prevalence of overweight and obesity in United Arab Emirates Expatriates: The UAE national diabetes and lifestyle study. *Diabetol. Metab. Syndr.* **2017**, *9*, 88. [CrossRef]

43. Razzak, H.A.; El-Metwally, A.; Harbi, A.; Al-Shujairi, A.; Qawas, A. The prevalence and risk factors of obesity in the United Arab Emirates. *Saudi J. Obes.* **2017**, *5*, 57. [CrossRef]

44. Belal, A.M. Nutrition-related chronic diseases Epidemic in UAE: Can we stand to STOP it? *Sudan. J. Public Health* **2009**, *4*, 383–392.

45. Makansi, N.; Allison, P.; Awad, M.; Bedos, C. Fruit and vegetable intake among Emirati adolescents: A mixed methods study. *East. Mediterr. Health J.* **2018**, *24*. [CrossRef]

46. Díez, J.; Bilal, U.; Franco, M. Unique features of the Mediterranean food environment: Implications for the prevention of chronic diseases Rh: Mediterranean food environments. *Eur. J. Clin. Nutr.* **2019**, *72*, 71–75. [CrossRef]

47. Martínez-González, M.A.; Gea, A.; Ruiz-Canela, M. The Mediterranean diet and cardiovascular health: A critical review. *Circ. Res.* **2019**, *124*, 779–798. [CrossRef]

48. Becerra-Tomás, N.; Blanco Mejía, S.; Viguiliouk, E.; Khan, T.; Kendall, C.W.; Kahleova, H.; Rahelić, D.; Sievenpiper, J.L.; Salas-Salvadó, J. Mediterranean diet, cardiovascular disease and mortality in diabetes: A systematic review and meta-analysis of prospective cohort studies and randomized clinical trials. *Crit. Rev. Food Sci. Nutr.* **2020**, *60*, 1207–1227. [CrossRef] [PubMed]

49. Godos, J.; Zappala, G.; Bernardini, S.; Giambini, I.; Bes-Rastrollo, M.; Martinez-Gonzalez, M. Adherence to the Mediterranean diet is inversely associated with metabolic syndrome occurrence: A meta-analysis of observational studies. *Int. J. Food Sci. Nutr.* **2017**, *68*, 138–148. [CrossRef] [PubMed]

50. Germani, A.; Vitiello, V.; Giusti, A.M.; Pinto, A.; Donini, L.M.; del Balzo, V. Environmental and economic sustainability of the Mediterranean Diet. *Int. J. Food Sci. Nutr.* **2014**, *65*, 1008–1012. [CrossRef] [PubMed]

51. Giugliano, D.; Esposito, K. Mediterranean diet and metabolic diseases. *Curr. Opin. Lipidol.* **2008**, *19*, 63–68. [CrossRef] [PubMed]

52. Hassapidou, M.; Tziomalos, K.; Lazaridou, S.; Pagkalos, I.; Papadimitriou, K.; Kokkinopoulou, A.; Tzotzas, T. The Nutrition Health Alliance (NutriHeAl) Study: A Randomized, Controlled, Nutritional Intervention Based on Mediterranean Diet in Greek Municipalities. *J. Am. Coll. Nutr.* **2020**, *39*, 338–344. [CrossRef] [PubMed]

53. Sánchez-Villegas, A.; Bes-Rastrollo, M.; Martínez-González, M.A.; Serra-Majem, L. Adherence to a Mediterranean dietary pattern and weight gain in a follow-up study: The SUN cohort. *Int. J. Obes.* **2006**, *30*, 350–358. [CrossRef]

54. Serra-Majem, L.; Roman-Vinas, B.; Sanchez-Villegas, A.; Guasch-Ferre, M.; Corella, D.; La Vecchia, C. Benefits of the Mediterranean diet: Epidemiological and molecular aspects. *Mol. Asp. Med.* **2019**, *67*, 1–55. [CrossRef]

55. Martínez-González, M.A.; Salas-Salvadó, J.; Estruch, R.; Corella, D.; Fitó, M.; Ros, E. Benefits of the Mediterranean Diet: Insights From the PREDIMED Study. *Prog. Cardiovasc. Dis.* **2015**, *58*, 50–60. [CrossRef]

56. Turk-Adawi, K.; Sarrafzadegan, N.; Fadhil, I.; Taubert, K.; Sadeghi, M.; Wenger, N.K.; Tan, N.S.; Grace, S.L. Cardiovascular disease in the Eastern Mediterranean region: Epidemiology and risk factor burden. *Nat. Rev. Cardiol.* **2018**, *15*, 106–119. [CrossRef]

57. Mahmoud, I.; Sulaiman, N. Dyslipidaemia prevalence and associated risk factors in the United Arab Emirates: A population-based study. *BMJ Open* **2019**, *9*, e031969. [CrossRef]

58. Taha, Z.; Eltom, S.E. The Role of Diet and Lifestyle in Women with Breast Cancer: An Update Review of Related Research in the Middle East. *Biores. Open Access* **2018**, *7*, 73–80. [CrossRef] [PubMed]

59. Musaiger, A.O.; Al-Hazzaa, H.M. Prevalence and risk factors associated with nutrition-related noncommunicable diseases in the Eastern Mediterranean region. *Int. J. Gen. Med.* **2012**, *5*, 199–217. [CrossRef]
60. Galal, O. Nutrition-related health patterns in the Middle East. *Asia Pac. J. Clin. Nutr.* **2003**, *12*, 337–343.
61. Gombart, A.F.; Pierre, A.; Maggini, S. A review of micronutrients and the immune System–Working in harmony to reduce the risk of infection. *Nutrients* **2020**, *12*, 236. [CrossRef] [PubMed]
62. Ipsos. 5 Ways COVID-19 Has Impacted MENA's Food Habits. Available online: https://www.ipsos.com/sites/default/files/ct/news/documents/2020-06/5_ways_covid-19_impacted_menas_food_habits_-_ipsos_mena_0.pdf (accessed on 16 August 2020).
63. Ammar, A.; Brach, M.; Trabelsi, K.; Chtourou, H.; Boukhris, O.; Masmoudi, L.; Bouaziz, B.; Bentlage, E.; How, D.; Ahmed, M. Effects of COVID-19 home confinement on physical activity and eating behaviour Preliminary results of the ECLB-COVID19 international online-survey. *medRxiv* **2020**. [CrossRef]
64. Abbas, A.M.; Fathy, S.K.; Fawzy, A.T.; Salem, A.S.; Shawky, M.S. The mutual effects of COVID-19 and obesity. *Obes. Med.* **2020**. [CrossRef] [PubMed]
65. Burtscher, J.; Burtscher, M.; Millet, G.P. (Indoor) isolation, stress and physical inactivity: Vicious circles accelerated by Covid-19? *Scand. J. Med. Sci. Sports* **2020**. [CrossRef]
66. Jiménez-Pavón, D.; Carbonell-Baeza, A.; Lavie, C.J. Physical exercise as therapy to fight against the mental and physical consequences of COVID-19 quarantine: Special focus in older people. *Prog. Cardiovasc. Dis.* **2020**. [CrossRef] [PubMed]
67. Czosnek, L.; Lederman, O.; Cormie, P.; Zopf, E.; Stubbs, B.; Rosenbaum, S. Health benefits, safety and cost of physical activity interventions for mental health conditions: A meta-review to inform translation efforts. *Ment. Health Phys. Act.* **2019**, *16*, 140–151. [CrossRef]
68. Shigemura, J.; Ursano, R.J.; Morganstein, J.C.; Kurosawa, M.; Benedek, D.M. Public responses to the novel 2019 coronavirus (2019-nCoV) in Japan: Mental health consequences and target populations. *Psychiatry Clin. Neurosci.* **2020**, *74*, 281–282. [CrossRef] [PubMed]
69. Wang, C.; Pan, R.; Wan, X.; Tan, Y.; Xu, L.; Ho, C.S.; Ho, R.C. Immediate psychological responses and associated factors during the initial stage of the 2019 coronavirus disease (COVID-19) epidemic among the general population in China. *Int. J. Environ. Res. Public Health* **2020**, *17*, 1729. [CrossRef]
70. Zandifar, A.; Badrfam, R. Iranian mental health during the COVID-19 epidemic. *Asian J. Psychiatry* **2020**, *51*. [CrossRef] [PubMed]
71. World Health Organization. *Mental Health and Psychosocial Considerations during the COVID-19 Outbreak, 18 March 2020*; World Health Organization: Geneva, Switzerland, 2020.
72. Cinelli, M.; Quattrociocchi, W.; Galeazzi, A.; Valensise, C.M.; Brugnoli, E.; Schmidt, A.L.; Zola, P.; Zollo, F.; Scala, A. The covid-19 social media infodemic. *arXiv* **2020**, arXiv:2003.05004. [CrossRef] [PubMed]
73. Gao, J.; Zheng, P.; Jia, Y.; Chen, H.; Mao, Y.; Chen, S.; Wang, Y.; Fu, H.; Dai, J. Mental health problems and social media exposure during COVID-19 outbreak. *PLoS ONE* **2020**, *15*, e0231924. [CrossRef]
74. Xiao, H.; Zhang, Y.; Kong, D.; Li, S.; Yang, N. The effects of social support on sleep quality of medical staff treating patients with coronavirus disease 2019 (COVID-19) in January and February 2020 in China. *Med. Sci. Monit. Int. Med. J. Exp. Clin. Res.* **2020**, *26*, e923549. [CrossRef]
75. Zhou, X.; Snoswell, C.L.; Harding, L.E.; Bambling, M.; Edirippulige, S.; Bai, X.; Smith, A.C. The role of telehealth in reducing the mental health burden from COVID-19. *Telemed. e-Health* **2020**, *26*, 377–379. [CrossRef]
76. Rosato, V.; Temple, N.J.; La Vecchia, C.; Castellan, G.; Tavani, A.; Guercio, V. Mediterranean diet and cardiovascular disease: A systematic review and meta-analysis of observational studies. *Eur. J. Nutr.* **2019**, *58*, 173–191. [CrossRef]
77. Salvatore, F.P.; Relja, A.; Filipčić, I.Š.; Polašek, O.; Kolčić, I. Mediterranean diet and mental distress:"10,001 Dalmatians" study. *Br. Food J.* **2019**, *121*, 1314–1326. [CrossRef]
78. Godos, J.; Ferri, R.; Caraci, F.; Cosentino, F.I.I.; Castellano, S.; Galvano, F.; Grosso, G. Adherence to the mediterranean diet is associated with better sleep quality in Italian adults. *Nutrients* **2019**, *11*, 976. [CrossRef]

79. Muñoz, M.A.; Fíto, M.; Marrugat, J.; Covas, M.I.; Schröder, H. Adherence to the Mediterranean diet is associated with better mental and physical health. *Br. J. Nutr.* **2008**, *101*, 1821–1827. [CrossRef]

80. Smith, G. *Does Gender Influence Online Survey Participation: A Record-Linkage Analysis of University Faculty Online Survey Response Behavior*; ERIC Document Reproduction Service No. ED 501717; San Jose State University, ScholarWorks: San Jose, CA, USA, 2008.

6

Validation of Surrogate Anthropometric Indices in Older Adults: What is the Best Indicator of High Cardiometabolic Risk Factor Clustering?

Robinson Ramírez-Vélez [1,*], Miguel Ángel Pérez-Sousa [2], Mikel Izquierdo [1,3], Carlos A. Cano-Gutierrez [4], Emilio González-Jiménez [5], Jacqueline Schmidt-RioValle [5], Katherine González-Ruíz [6] and María Correa-Rodríguez [5]

[1] Department of Health Sciences, Public University of Navarra, Navarrabiomed-Biomedical Research Centre, IDISNA-Navarra's Health Research Institute, C/irunlarrea 3, Complejo Hospitalario de Navarra, 31008 Pamplona, Navarra, Spain

[2] Faculty of Sport Sciences, University of Huelva, Avenida de las Fuerzas Armadas s/n, 21007 Huelva, Spain

[3] Centro de Investigación Biomédica en Red de Fragilidad y Envejecimiento Saludable (CIBERFES), Instituto de Salud Carlos III, 28029 Madrid, Spain

[4] Hospital Universitario San Ignacio – Aging Institute, Pontificia Universidad Javeriana, Bogotá 110111, Colombia

[5] Department of Nursing, Faculty of Health Sciences, University of Granada, Av. Ilustración, 60, 18016 Granada, Spain

[6] Grupo de Ejercicio Físico y Deportes, Vicerrectoría de Investigaciones, Facultad de Salud, Universidad Manuela Beltrán, Bogotá 110231, DC, Colombia

* Correspondence: robin640@hotmail.com

Abstract: The present study evaluated the ability of five obesity-related parameters, including a body shape index (ABSI), conicity index (CI), body roundness index (BRI), body mass index (BMI), and waist-to-height ratio (WtHR) for predicting increased cardiometabolic risk in a population of elderly Colombians. A cross-sectional study was conducted on 1502 participants (60.3% women, mean age 70 ± 7.6 years) and subjects' weight, height, waist circumference, serum lipid indices, blood pressure, and fasting plasma glucose were measured. A cardiometabolic risk index (CMRI) was calculated using the participants' systolic and diastolic blood pressure, triglycerides, high-density lipoprotein and fasting glucose levels, and waist circumference. Following the International Diabetes Federation definition, metabolic syndrome was defined as having three or more metabolic abnormalities. All surrogate anthropometric indices correlated significantly with CMRI ($p < 0.01$). Receiver operating characteristic curve analysis of how well the anthropometric indices identified high cardiometabolic risk showed that WtHR and BRI were the most accurate indices. The best WtHR and BRI cut-off points in men were 0.56 (area under curve, AUC 0.77) and 4.71 (AUC 0.77), respectively. For women, the WtHR and BRI cut-off points were 0.63 (AUC 0.77) and 6.20 (AUC 0.77), respectively. In conclusion, BRI and WtHR have a moderate discriminating power for detecting high cardiometabolic risk in older Colombian adults, supporting the idea that both anthropometric indices are useful screening tools for use in the elderly.

Keywords: anthropometric indices; diagnosis criteria; metabolic syndrome; cardiometabolic risk; elderly

1. Introduction

Metabolic syndrome (MetS) is a complex cluster of cardiovascular risk factors associated with a sedentary lifestyle, poor nutrition, and consequent overweight. It is also strongly associated with other abnormalities linked to cardiovascular disease (CVD), including glucose intolerance (type 2 diabetes, impaired glucose tolerance, or impaired fasting glycemia), insulin resistance, abdominal obesity, dyslipidemia, and hypertension [1]. Accordingly, MetS increases the risk of developing diseases of cardiovascular origin, such as acute myocardial infarction, ischemic stroke, or coronary heart disease [2]. Indeed, the prevalence of CVD attributable to MetS is estimated at around 12–17% [3]. Several studies have examined the presence of MetS in Latin America, reporting associated factors including advanced age, having Hispanic or indigenous heritage, physical inactivity, high alcohol intake, smoking, history of hypertension or type 2 diabetes (first-degree family members), and having a low socioeconomic status (reviewed in [4]). The general prevalence of MetS in Latin-American countries has been established as 24.9% (range: 18.8–43.3%) and is slightly more frequent in women (25.3%) than in men (23.2%).

The clinical utility of identifying MetS in older adults has been much debated because, among the issues raised, it has been argued that there is no consensus on the clinical criteria for screening the elderly population to identify patients likely to be characterized with MetS. In this line, several clinical criteria and cut-off points have been proposed. For instance, the cardiometabolic risk index (CMRI) in older adults, measured as a continuous summary score, might represent an important intermediate or preclinical outcome that can be measured prior to the onset of disease, and could provide opportunities for prevention. As a marker of cardiometabolic disease risk, the use of adult CMRI severity z-scores has been suggested as an accurate method to detect overall metabolic changes [5]. This continuous score would be more sensitive to small and large changes that do not modify the most recent Joint Interim Statement of the International Diabetes Federation (IDF) Task Force on Epidemiology and Prevention criteria [6]. Thus, an increase in cholesterol from 150 to 250 mg/dl would have no impact on the IDF score, but would be reflected as a non-trivial change in the continuous CMRI [7]. Nevertheless, there is no validated or harmonized consensus for defining CMRI in older adults, and several continuous CMRI scores have been reported in the literature, as described in previous narrative reviews.

Measurements of anthropometric indices are inexpensive and non-invasive, and are easily conducted as part of normal health exams. Interestingly, anthropometric measurements such as body mass index (BMI), waist circumference (WC), and waist-to-height ratio (WtHR) show a close correlation with MetS components and could thus be useful surrogate markers for predicting MetS [8–10]. That being said, there remains controversy over which anthropometric indices [11] are the most appropriate predictors of cardiometabolic disease [12]. In 2012, Krakauer and Krakauer developed "A Body Shape Index" (ABSI), based on WC adjusted for height and weight [13], and demonstrated that a high ABSI is associated with the accumulation of excess abdominal adipose tissue and seems to be a substantial risk factor for premature mortality in the general population [13]. In a similar vein, the conicity index (CI), an index of abdominal obesity, has been considered useful for detecting central obesity, and has been studied as a predictor for alterations in fasting insulin, blood pressure, and triglyceride levels [14]. Lastly, in 2013, Thomas and colleagues [15] developed the body roundness index (BRI), which combines height and WC to predict the percentage of body fat. When compared with other anthropometric indices, BRI was optimal for identifying MetS, insulin resistance, inflammatory factors [16], and arterial stiffness [17] in obese and overweight populations. However, to date, few studies have evaluated the predictive ability of BRI, ABSI, or CI compared with traditional metrics, such as BMI and WtHR, with regard to CMRI in older adults [18–20].

South America has undergone a rapid epidemiologic transition, including a non-communicable disease epidemic [21] and adverse lifestyle changes that could contribute to increase a cluster of cardiometabolic risk factors such as MetS [4]. To the best of our knowledge, the predictive power of anthropometric measurements, which can be measured easily in a routine health exam, has not been assessed in elderly Latin-American individuals with high cardiovascular risk, for whom the early detection of risk factors is essential for prevention of CVD. This is particularly true in Colombia, where anthropometric index measurements and blood collection are not usually standard in the annual health exam, and, to date, there have been few studies conducted in the general older population.

For these reasons, the aim of the present study was to evaluate the prevalence of MetS using a CMRI among older adults from Colombia, and validate the associated anthropometric surrogate markers. We also compared the predictive ability of BRI, ABSI, CI, BMI, and WtHR to determine whether there is a single best CMRI predictor.

2. Materials and Methods

2.1. Study Design and Participants

The data for this secondary cross-sectional study was obtained from the 2015 Colombian Health, Well-Being and Aging Survey (SABE 2015, from the Spanish: SAlud, Bienestar and Envejecimiento, 2015), a multicenter project conducted from 2014 to 2015 by the Pan-American Health Organization and supported by the Epidemiological Office of the Ministry of Health and Social Protection of Colombia (https://www.minsalud.gov.co/). The survey is a cross-sectional tool for exploring and evaluating several aspects that intervene in the phenomenon of aging and old age in the Colombian population [19]. Details of the survey have been previously published [19]. SABE 2015 was a joint venture between the Ministry of Health and Social Protection and the Administrative Department of Science, Technology and Innovation in Colombia.

The sample was regionally representative and involved self-representation in large cities, with urban-rural stratification of the sample and stage selection in accordance with the municipal map available from the Ministry of Health and Social Protection, with the following hierarchy: municipalities, urban/rural segments, homes or sidewalks, homes, and people. The study included the Colombian population ≥60 years old, and the indicators were disaggregated by age range, sex, ethnicity, and socioeconomic level. To calculate the original sample size, the non-institutionalized Colombian population aged ≥60 years was considered, and the following parameters were used: minimum estimable proportion = 0.03, design effect = 1.2, and Relative Standard Error = 0.05 (1.2). The universe of study comprised 99% of the population residing in private homes in both urban and rural areas.

A total of 23,694 surveys were conducted across the country and 6365 total population segments were investigated in 246 municipalities. As Bogotá is the capital it was independently selected, with a total of 545 urban segments and one rural segment. The average number of adults per segment was 4.2. The estimation of means or proportions was conducted to a level of precision of up to 6% of the maximum expected error, at a level of national disaggregation only. The basic procedure for the population survey was a face-to-face interview using a structured questionnaire. The interviewers visited the selected homes, carrying the appropriate identification. At each home visited, the standardized process involved the following: identifying the participants, registering the demographic data, obtaining the signed informed consent, applying the established filters and selection criteria, obtaining a signed assent form when necessary, and completion of the questionnaire by the interviewer. A total of 1502 participants from 86 municipalities were included in this analysis.

The institutional review boards involved in developing the SABE 2015 study (the University of Caldas, ID protocol CBCS-021-14, and the University of Valle, ID protocol 09-014 and O11-015) reviewed and approved the study protocol. Written informed consent was obtained from each individual before inclusion and completion of the first examination. One of the authors (C.A.C.-G.) applied to the Ministry of Health and Social Protection of Colombia and obtained permission to use publicly available data for research and teaching purposes (permission and details available at https://www.minsalud.gov.co/). The study protocol for the secondary analysis was approved by the Human Subjects Committee at the Pontificia Universidad Javeriana (ID protocol 20/2017-2017/180, FM-CIE-0459-17) in accordance with the Declaration of Helsinki (World Medical Association) and Resolution 8430 from 1993, of the then Colombian Ministry of Health, on technical, scientific, and administrative standards for conducting research with humans.

2.2. Anthropometric Measurements

The research teams of the coordinating centers (Caldas and Valle universities, Colombia) trained the data collection staff to carry out the face-to-face interviews and physical measurements. Anthropometric measurements included height and body weight, which were measured using a portable stadiometer (SECA 213®, Hamburg, Germany) and an electronic scale (Kendall graduated platform scale), respectively. BMI was estimated in kg/m^2 from the measured body weight and height. WC was measured using inextensible anthropometric tape with the subjects standing erect and relaxed, with their arms at their sides and their feet positioned close together, parallel to the floor. WtHR was calculated as the ratio of WC (cm) to height (cm). The other anthropometric indexes (BRI, ABSI, and CI) were calculated using the following formulas: $BRI = 364.2 - 365.5 (1 - \pi^{-2} WC^2 (m) Height^{-2} (m))^{1/2}$ [15]; $ABSI = WC (m)/(BMI^{2/3}(kg/m^2)Height^{1/2} (m))$ [13]; $CI = 0.109^{-1} WC (m) (Weight (kg)/Height (m))^{-1/2}$ [22].

2.3. Serum Biochemical Examination

After an overnight fast, blood was collected in the morning. Blood samples were centrifuged for 10 min at 3000 rpm, 30 min after sampling. All samples were delivered to a single central laboratory (Dinamica Laboratories, Bogotá, Colombia) for analysis within 24 h. Serum fasting glucose, low-density lipoprotein cholesterol (LDL-C), high-density lipoprotein cholesterol (HDL-C), total cholesterol, and triglycerides (TG) were analyzed using enzymatic colorimetric methods (Olympus AU5200, Melville, NY, USA). Low-density lipoprotein cholesterol (LDL-C) was estimated using the Friedewald equation ((LDL-C) = (Total Cholesterol) − (HDL-C) − ((TG)/5)).

2.4. Blood Pressure Determination

We measured systolic (SBP) and diastolic (DBP) blood pressure levels using an automatic blood pressure monitor (OMRON HEM-705, Omron Healthcare Co., Ltd., Kyoto, Japan), following the recommendations of the American College of Cardiology Foundation/American Heart Association 2011 Expert Consensus Document on Hypertension in the Elderly [23]. Values were recorded after 5 min of rest in the sitting position and three consecutive measures were obtained, waiting for at least 30 s between readings. The average of the three values for each measurement were used in the analysis.

2.5. Diagnostic Criteria of Metabolic Syndrome

MetS was defined according to the most recent Joint Interim Statement of the IDF [6] by adopting the Ethnic Central and South American criteria for WC. Participants were classified as having MetS if they had at least three of following metabolic risk factors or components (MetS-components): abdominal obesity (WC ≥90 cm for Latin-American males and ≥80 cm for Latin-American females), elevated TG (fasting serum TG ≥150 mg/dL or taking medication for abnormal lipid levels), low HDL-C (fasting serum HDL-C <40 mg/dL in males and <50 mg/dL in females, or specific treatment for this lipid abnormality), elevated blood pressure (SBP ≥130 mmHg or DBP ≥85 mmHg or taking hypertension medication), or elevated fasting glucose (serum glucose level ≥100 mg/dL or taking diabetes medication).

2.6. Definition of Cardiometabolic Risk Index

We calculated the CMRI as a continuous score of the MetS risk factors. The CMRI was calculated using sex- and race-specific algorithms for the IDF criteria cut-off values, using the values of the participants' SBP and DBP, TG, HDL-C, fasting glucose, and WC. For each of these variables, a z-score was computed as the number of standard deviation (SD) units from the sample mean after normalization of the variables, that is, z-score = ((value − sample mean)/sample SD)). The HDL-C z-score was multiplied by −1 to indicate higher cardiovascular risk with increasing value. Individuals with a

CMRI ≥ 1 SD above the mean were identified as having increased cardiometabolic risk, and a lower CMRI (<1 SD) being indicative of a healthier risk profile.

2.7. Co-Variables

For lifestyle characteristics, personal habits regarding alcohol intake (participants were categorized as those who do not drink and those who drink less than one day per week, two to six days a week, or every day) and cigarette smoking (participants were categorized as those who do not smoke and those who have never-smoked, those who currently smoke or those who previously smoked) were recorded. A "proxy physical activity" report was conducted by the following questions: (i) "Have you regularly exercised, such as jogging or dancing, or performed rigorous physical activity at least three times a week for the past year?"; (ii) "do you walk at least three times a week between nine and 20 blocks (1.6 km) without resting?"; (iii) "do you walk at least three times a week eight blocks (0.5 km) without resting?". Participants were considered physically active if they responded affirmatively to two of the three questions [24].

Medical information including multimorbidity, as well as chronic conditions adapted from the original SABE study, was assessed by asking the participants if they had been medically diagnosed with hypertension, type 2 diabetes mellitus, chronic obstructive pulmonary disease, CVD (heart attack, angina), stroke, cancer, arthritis, osteoporosis, or sensory impairments (vision and hearing loss).

Race/ethnicity was self-reported and grouped into indigenous (people belonging to various indigenous groups such as Ika, Kankuamo, Emberá, Misak, Nasa, Wayuu, Awuá, and Mokane); black, "mulatto", or Afro-Colombian; white; and other (mestizo, gypsy, etc.).

Socioeconomic status was determined on a scale of one to six based on the housing stratum, with one representing the highest level of poverty and six the greatest wealth. This classification was developed by the National Government of Colombia and considers the physical characteristics of the dwellings as well as their surroundings. Classification into one of the six strata was taken to approximate the hierarchical socioeconomic differences from poverty to wealth.

2.8. Statistical Analysis

Descriptive analyses using the mean ± SD or standard error (SE) for the continuous variables, median and interquartile range for the skewed continuous variables, and the frequency distribution of the categorical variables were used to determine the characteristics of the sample. Data normality was examined using the Kolmogorov–Smirnoff test. Significant differences between men and women were analyzed using Student's t-test, Wilcoxon rank-sum test, or chi-square (χ^2) post-hoc test. To visualize the relationship between CMRI and anthropometric indices, Spearman and Pearson correlation and linear regression analysis were applied to the total sample and individual genders. The linear regression analysis was adjusted by age as a covariate.

The area under receiver operating characteristic (ROC) curves was calculated to evaluate the abilities of the anthropometric indices to predict high CMRI. Cut-off points were proposed after calculation of Youden's Index (sensitivity + specificity − 1) [25]. The DeLong et al. [26] non-parametric approach was used to compare the areas under the ROC curves. Since abdominal obesity is a component of CMRI, we conducted a multicollinearity test for the anthropometric indices that included WC (WtHR, CI, BRI, and ABSI), and the variance inflation factor (VIF) was calculated. Each cardiometabolic risk factor among BMI, WtHR, BRI, ABSI, and CI was determined using analysis of variance without any adjustment and then after adjusting (analysis of covariance, ANCOVA) for ethnicity, socio-economic status, smoking status, alcohol intake, physical activity "proxy", and medical conditions (i.e., presence or absence of osteoporosis, CVD, hypertension, type 2 diabetes, cancer, or respiratory diseases) as covariates, followed by Tukey's test. Collinearity was tested between all anthropometric indexes that included WC; a VFI > 10, was interpreted as high collinearity [27].

Statistical analyses were performed using SPSS v24.0 (IBM, Armonk, NY, USA) and JASP v0.9 (JASP Team, Amsterdam, The Netherlands). Statistical significance was defined as $p < 0.05$.

3. Results

3.1. Baseline Characteristics of the Participants

The participants' characteristics are summarized in Table 1. Of the 1502 older adults studied, 60.3% were women, and the mean age was 70 ± 7.6 years. The prevalence of smoking (9.7%), alcohol intake (12.7%), and a physical activity proxy (17.7%) was relatively low, but significantly higher in CMRI ≥ 1 SD than in CMRI < 1 SD (alcohol: 13.1% vs. 12.6%, $p < 0.001$). The means (SD or range interquartile) of the WtHR, BMI, BRI, ABSI, and CI in the overall sample were 0.59 (0.1), 27.3 (24–30) kg/m^2, 5.2 (4.1–6.3), 0.081 (0.078–0.085), and 22.2 (20.9–23.8), respectively. The overall prevalence of MetS was 58.7%. Significant differences were found between the high/low CMRI status groups for almost all characteristics, with the exception of height, LDL-C and HDL-C levels.

Table 1. Characteristics of study participants according to high (≥ 1 SD) and low (< 1 SD) cardiometabolic risk index (CMRI) status among Colombian older adults.

Characteristics	Total Sample (n = 1502)	High CMRI ≥ 1 SD (n = 397)	Low CMRI < 1 SD (n = 1105)	p-Value
Sex, n (%)				
Men	596 (39.7)	141 (23.7)	455 (76.3)	<0.001
Women	906 (60.3)	254 (28.0)	652 (72.0)	<0.001
Socioeconomic status				
1	456 (30.4)	121 (30.5)	335 (32.1)	<0.001
2	635 (42.3)	176 (44.3)	459 (41.5)	<0.001
3	375 (25.0)	98 (24.7)	277 (25.1)	<0.001
4	29 (1.9)	2 (0.5)	27 (2.4)	<0.001
>5	7 (0.5)	0 (0.0)	7 (0.6)	N.A
Ethnic group				
Indigenous	78 (5.2)	25 (6.3)	53 (4.8)	0.002
Black	119 (7.9)	28 (7.1)	91 (8.2)	<0.001
White	396 (26.4)	106 (26.7)	290 (26.2)	<0.001
Others	909 (60.5)	194 (48.9)	512 (46.3)	<0.001
Smoking status, n (%)				
Yes	145 (9.7)	29 (7.3)	116 (10.5)	<0.001
No	1357 (90.3)	368 (92.7)	989 (89.5)	<0.001
Alcohol intake, n (%)				
Yes	191 (12.7)	52 (13.1)	139 (12.6)	<0.001
No	1310 (87.2)	345 (86.9)	965 (87.3)	<0.001
Physical Activity "proxy", n (%)				
Physically active	266 (17.7)	70 (17.6)	196 (17.7)	0.980
Non-Physically active	1231 (82.0)	323 (81.4)	908 (82.2)	<0.001
Anthropometric measures/indices				
Height (m)	1.55 (1.49–1.62)	1.54 (1.49–1.62)	1.55 (1.49–1.62)	0.170
Weight (kg)	64 (57–72)	71 (63–79)	62 (55–69)	<0.001
Waist circumference (cm)	92 (85–100)	101 (93–107)	89 (83–97)	<0.001
Body mass index (kg/m^2)	27 (24–30)	29.7 (26.7–33)	26.1 (23.3–29)	<0.001
WtHR	0.59 (0.1)	0.64 (0.06)	0.57 (0.06)	<0.001
BRI	5.2 (4.1–6.3)	6.4 (5.3–7.7)	4.8 (3.9–5.9)	<0.001
ABSI (m$^{11/6} \cdot$ kg$^{-2/3}$)	0.081 (0.078–0.085)	0.083 (0.080–0.086)	0.081 (0.077–0.084)	<0.001
CI	22.2 (20.9–23.8)	21.1 (19.8–22.4)	22.6 (21.4–24.1)	<0.001
Metabolic syndrome components, n (%)				
Prevalence of MetS	811 (58.7)	308 (77.6)	503 (45.5)	<0.001
Abdominal obesity	1177 (78.4)	374 (94.2)	803 (72.7)	<0.001
Hypertension	790 (52.6)	304 (76.6)	486 (44.0)	<0.001
High levels of fasting glucose	465 (31.0)	220 (55.4)	245 (22.2)	<0.001
High levels of triglycerides	696 (46.3)	253 (63.7)	443 (40.1)	<0.001
Low levels of HDL-C	821 (54.7)	219 (55.2)	602 (54.5)	0.393

Table 1. em Cont.

Characteristics	Total Sample (n = 1502)	High CMRI ≥ 1 SD (n = 397)	Low CMRI < 1 SD (n = 1105)	p-Value
Cardiometabolic measurements				
SBP (mmHg)	130 (117–145)	142 (130–163)	126 (114–140)	**<0.001**
DBP (mmHg)	72 (65–79)	78 (72–86)	70 (64–77)	**<0.001**
MBP (mmHg)	92 (84–101)	100 (91–111)	89 (81–97)	**<0.001**
Total cholesterol (mg/dL)	193 (166–221)	202 (171–232)	190 (164–216)	**<0.001**
Triglycerides (mg/dL)	144 (105–192)	174 (134–252)	134 (101–180)	**<0.001**
LDL-C (mg/dL)	126 (102–149)	127 (103–152)	125 (102–147)	0.116
HDL-C (mg/dL)	43 (36–53)	43 (36–54)	44 (36–53)	0.740
Glucose (mg/dL)	94 (86–102)	102 (93–121)	91 (84–98)	**<0.001**
CMRI	−0.21 (−1.41–1.07)	2.00 (1.44–2.84)	−0.83 (−1.83–0.05)	**<0.001**
Self-report comorbid chronic diseases, n (%)				
Hypertension	826 (55.0)	249 (62.7)	577 (52.2)	**<0.001**
Diabetes	245 (16.3)	113 (28.5)	132 (11.9)	**<0.001**
Respiratory diseases	165 (11.0)	49 (12.3)	116 (10.5)	**<0.001**
Cardiovascular diseases	213 (14.2)	155 (39.0)	58 (5.2)	**<0.001**
Stroke	70 (4.7)	22 (5.5)	48 (4.3)	**<0.001**
Osteoporosis	184 (12.3)	66 (16.6)	118 (10.7)	**<0.001**
Cancer	80 (5.3)	56 (14.1)	24 (2.2)	**<0.001**
Hearing loss	360 (24.1)	89 (22.4)	271 (24.5)	**<0.001**
Vision loss	851 (56.7)	228 (57.4)	623 (56.4)	**<0.001**

Skewed continuous variables are reported as median and interquartile range (Q3-Q1), for non-skewed continuous variables mean values (standard deviations (SD)) are given, and categorical variables are reported as numbers and percentages in brackets. Significant between-sex differences (Student's t-test, Wilcoxon rank-sum test or χ2). BMI: body mass index; WtHR: waist-to-height ratio; BRI: body roundness index; ABSI: a body shape index; CI: conicity index; LDL-C: low-density lipoprotein cholesterol; HDL-C: high-density lipoprotein cholesterol; CMRI: cardiometabolic risk index. p-values marked in bold are significant.

3.2. Association between Surrogate Anthropometric Indices with CMRI

Linear regression analyses of surrogate anthropometric indices and CMRI on the total sample and also stratified by sex are shown in Figure 1. Overall, we found an acceptable-to-moderate positive correlation of CMRI with WtHR ($r = 0.52$, $p < 0.001$), ABSI ($r = 0.17$, $p < 0.001$), BMI ($r = 0.46$, $p < 0.001$), and BRI ($r = 0.52$, $p < 0.001$), whereas CI was negatively correlated with CMRI ($r = -0.42$, $p < 0.001$). When analyzing by sex, the decreasing order of the correlation coefficients in men was WtHR ($r = 0.50$, $p < 0.001$), BRI ($r = 0.50$, $p < 0.001$), BMI ($r = 0.49$, $p < 0.001$), CI ($r = -0.46$, $p < 0.001$), and ABSI ($r = 0.16$, $p < 0.001$), while in women the decreasing order of the correlation coefficients was WtHR ($r = 0.55$, $p < 0.001$), BRI ($r = 0.54$, $p < 0.001$), BMI ($r = 0.45$, $p < 0.01$), CI ($r = -0.44$, $p < 0.001$), and ABSI ($r = 0.22$, $p < 0.001$).

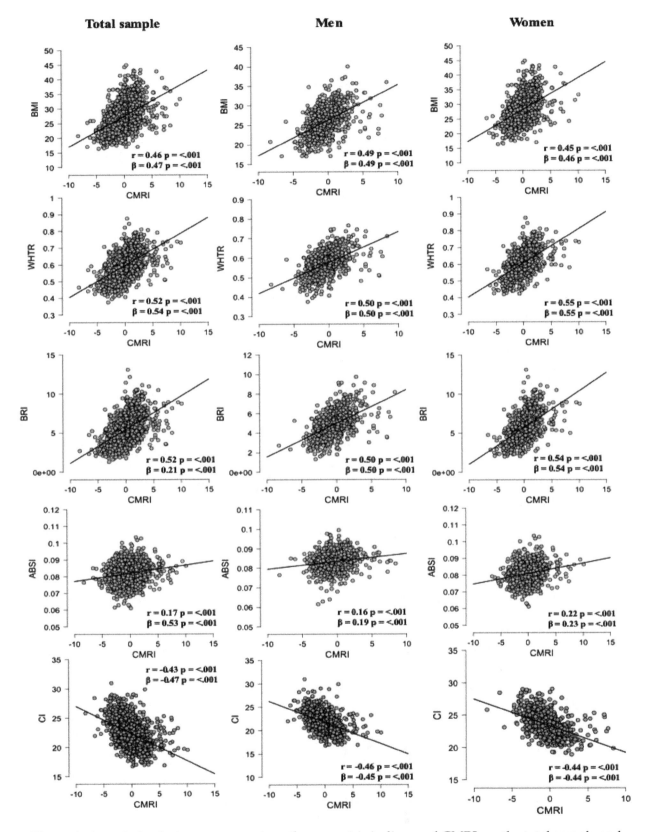

Figure 1. Association between surrogate anthropometric indices and CMRI, on the total sample and stratified by sex. BMI: body mass index; WtHR: waist to height ratio; BRI: body roundness index; ABSI: a body shape index; CI: conicity index; CMRI: cardiometabolic risk index.

3.3. Optimal Cut-Offs for Screening for CMRI by Sex

The ROC curve analyses of the diagnostic performance of BMI, WtHR, BRI, ABSI, and CI in identifying a high cardiometabolic risk are shown in Table 2 and Figure 2. In men, when considering the full sample, the best cut-off vales of BMI, WtHR, BRI, ABSI, and CI for detecting high cardiometabolic risk (CMRI ≥ 1 SD) were 25.2 (area under curve, AUC 0.76, sensitivity 84.4% and specificity 54.7%), 0.56 (AUC 0.77, sensitivity 83.6% and specificity 58.9%), 4.71 (AUC 0.77, sensitivity 83.6% and specificity 58.9%), 0.083 (AUC 0.60, sensitivity 69.5% and specificity 53.6%), and 22.9 (AUC 0.75, sensitivity 72.3% and specificity 65.9%), respectively. For women, the best cut-off values of BMI, WtHR, BRI, ABSI, and CI for detecting high cardiometabolic risk (CMRI ≥ 1 SD) were 28.4 (AUC 0.71, sensitivity 69.5% and specificity 64.1%), 0.63 (AUC 0.77, sensitivity 64.4% and specificity 76.7%), 6.20 (AUC 0.77, sensitivity 65.2% and specificity 76.1%), 0.080 (AUC 0.62, sensitivity 68.7% and specificity 51.6%), and 21.0 (AUC 0.71, sensitivity 63.6% and specificity 70.2%), respectively.

Table 2. Cut-off points, area under curve, sensitivity and specificity for BMI, WtHR, BRI, ABSI, and CI to detect high cardiometabolic risk (CMRI ≥ 1 SD) by sex.

Parameters	BMI		WtHR		BRI		ABSI		CI	
	Men	Women	Men	Women	Men	Women	Men	Women	Men	Women
Area under curve	0.76	0.71	0.77	0.77	0.77	0.77	0.60	0.62	0.75	0.71
p-value	<0.0001	<0.0001	<0.0001	<0.0001	<0.0001	<0.0001	<0.0001	<0.0001	<0.0001	<0.0001
Optimal cut-off	25.2	28.4	0.56	0.63	4.71	6.20	0.083	0.080	22.9	21.0
Youden index J	0.39	0.33	0.42	0.41	0.42	0.41	0.23	0.20	0.38	0.33
Sensitivity (%)	84.4	69.5	83.6	64.4	83.6	65.2	69.5	68.7	72.3	63.6
Specificity (%)	54.7	64.1	58.9	76.7	58.9	76.1	53.6	51.6	65.9	70.2
(+) Likelihood ratio	1.83	1.93	2.00	2.70	2.04	2.74	1.50	1.42	2.12	2.14
(−) Likelihood ratio	0.29	0.48	0.28	0.47	0.28	0.46	0.57	0.60	0.42	0.52

BMI: body mass index; WtHR: waist to height ratio; BRI: body roundness index; ABSI: a body shape index; CI: conicity index.

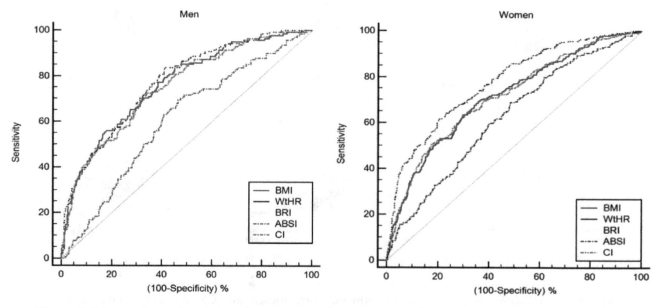

Figure 2. Diagnostic performance of surrogate anthropometric indices to detect high risk of CMRI by gender. BMI: body mass index; WtHR: waist-to-height ratio; BRI: body roundness index; ABSI: a body shape index; CI: conicity index.

The ROC curves were compared using a pairwise comparison method and the differences between the five methods are shown in Table 3. Independently of sex, the ROC-AUC of WtHR did not significantly differ from that of BRI. The results indicated that WtHR and BRI seem to provide the best results in Colombian older adults, owing to their greater precision in identifying subjects with a high cardiometabolic risk.

Table 3. Pairwise comparison for receiver operating characteristic (ROC) curves among Colombian older adults by sex.

Parameters	BMI–WtHR	BMI–BRI	BMI–ABSI	BMI–CI	WtHR–BRI	WtHR–ABSI	WtHR–CI	BRI–ABSI	BRI–CI	ABSI–CI
				Men						
Diff. AUC	0.000	0.00	0.15	0.01	0.00	0.16	0.01	0.16	0.02	0.14
SE	0.01	0.01	0.03	0.00	0.00	0.02	0.01	0.02	0.01	0.03
p-value	0.542	0.540	**0.001**	0.220	0.090	**0.001**	0.100	**0.001**	0.090	**0.001**
				Women						
Diff. AUC	0.06	0.06	0.08	0.00	0.00	0.15	0.06	0.15	0.06	0.08
SE	0.01	0.01	0.03	0.00	0.00	0.02	0.01	0.02	0.01	0.03
p-value	**0.001**	**0.001**	**0.001**	0.99	0.97	**0.001**	**0.001**	**0.001**	**0.001**	**0.001**

AUC: area under curve; SE: standard error; BMI: body mass index; WtHR: waist to height ratio; BRI: body roundness index; ABSI: a body shape index; CI: conicity index. P-values marked in bold are significant.

3.4. Sex Thresholds for Surrogate Anthropometric Indices to Screen for CMRI

Thresholds were determined for each of the surrogate anthropometric indices for the low/high CMRI in males and females, with corresponding differences in cardiometabolic parameters (Figure 2 and Table 4). In all groups (healthy/unhealthy) thresholds may be used to categorize individuals into one of two risk categories (i.e., low and high), on the combined basis of sex and surrogate anthropometric indices. In both sexes, after adjusting for ethnicity, socioeconomic status, smoking status, alcohol intake, physical activity proxy, and medical conditions (presence or absence of osteoporosis, CVD, hypertension, diabetes, cancer, and respiratory disease), the ANCOVA revealed that there were differences in blood pressure, HDL-C, and glucose in the BMI and CI parameters. By contrast, diagnostic performance results for CMRI without the central obesity component (i.e., WC) revealed lower accuracy (AUC) in all thresholds for surrogate anthropometric indices (Supplementary Material Table S1).

Finally, the collinearity test for all anthropometric indices that included WC in their calculation was found to be negative for BRI (VFI: 9.3), ABSI (VFI: 3.5), and WtHR (VFI: 9.1) and positive for CI (VFI: 10.9).

Table 4. Adjusted thresholds for surrogate anthropometric indices with cardiometabolic measurements among Colombian older adults by sex.

Variables	Cut-Off	BMI		WtHR		BRI		ABSI		CI	
		Mean (SE)	p-Value	Mean (SE)	p-Value	Mean (SE)	p-Value	Mean (SE)	p-Value	Mean (SE)	p-Value
Men											
SBP (mmHg)	healthy	130.1 (1.5)	**0.001**	131.7 (1.5)	0.107	131.5 (1.4)	**0.045**	134.7 (2.1)	0.477	131.3 (1.3)	0.005
	unhealthy	136.1 (1.3)		135.0 (1.3)		135.6 (1.4)		133.3 (1.1)		136.6 (1.5)	
DBP (mmHg)	healthy	72.3 (0.8)	**0.001**	73.8 (0.8)	0.250	73.7 (0.7)	0.131	76.1 (13.4)	0.176	73.1 (0.7)	**0.003**
	unhealthy	76.3 (0.7)		75.3 (0.7)		75.4 (0.7)		74.1 (0.6)		76.5 (0.8)	
MBP (mmHg)	healthy	91.5 (1.0)	**0.001**	93.1 (0.9)	0.148	92.9 (0.9)	0.064	95.5 (1.3)	0.282	92.4 (0.8)	**0.003**
	unhealthy	96.1 (0.8)		95.0 (0.8)		95.4 (0.9)		93.8 (0.7)		96.4 (0.9)	
Total cholesterol (mg/dL)	healthy	189.5 (2.0)	**0.011**	190.0 (2.5)	**0.010**	188.0 (2.4)	0.099	186.6 (3.5)	0.947	186.6 (2.2)	0.224
	unhealthy	181.8 (2.2)		181.2 (2.2)		182.4 (2.3)		184.7 (1.9)		183.1 (2.5)	
Triglycerides (mg/dL)	healthy	149.6 (5.7)	0.22	149.4 (5.6)	0.088	151.4 (5.3)	0.176	147.7 (7.8)	00.085	150.7 (4.9)	00.054
	unhealthy	162.7 (4.9)		163.2 (4.9)		162.5 (5.2)		160.0 (4.2)		165.4 (5.6)	
LDL-C (mg/dL)	healthy	123.5 (2.2)	0.055	123.7 (2.1)	0.058	122.5 (2.0)	0.211	119.8 (3.0)	0.511	121.3 (1.9)	0.467
	unhealthy	118.4 (1.8)		118.1 (1.9)		118.8 (1.9)		120.8 (1.6)		119.6 (2.1)	
HDL-C (mg/dL)	healthy	45.1 (0.7)	**0.001**	44.3 (0.7)	**0.001**	44.3 (12.4)	**0.001**	45.4 (1.0)	**0.001**	43.9 (0.6)	**0.001**
	unhealthy	39.5 (0.6)		39.6 (0.6)		39.3 (9.5)		40.8 (0.5)		39.2 (0.7)	
Glucose (mg/dL)	healthy	93.7 (1.5)	**0.005**	93.9 (1.5)	**0.009**	93.6 (1.4)	**0.002**	98.0 (2.1)	0.519	95.0 (1.3)	**0.028**
	unhealthy	99.1 (1.3)		99.0 (1.3)		99.8 (1.4)		96.4 (1.1)		99.0 (1.5)	
CMRI	healthy	-1.09 (0.1)	**0.001**	-1.05 (0.1)	**0.001**	-1.05 (0.1)	**0.001**	-0.66 (0.18)	**0.010**	-0.87 (0.11)	**0.001**
	unhealthy	0.36 (0.1)		0.36 (0.1)		0.50 (0.1)		-0.13 (0.09)		0.53 (0.12)	
Women											
SBP (mmHg)	healthy	130.4 (1.1)	0.530	130.6 (1.0)	0.942	130.6 (1.0)	0.935	129.8 (1.2)	0.639	130.4 (1.0)	0.537
	unhealthy	131.1 (1.1)		130.8 (1.3)		130.8 (1.3)		131.4 (1.0)		131.1 (1.2)	
DBP (mmHg)	healthy	70.9 (0.5)	**0.021**	71.6 (0.5)	0.458	71.6 (0.5)	0.414	72.0 (0.6)	0.993	71.1 (0.5)	**0.034**
	unhealthy	72.9 (10.5)		72.3 (0.6)		72.3 (0.6)		71.8 (0.5)		73.1 (0.6)	
MBP (mmHg)	healthy	90.6 (0.6)	0.097	91.2 (0.6)	0.721	91.2 (0.6)	0.691	91.2 (0.7)	0.823	90.8 (0.6)	0.139
	unhealthy	92.3 (0.7)		91.7 (0.8)		91.8 (0.8)		91.6 (0.6)		92.4 (0.7)	
Total cholesterol (mg/dL)	healthy	203.7 (1.9)	0.233	204.1 (1.8)	0.098	203.9 (1.8)	0.149	202.0 (2.1)	0.572	203.2 (1.8)	0.376
	unhealthy	200.4 (2.1)		198.8 (2.3)		199.0 (2.4)		202.2 (1.9)		200.5 (2.2)	
Triglycerides (mg/dL)	healthy	161.1 (4.0)	0.111	160.8 (3.7)	0.059	161.2 (3.7)	0.068	157.0 (4.4)	**0.044**	162.3 (3.8)	0.159
	unhealthy	170.8 (4.3)		173.5 (4.8)		173.4 (4.9)		172.4 (3.9)		170.7 (4.7)	
LDL-C (mg/dL)	healthy	132.3 (1.7)	0.258	132.6 (1.6)	0.164	132.5 (1.5)	0.132	132.0 (34.8)	0.812	132.0 (1.6)	0.381
	unhealthy	129.8 (1.8)		128.8 (2.0)		128.8 (2.1)		131.1 (37.4)		129.9 (2.0)	
HDL-C (mg/dL)	healthy	48.8 (0.6)	**0.009**	48.8 (0.5)	**0.001**	48.6 (0.5)	**0.007**	48.7 (13.9)	0.104	48.5 (0.5)	**0.018**
	unhealthy	46.1 (0.6)		45.4 (0.7)		45.6 (0.7)		46.9 (12.3)		46.1 (0.7)	
Glucose (mg/dL)	healthy	97.3 (1.1)	**0.016**	96.8 (1.0)	**0.001**	96.6 (1.0)	**0.001**	98.1 (1.2)	0.241	97.0 (1.0)	**0.002**
	unhealthy	101.2 (1.2)		102.9 (1.3)		103.5 (1.3)		99.9 (1.1)		102.3 (1.3)	
CMRI	healthy	-0.61 (0.09)	**0.001**	-0.57 (0.08)	**0.001**	-0.56 (0.08)	**0.001**	-0.32 (0.10)	**0.001**	-0.52 (0.08)	**0.001**
	unhealthy	0.82 (0.09)		1.09 (0.10)		1.16 (0.01)		0.36 (0.09)		0.94 (0.10)	

Data reported as mean and standard error (SE). BMI: body mass index; WtHR: waist-to-height ratio; BRI: body roundness index; ABSI: a body shape index; CI: conicity index; SBP: systolic blood pressure; DBP: diastolic blood pressure; MBP: mean blood pressure. p-value from ANCOVA analysis performed with ethnicity, socio-economic status, smoking status, alcohol intake, physical activity "proxy", and medical conditions (i.e., presence or absence of osteoporosis, cardiovascular diseases, hypertension, diabetes, cancer, or respiratory disease) as covariates. p-values marked in bold are significant.

4. Discussion

Metabolic abnormalities including elevated blood pressure, hypertriglyceridemia, low levels of HDL-C, impaired glucose tolerance and central obesity, have been proposed as cardiometabolic risk factors for CVD and all-cause mortality [28,29]. For this reason, identifying a screening tool for detecting high cardiometabolic risk in older adults is particularly important, as this might facilitate the early implementation of effective strategies to those at high risk. This study investigated multiple anthropometric measurements for predicting cardiometabolic risk in a large population of older Colombian adults. Firstly, we demonstrated that all the surrogate anthropometric indices including BMI, WtHR, BRI, ABSI, and CI significantly correlated with CMRI. Secondly, we showed that WtHR and BRI are the most accurate anthropometric indices for identifying adults at high cardiometabolic risk, supporting the hypothesis that these two indices could effectively predict cardiometabolic risk in the elderly Colombian population.

In the present study, conducted on a representative cohort of older adults, the overall prevalence of MetS was 58.7% according to IDF criteria. These findings differ slightly from the results of Davila et al., who showed that the prevalence of MetS among adults from Medellin (Colombia) aged 25–64 was 41% [30]. Furthermore, the Cardiovascular Risk Factor Multiple Evaluation in Latin America (CARMELA) study estimated a prevalence of 30.1% in men and 48.6% in women, respectively, in the 55–64 age group in Bogotá [31]. The differences in prevalence could be explained by either the MetS cluster used, since the CARMELA study defined MetS according to the National Cholesterol Education Program Adult Treatment Panel III, or the age range of the target populations (55–64 vs. ≥60). Nonetheless, there is a high prevalence of MetS in Latin American populations and, accordingly, there is growing interest in developing accurate tools for identifying subjects at high risk and defining cut-off points for anthropometric indices for detecting high CMRI.

BRI is a novel body index that has recently shown promise for clinical use [15]. We found that BRI has a moderate discriminating power for detecting high cardiometabolic risk in older Colombian adults, supporting the diagnostic potential of this new shape measure. We found that BRI performed better as a predictor of a high CMRI than BMI, the standard measure. Similarly, Tian et al. observed that BRI was suitable for use as a single anthropometric measure for identifying a cluster of cardiometabolic abnormalities, as compared with BMI and WtHR, using data from the 2009 wave of the China Health and Nutrition Survey [32]. Likewise, a recent study assessing the ability of BRI to predict the risk of MetS and its components in Peruvian adults concluded that BRI is a potentially useful clinical predictor of MetS that performs better than BMI [18]. BRI also showed potential for use as an alternative obesity measure in type 2 diabetes mellitus assessment among a rural population from northeastern China, although it performed similarly to BMI [33]. Additionally, Maessen et al. found that BRI could identify both the presence of CVD and cardiovascular risk factors in a population-based study in Nijmegen, the Netherlands, although the authors indicated that its capacity did not exceed that of BMI [19]. The heterogeneity of the population characteristics (ethnicity and age range) might explain the differences between these studies.

We demonstrated that WtHR is also an accurate screening tool for detecting a high cardiometabolic risk in older Colombian adults. Indeed, we found that WtHR was a better predictor of cardiometabolic risk than other anthropometric indices (BMI, CI, and ABSI). Wang et al. [34] also indicated that when evaluating cardiometabolic risk factors among non-obese adults, WtHR functioned as a simple but effective index for Chinese adults and, similarly, Amirabdollahian et al. [35] concluded that WtHR was the best predictor of cardiometabolic risk in a population of young adults from northwestern England. Comparable results were reported in a previous systematic review and meta-analysis involving 300,000 adults from several ethnic groups [36], showing the superiority of WtHR over BMI for detecting cardiometabolic risk factors in both sexes. However, it should be noted that the aforementioned studies did not compare WtHR with ABSI or BRI.

Interestingly, it should be noted that the greatest AUC values were observed for WtHR and BRI in men and women, suggesting that both body indices are capable of detecting a high cardiometabolic risk in the elderly. In addition, the AUC of WtHR did not differ significantly from that of BRI. This highlights the similar diagnostic capabilities of the two anthropometric indices. Furthermore, the AUC value of BRI for identifying metabolic risk factors was very close to that of WtHR in a Chinese population of adults [37]. In fact, Wang et al. concluded that although BRI does not exhibit a significantly better predictive ability than WtHR, it could be used as an alternative body index [34].

Our results showed that ABSI presented the lowest AUC for high cardiometabolic risk in men and women. These observations are consistent with previous studies [18–20,35,37,38]. Tian et al. reported that ABSI had the weakest discriminative power for identifying a cluster of cardiometabolic abnormalities [32]. Similarly, ABSI exhibited the lowest AUC value for identifying cardiometabolic risk factors compared with WtHR and BRI in Chinese adults [37], and a study involving an Iranian population also reported that ABSI was a weak predictor of CVD risk and MetS [38]. In the same line, Stefanescu et al. found that ABSI underperformed against other measures such as BMI and BRI for predicting MetS and its components [18], and Maessen et al. reported that ABSI was incapable of determining the presence of CVD in a Dutch population [19]. Thus, based on both our results and those of previous research, it can be concluded that ABSI does not seem to be a useful anthropometric index for predicting cardiometabolic risk.

The present study has some limitations and strengths that should be mentioned. Firstly, the cross-sectional design of the study meant that causality could not be inferred. Secondly, all of the study participants were of Latin-American ethnicity and resident in Colombia. This may therefore limit the generalizability of our results to other ethnic groups. Further studies involving other populations are therefore warranted. By contrast, the main strength of our study is that we provide gender-specific thresholds for various surrogate anthropometric indices (BMI, WtHR, BRI, ABSI, and CI) with cardiometabolic measurements among older Colombian adults. To our knowledge, no research has previously been published assessing the efficacy of these anthropometric indices for predicting a high CMRI in a Latin-American population. Lastly, the large sample size and the highly standardized procedures of the SABE project, which minimized measurement bias, were also major strengths of this study [39,40].

5. Conclusions

In conclusion, BRI and WtHR have a moderate discriminating power for determining a high cardiometabolic risk in a Colombian population of older adults, supporting the notion that both anthropometric indices should be considered as screening tools for the elderly. Both anthropometric indices were the most accurate among those tested for identifying men and women at a high cardiometabolic risk. In addition, we provide the first BMI, WtHR, BRI, ABSI, and CI thresholds for predicting a high CRMI in older Colombian adults. These data are clinically significant, as anthropometric index reference thresholds can be used to identify those adults who are at high cardiometabolic risk. Further investigation is required to provide reference values applicable to different populations.

Author Contributions: Data curation, R.R.-V., and M.Á.P.-S.; Formal analysis, R.R.-V., and M.Á.P.-S.; Investigation, R.R.-V., C.A.C.-G., J.S.-R., K.G.-R. and M.C.-R.; Methodology, R.R.-V., E.G.-J., J.S.-R., K.G.-R. and M.C.-R.; Project administration, C.A.C.-G.; Resources, C.A.C.-G. and K.G.-R; Supervision, C.A.C.-G. and E.G.-J.; Validation, M.I., K.G.-R. and M.C.-R.; Writing—original draft, R.R.-V., M.Á.P.-S., K.G.-R. and M.C.-R.; Writing—review and editing, R.R.-V., M.I., E.G.-J., J.S.-R. and M.C.-R.

Acknowledgments: We would like to thank the staff, scientists, and participants of the Colombian Health, Well-Being and Aging study (SABE, 2015) Survey for making this work possible.

References

1. Mente, A.; Yusuf, S.; Islam, S.; McQueen, M.J.; Tanomsup, S.; Onen, C.L.; Rangarajan, S.; Gerstein, H.C.; Anand, S.S. INTERHEART Investigators Metabolic Syndrome and Risk of Acute Myocardial Infarction. *J. Am. Coll. Cardiol.* **2010**, *55*, 2390–2398. [CrossRef] [PubMed]

2. Chien, K.-L.; Hsu, H.-C.; Sung, F.-C.; Su, T.-C.; Chen, M.-F.; Lee, Y.-T. Metabolic syndrome as a risk factor for coronary heart disease and stroke: An 11-year prospective cohort in Taiwan community. *Atherosclerosis* **2007**, *194*, 214–221. [CrossRef] [PubMed]

3. Boden-Albala, B.; Sacco, R.L.; Lee, H.-S.; Grahame-Clarke, C.; Rundek, T.; Elkind, M.V.; Wright, C.; Giardina, E.-G.V.; DiTullio, M.R.; Homma, S.; et al. Metabolic Syndrome and Ischemic Stroke Risk. *Stroke* **2008**, *39*, 30–35. [CrossRef] [PubMed]

4. Márquez-Sandoval, F.; Macedo-Ojeda, G.; Viramontes-Hörner, D.; Fernández Ballart, J.; Salas Salvadó, J.; Vizmanos, B. The prevalence of metabolic syndrome in Latin America: A systematic review. *Public Health Nutr.* **2011**, *14*, 1702–1713. [CrossRef] [PubMed]

5. DeBoer, M.D.; Gurka, M.J.; Woo, J.G.; Morrison, J.A. Severity of the metabolic syndrome as a predictor of type 2 diabetes between childhood and adulthood: The Princeton Lipid Research Cohort Study. *Diabetologia* **2015**, *58*, 2745–2752. [CrossRef] [PubMed]

6. Alberti, K.G.M.M.; Eckel, R.H.; Grundy, S.M.; Zimmet, P.Z.; Cleeman, J.I.; Donato, K.A.; Fruchart, J.-C.; James, W.P.T.; Loria, C.M.; Smith, S.C.; et al. Harmonizing the Metabolic Syndrome. *Circulation* **2009**, *120*, 1640–1645. [CrossRef] [PubMed]

7. Correa-Rodríguez, M.; Ramírez-Vélez, R.; Correa-Bautista, J.; Castellanos-Vega, R.; Arias-Coronel, F.; González-Ruíz, K.; Alejandro Carrillo, H.; Schmidt-RioValle, J.; González-Jiménez, E. Association of Muscular Fitness and Body Fatness with Cardiometabolic Risk Factors: The FUPRECOL Study. *Nutrients* **2018**, *10*, 1742. [CrossRef]

8. Ramírez-Vélez, R.; Correa-Bautista, J.; Carrillo, H.; González-Jiménez, E.; Schmidt-RioValle, J.; Correa-Rodríguez, M.; García-Hermoso, A.; González-Ruíz, K. Tri-Ponderal Mass Index vs. Fat Mass/Height3 as a Screening Tool for Metabolic Syndrome Prediction in Colombian Children and Young People. *Nutrients* **2018**, *10*, 412. [CrossRef]

9. Ramírez-Vélez, R.; Correa-Bautista, J.; González-Ruíz, K.; Tordecilla-Sanders, A.; García-Hermoso, A.; Schmidt-RioValle, J.; González-Jiménez, E. The Role of Body Adiposity Index in Determining Body Fat Percentage in Colombian Adults with Overweight or Obesity. *Int. J. Environ. Res. Public Health* **2017**, *14*, 1093. [CrossRef] [PubMed]

10. Knowles, K.M.; Paiva, L.L.; Sanchez, S.E.; Revilla, L.; Lopez, T.; Yasuda, M.B.; Yanez, N.D.; Gelaye, B.; Williams, M.A. Waist Circumference, Body Mass Index, and Other Measures of Adiposity in Predicting Cardiovascular Disease Risk Factors among Peruvian Adults. *Int. J. Hypertens.* **2011**, *2011*. [CrossRef]

11. Browning, L.M.; Hsieh, S.D.; Ashwell, M. A systematic review of waist-to-height ratio as a screening tool for the prediction of cardiovascular disease and diabetes: 0·5 could be a suitable global boundary value. *Nutr. Res. Rev.* **2010**, *23*, 247–269. [CrossRef] [PubMed]

12. Dobbelsteyn, C.; Joffres, M.; MacLean, D.; Flowerdew, G. A comparative evaluation of waist circumference, waist-to-hip ratio and body mass index as indicators of cardiovascular risk factors. The Canadian Heart Health Surveys. *Int. J. Obes.* **2001**, *25*, 652–661. [CrossRef] [PubMed]

13. Krakauer, N.Y.; Krakauer, J.C. A New Body Shape Index Predicts Mortality Hazard Independently of Body Mass Index. *PLoS ONE* **2012**, *7*, e39504. [CrossRef] [PubMed]

14. Mantzoros, C.; Evagelopoulou, K.; Georgiadis, E.; Katsilambros, N. Conicity Index as a Predictor of Blood Pressure Levels, Insulin and Triglyceride Concentrations of Healthy Premenopausal Women. *Horm. Metab. Res.* **1996**, *28*, 32–34. [CrossRef] [PubMed]

15. Thomas, D.M.; Bredlau, C.; Bosy-Westphal, A.; Mueller, M.; Shen, W.; Gallagher, D.; Maeda, Y.; McDougall, A.; Peterson, C.M.; Ravussin, E.; et al. Relationships between body roundness with body fat and visceral adipose tissue emerging from a new geometrical model. *Obesity* **2013**, *21*, 2264–2271. [CrossRef] [PubMed]

16. Li, G.; Wu, H.; Wu, X.; Cao, Z.; Tu, Y.; Ma, Y.; Li, B.; Peng, Q.; Cheng, J.; Wu, B.; et al. The feasibility of two anthropometric indices to identify metabolic syndrome, insulin resistance and inflammatory factors in obese and overweight adults. *Nutrition* **2019**, *57*, 194–201. [CrossRef] [PubMed]

17. Li, G.; Yao, T.; Wu, X.-W.; Cao, Z.; Tu, Y.-C.; Ma, Y.; Li, B.-N.; Peng, Q.-Y.; Wu, B.; Hou, J. Novel and traditional anthropometric indices for identifying arterial stiffness in overweight and obese adults. *Clin. Nutr.* **2019**. [CrossRef] [PubMed]

18. Stefanescu, A.; Revilla, L.; Lopez, T.; Sanchez, S.E.; Williams, M.A.; Gelaye, B. Using A Body Shape Index (ABSI) and Body Roundness Index (BRI) to predict risk of metabolic syndrome in Peruvian adults. *J. Int. Med. Res.* **2019**. [CrossRef]

19. Maessen, M.F.H.; Eijsvogels, T.M.H.; Verheggen, R.J.H.M.; Hopman, M.T.E.; Verbeek, A.L.M.; de Vegt, F. Entering a New Era of Body Indices: The Feasibility of a Body Shape Index and Body Roundness Index to Identify Cardiovascular Health Status. *PLoS ONE* **2014**, *9*, e107212. [CrossRef] [PubMed]

20. Krakauer, N.Y.; Krakauer, J.C. Untangling Waist Circumference and Hip Circumference from Body Mass Index with a Body Shape Index, Hip Index, and Anthropometric Risk Indicator. *Metab. Syndr. Relat. Disord.* **2018**, *16*, 160–165. [CrossRef] [PubMed]

21. Popkin, B.M.; Reardon, T. Obesity and the food system transformation in Latin America. *Obes. Rev.* **2018**, *19*, 1028–1064. [CrossRef] [PubMed]

22. Valdez, R. A simple model-based index of abdominal adiposity. *J. Clin. Epidemiol.* **1991**, *44*, 955–956. [CrossRef]

23. Aronow, W.S.; Banach, M. Ten most important things to learn from the ACCF/AHA 2011 expert consensus document on hypertension in the elderly. *Blood Press.* **2012**, *21*, 3–5. [CrossRef] [PubMed]

24. Ramírez-Vélez, R.; Correa-Bautista, J.E.; García-Hermoso, A.; Cano, C.A.; Izquierdo, M. Reference values for handgrip strength and their association with intrinsic capacity domains among older adults. *J. Cachexia Sarcopenia Muscle* **2019**, *10*, 278–286. [CrossRef] [PubMed]

25. Bewick, V.; Cheek, L.; Ball, J. Statistics review 13: Receiver operating characteristic curves. *Crit. Care* **2004**, *8*, 508–512. [CrossRef] [PubMed]

26. DeLong, E.R.; DeLong, D.M.; Clarke-Pearson, D.L. Comparing the areas under two or more correlated receiver operating characteristic curves: A nonparametric approach. *Biometrics* **1988**, *44*, 837–845. [CrossRef] [PubMed]

27. Kutner, M.H.; Nachtsheim, C.; Neter, J. *Applied Linear Regression Models*; McGraw-Hill/Irwin: New York, NY, USA, 2004; ISBN 0073014664.

28. Tune, J.D.; Goodwill, A.G.; Sassoon, D.J.; Mather, K.J. Cardiovascular consequences of metabolic syndrome. *Transl. Res.* **2017**, *183*, 57–70. [CrossRef] [PubMed]

29. Hamer, M.; Stamatakis, E. Metabolically healthy obesity and risk of all-cause and cardiovascular disease mortality. *J. Clin. Endocrinol. Metab.* **2012**, *97*, 2482–2488. [CrossRef]

30. Davila, E.P.; Quintero, M.A.; Orrego, M.L.; Ford, E.S.; Walke, H.; Arenas, M.M.; Pratt, M. Prevalence and risk factors for metabolic syndrome in Medellin and surrounding municipalities, Colombia, 2008–2010. *Prev. Med.* **2013**, *56*, 30–34. [CrossRef]

31. Escobedo, J.; Schargrodsky, H.; Champagne, B.; Silva, H.; Boissonnet, C.P.; Vinueza, R.; Torres, M.; Hernandez, R.; Wilson, E. Prevalence of the Metabolic Syndrome in Latin America and its association with sub-clinical carotid atherosclerosis: The CARMELA cross sectional study. *Cardiovasc. Diabetol.* **2009**, *8*, 52. [CrossRef]

32. Tian, S.; Zhang, X.; Xu, Y.; Dong, H. Feasibility of body roundness index for identifying a clustering of cardiometabolic abnormalities compared to BMI, waist circumference and other anthropometric indices: The China Health and Nutrition Survey, 2008 to 2009. *Medicine* **2016**, *95*, e4642. [CrossRef] [PubMed]

33. Chang, Y.; Guo, X.; Chen, Y.; Guo, L.; Li, Z.; Yu, S.; Yang, H.; Sun, Y. A body shape index and body roundness index: Two new body indices to identify diabetes mellitus among rural populations in northeast China. *BMC Public Health* **2015**, *15*, 794. [CrossRef] [PubMed]

34. Wang, H.; Liu, A.; Zhao, T.; Gong, X.; Pang, T.; Zhou, Y.; Xiao, Y.; Yan, Y.; Fan, C.; Teng, W.; et al. Comparison of anthropometric indices for predicting the risk of metabolic syndrome and its components in Chinese adults: A prospective, longitudinal study. *BMJ Open* **2017**, *7*, e016062. [CrossRef] [PubMed]

35. Amirabdollahian, F.; Haghighatdoost, F. Anthropometric Indicators of Adiposity Related to Body Weight and Body Shape as Cardiometabolic Risk Predictors in British Young Adults: Superiority of Waist-to-Height Ratio. *J. Obes.* **2018**, *2018*, 8370304. [CrossRef] [PubMed]

36. Ashwell, M.; Gunn, P.; Gibson, S. Waist-to-height ratio is a better screening tool than waist circumference and BMI for adult cardiometabolic risk factors: Systematic review and meta-analysis. *Obes. Rev.* **2012**, *13*, 275–286. [CrossRef] [PubMed]

37. Liu, P.J.; Ma, F.; Lou, H.P.; Zhu, Y.N. Comparison of the ability to identify cardiometabolic risk factors between two new body indices and waist-to-height ratio among Chinese adults with normal BMI and waist circumference. *Public Health Nutr.* **2017**, *20*, 984–991. [CrossRef] [PubMed]

38. Haghighatdoost, F.; Sarrafzadegan, N.; Mohammadifard, N.; Asgary, S.; Boshtam, M.; Azadbakht, L. Assessing body shape index as a risk predictor for cardiovascular diseases and metabolic syndrome among Iranian adults. *Nutrition* **2014**, *30*, 636–644. [CrossRef] [PubMed]

39. Perez-Sousa, M.A.; Venegas-Sanabria, L.C.; Chavarro-Carvajal, D.A.; Cano-Gutierrez, C.A.; Izquierdo, M.; Correa-Bautista, J.E.; Ramírez-Vélez, R. Gait speed as a mediator of the effect of sarcopenia on dependency in activities of daily living. *J. Cachexia Sarcopenia Muscle* **2019**. [CrossRef] [PubMed]

40. Gomez, F.; Corchuelo, J.; Curcio, C.L.; Calzada, M.T.; Mendez, F. SABE Colombia: Survey on Health, Well-Being, and Aging in Colombia-Study Design and Protocol. *Curr. Gerontol. Geriatr. Res.* **2016**, *2016*. [CrossRef]

7

Association of the Modified Mediterranean Diet Score (mMDS) with Anthropometric and Biochemical Indices in US Career Firefighters

Maria Romanidou [1,*], Grigorios Tripsianis [1], Maria Soledad Hershey [2],
Mercedes Sotos-Prieto [3,4,5], Costas Christophi [3,6], Steven Moffatt [7], Theodoros C. Constantinidis [8] and Stefanos N. Kales [3,9]

[1] Department of Medical Statistics, Medical Faculty, Democritus University of Thrace,
    68100 Alexandroupolis, Greece; gtryps@med.duth.gr
[2] Department of Preventive Medicine and Public Health, Navarra Institute for Health Research,
    University of Navarra, 31008 Pamplona, Spain; mhershey@alumni.unav.es
[3] Department of Environmental Health, T.H. Chan School of Public Health, Harvard University,
    Boston, MA 02215, USA; msotosp@hsph.harvard.edu or Mercedes.sotos@uam.es (M.S.-P.);
    costas.christophi@cut.ac.cy (C.C.); skales@hsph.harvard.edu (S.N.K.)
[4] Department of Preventive Medicine and Public Health, School of Medicine, Universidad Autónoma
    de Madrid, IdiPaz (Instituto de Investigación Sanitaria Hospital Universitario La Paz), Calle del Arzobispo
    Morcillo 4, 28029 Madrid, Spain
[5] Biomedical Research Network Centre of Epidemiology and Public Health (CIBERESP), Carlos III
    Health Institute, 28029 Madrid, Spain
[6] Cyprus International Institute for Environmental and Public Health, Cyprus University of Technology,
    30 Archbishop Kyprianou Str., Lemesos 3036, Cyprus
[7] National Institute for Public Safety Health, IN 324 E New York Street, Indianapolis, IN 46204, USA;
    steven.moffatt@ascension.org
[8] Laboratory of Hygiene and Environmental Protection, Medical School, Democritus University of Thrace,
    68100 Alexandroupolis, Greece; tconstan@med.duth.gr
[9] Occupational Medicine, Cambridge Health Alliance/Harvard Medical School, Cambridge, MA 02319, USA
*   Correspondence: mromanid@med.duth.gr

Abstract: The Mediterranean diet is associated with multiple health benefits, and the modified Mediterranean Diet Score (mMDS) has been previously validated as a measure of Mediterranean diet adherence. The aim of this study was to examine associations between the mMDS and anthropometric indices, blood pressure, and biochemical parameters in a sample of career firefighters. The participants were from Indiana Fire Departments, taking part in the "Feeding America's Bravest" study, a cluster-randomized controlled trial that aimed to assess the efficacy of a Mediterranean diet intervention. We measured Mediterranean diet adherence using the mMDS. Anthropometric, blood pressure, and biochemical measurements were also collected. Univariate and multivariate linear regression models were used. In unadjusted analyses, many expected favorable associations between the mMDS and cardiovascular disease risk factors were found among the 460 firefighters. After adjustment for age, gender, ethnicity, physical activity, and smoking, a unitary increase in the mMDS remained associated with a decrease of the total cholesterol/HDL ratio (β-coefficient −0.028, $p = 0.002$) and an increase of HDL-cholesterol (β-coefficient 0.254, $p = 0.004$). In conclusion, greater adherence to the Mediterranean diet was associated with markers of decreased cardiometabolic risk. The mMDS score is a valid instrument for measuring adherence to the Mediterranean diet and may have additional utility in research and clinical practice.

Keywords: Mediterranean diet; Mediterranean diet scores; anthropometrics; lipids; cardiometabolic risk

1. Introduction

Obesity, metabolic syndrome, and cardiovascular disease (CVD) have major impacts on US emergency responders, such as firefighters. These non-communicable, lifestyle-influenced conditions can put firefighters' career and life at risk [1–6]. The hazardous working environment, with risks of burns and physical trauma, air pollutants, physical and emotional stress, and shiftwork, causes additional stress to the cardiovascular system and may put firefighters at a higher cardiovascular disease risk with respect to the general population [7,8]. In fact, among US firefighters, sudden cardiac death is the leading cause of on-duty death, is, in most cases, due to underlying coronary heart disease and cardiomegaly, and is responsible for over 40% of duty-related deaths [9,10].

The number and proportion of CVD fatalities have remained relatively similar over the years, which suggests the need for more aggressive lifestyle-related interventions [11]. A recent study in older firefighters suggested that wellness programs can improve the cardiorespiratory function [12]. The eating and lifestyle patterns of firefighters often lead to obesity and have negative impacts on society by contributing to an increased rate of sick leave and increased healthcare expenses [13,14]. On the other hand, firefighters who follow a healthy lifestyle by exercising and maintaining a healthy weight are more likely to maintain high levels of cardiorespiratory fitness during aging [15].

The Mediterranean diet has been shown to reduce the risk of CVD and promote longevity in a variety of international settings [16–18]. There is also an increasing trend to introduce the Mediterranean diet at work as an intervention to prevent non-communicable diseases [19]. The existing evidence also suggests that adherence to the Mediterranean diet not only improves the physical health and wellbeing of workers but also may reduce work stress and blood pressure [20–22]. In two recent meta-analyses of Randomized Control Trials (RCT), the Mediterranean diet, also in combination with physical activity, was the only eating pattern which showed significant and beneficial effects on weight, body mass index (BMI) waist circumference, total cholesterol, high-density lipoprotein (HDL)-cholesterol, glucose, and blood pressure, without any evidence of adverse associations [23,24].

Various Mediterranean diet scores have been developed worldwide to quantify adherence to the Mediterranean diet [25–29]. In the ATTICA intervention in Greece, adherence was measured with the MedDietScore (0–55 items) [30,31], while the European Prospective Investigation into Cancer Nutrition (EPIC) group used the MED score (0–9 scale) [32,33]. Other adaptations include the Italian alternative Mediterranean diet score aMED (0–9 scale) [34] and the I-MEDAS from Israel (17-item questionnaire) [35]. The PREDIMED score, which is based on 14 items from the Prevención con Dieta Mediterránea in Spain, is also widely used [36,37]. However, the use of these scores in different populations, cultures, and ethnicities has been questioned, as they may not be directly adaptable to different ethnic and social groups [38].

In the US, a Mediterranean diet score was constructed specifically to measure adherence to the Mediterranean diet in career firefighters and is known as the modified Mediterranean Diet Score (mMDS) [39].

"Feeding America's Bravest" is a cluster-randomized-controlled trial that aimed to assess the efficacy of a Mediterranean Diet intervention in 60 fire stations in two Indiana (USA) Fire Departments [40]. To assess Mediterranean diet adherence, the aforementioned mMDS was used. Its validity versus previously validated questionnaires [41,42] was established using a sample of firefighters participating in "Feeding America's Bravest" [43]. The aim of the present study was to further corroborate the validity of the mMDS as a measure of Mediterranean diet adherence by examining its cross-sectional associations with anthropometric indices, blood pressure, and biochemical parameters in participants of the "Feeding America's Bravest" study.

2. Materials and Methods

2.1. Study Population

In this cross-sectional study, we used baseline nutrition surveys to calculate the mMDS from a total study base of 486 career firefighters (428 firefighters were recruited from the Indianapolis Fire Department's 44 stations and 58 from the Fishers, Indiana Fire Department's 6 stations) who consented to and enrolled in the ongoing study "Feeding America's Bravest": Mediterranean Diet-Based Interventions to change Firefighters' Eating Habits and Improve Cardiovascular Risk Profiles between 28 November 2016 and 16 April 2018 [34,39]. We excluded firefighters who did not complete baseline anthropometric measurements or if their biomarker indices were missing (Figure 1). Recruitment, consent, and study procedures were carried out by trained staff of the National Institute for Public Safety Health, who work regularly with both or the respective fire departments.

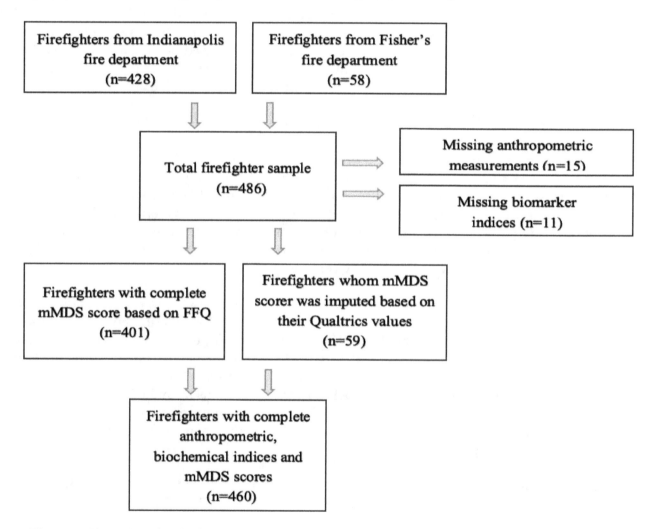

Figure 1. Flow chart for firefighters' sample selection. mMDS: modified Mediterranean Diet Score, FFQ: Food Frequency Questionnaire.

2.2. Dietary Assessment

A validated 131-item semi-quantitative Food Frequency Questionnaire (FFQ) [41] and the mMDS score [39] were used to quantify the firefighters' dietary intake patterns at baseline. The FFQ is a questionnaire previously developed by Yang et al. [39]. Two additional domains were added to the mMDS (nuts and legume consumption), and the score ranged between 0 = minimum adherence to the Mediterranean diet and 51 = maximum adherence to the Mediterranean diet. Because we had previously validated the mMDS in a Qualtrics survey with the Harvard FFQ [43] and more initial Indianapolis participants had complete FFQs, we calculated their mMDS score based on the FFQ and used a scaled value of the directly derived Qualtrics score for the Fishers firefighters who had not done an FFQ.

2.3. Physical Activity

Physical activity was calculated based on a 0–7 scale through a validated self-report scale (Self-Report of Physical Activity (SRPA)) embedded into our study questionnaire [44]. At baseline, the firefighters were asked to describe their physical activity levels over the past month using the following options: 0 = avoid walking or exertion (e.g., always use elevator, drive whenever possible instead of walking, biking, or rollerblading); 1 = walk for pleasure, routinely use stairs, occasionally exercise sufficiently to cause heavy breathing or perspiration; 2 = 10 to 60 min per week; 3 = over one hour per week; 4 = run less than 1 mile per week or spend less than 30 min per week in comparable physical activity; 5 = run 1 to 5 miles per week or spend 30 to 60 min per week in comparable physical activity; 6 = run 5 to 10 miles per week or spend 1 to 3 h per week in comparable physical activity; and 7 = run over 10 miles per week or spend over 3 h per week in comparable physical activity.

2.4. Outcome Assessments

At baseline recruitment, the participants underwent blood pressure and anthropometric assessments as part of the initial study visit. Resting blood pressure was measured using an appropriately sized cuff in seated position for each firefighter. BMI was recorded for all study subjects in kg/m² from measured height and weight. Body fat (%) was estimated by a Bioelectrical Impedance Analyzer (BIA) [40,45].

Separately, the firefighters had biochemical indices assessed at fire department-sponsored medical examinations. We used the biochemical measurements gathered at the closest date from the date of study consent within the same 12-month period. Blood samples were also collected after an overnight fast at baseline and at follow-up. Using EDTA collection tubes, up to 15 mL of blood was collected. Plasma and serum were aliquoted, frozen at −80 °C, stored, and run in batches. Automated high-throughput enzymatic analysis was used to determine the blood lipid profiles of the firefighters. This analysis achieved coefficients of variation ≤3% for cholesterol and ≤5% for triglycerides, using a cholesterol assay kit and reagents (Ref:7D62–21) and triglyceride assay kit and reagents (Ref:7D74–21) by the ARCHITECT c System, Abbott Laboratories, IL, USA. The lipid measures included total cholesterol, triglycerides, total cholesterol/HDL ratio, HDL-cholesterol, and low-density lipoprotein (LDL)-cholesterol.

2.5. Covariate Assessment

We collected sociodemographic characteristics, medical history, lifestyle habits, and dietary intake from the study's comprehensive lifestyle questionnaire [40].

2.6. Statistical Analysis

Statistical analysis was performed using IBM Statistical Package for the Social Sciences (SPSS), version 19.0 (IBM Corp., Armonk, NY, USA). The normality of the quantitative variables was tested with the Kolmogorov-Smirnov test. The quantitative variables were expressed as mean ± standard deviation (SD) or as median (Q1, Q3), as appropriate. The qualitative variables were expressed as absolute and relative (%) frequencies.

Multivariable linear regression models were used to examine the association of mMDS with anthropometric, blood pressure, and biochemical variables, after adjusting for age, gender, race, physical activity, and smoking. Beta coefficients were reported with the corresponding standard errors (SE) and p values. Component items of the mMDS were compared between firefighters with high and low values of biochemical parameters using the chi-square test.

All tests were two-tailed, and statistical significance was considered for p values < 0.05.

2.7. Ethics Statement

The overarching "Feeding America's Bravest" protocol was approved by the Harvard Institutional Review Board (IRB16-0170) ethics committee and is registered at Clinical Trials (NCT02941757). All participants provided signed informed consent for participation. The participants who met the criteria for enrollment in the intervention were all informed about their right to decline participation to the intervention or to withdraw at any time as per the Declaration of Helsinki, and the participants who decided to enroll gave full informed consent as per the protocol of the research [40].

3. Results

3.1. Sampling Procedure and Outcome

A sample of 460 firefighters from the two fire departments had complete data for analysis in the current study and represented 95% of all participants who consented to the parent clinical trial (Figure 1).

3.2. General Characteristics of the Firefighters

The majority of the firefighters were males (94.4%), with a mean age of 46.7 years (SD 8.3 years). Firefighters' personal characteristics are shown in Table 1. The mean mMDS in the study population was 21.88 (SD 6.68). The majority of the firefighters were overweight/obese, with an average body fat percentage of 28.10% (SD 6.55%).

Table 1. Characteristics of the participants.

Characteristic	N	
Male gender, n (%)	448	423 (94.4)
Age (years), mean (SD)	460	46.7 (8.3)
Race, n (%)	311	
Caucasian		266 (85.5)
African American		39 (12.5)
Other		6 (1.9)
Currently smoking, n (%)	314	15 (4.8)
Physical activity *, n (%)	307	
Low		39 (12.7)
Medium		65 (21.2)
High		203 (66.1)
Hours sitting per week, median (Q1–Q3)	300	15 (10–24)
Number of meals at the firehouse, median (Q1–Q3)	309	3 (2–3)
FFQ mMDS, mean (SD)	460	21.88 (6.68)
Anthropometric variables		
BMI (kg/m^2), mean (SD)	460	30.01 (4.39)
Normal weight	74	16%
Overweight	156	34%
Obese	230	50%
Waist circumference (cm), mean (SD)	459	99.7 (12.5)
Body fat percentage (%), mean (SD)	458	28.10 (6.55)
Blood pressure variables		
Resting SBP (mmHg), mean (SD)	460	125.5 (11.2)
Resting DBP (mmHg), mean (SD)	460	79.1 (6.8)

Table 1. *Cont.*

Characteristic	N	
Biochemical variables		
Total Cholesterol (mg/dL), mean (SD)	460	197.1 (37.7)
HDL-Cholesterol (mg/dL), mean (SD)	460	48.5 (11.4)
LDL-Cholesterol (mg/dL), mean (SD)	452	123.5 (32.6)
Total Cholesterol/HDL ratio, mean (SD)	460	4.26 (1.32)
Triglycerides (mg/dL), mean (SD)	459	126.0 (76.6)
Glucose (mg/dL), mean (SD)	460	99.5 (19.6)

* Physical activity. Low: did not participate regularly in programmed recreation, sport, or heavy physical activity. Medium: participated regularly in recreation requiring modest physical activity, such as golf, horseback riding, calisthenics, gymnastics, table tennis, bowling, weight-lifting, yard work. High: participated regularly in heavy physical exercise such as running or jogging, swimming, rowing, skipping rope, running in place, or engaging in vigorous aerobic activity such as tennis. basketball, or handball. FFQ: Food Frequency questionnaire, mMDS: modified Mediterranean Diet Score, SD: Standard Deviation, BMI: body mass index, SBP: systolic blood pressure, DBP: diastolic blood pressure, HDL: high-density lipoprotein, LDL: low-density lipoprotein.

3.3. Association of the Modified Mediterranean Diet Score with Anthropometric and Biochemical Indices

The association of mMDS with the participants' anthropometric measures, blood pressure, and biochemical variables is shown in Table 2. When the mMDS scores were categorized into quartiles, multivariate analysis adjusted for age and gender revealed statistically significant inverse associations of mMDS quartiles with BMI ($p = 0.030$), waist circumference ($p = 0.002$), body fat percentage ($p = 0.002$), and total cholesterol/HDL ratio ($p = 0.007$), whereas there was a positive association with HDL-cholesterol ($p = 0.002$).

Table 2. Association of the mMDS (categorized into quartiles) with anthropometric measures, blood pressure, and biochemical variables.

Risk Factor	mMDS				P Trend *	P Trend †	P Trend ‡
	1st Quartile	2nd Quartile	3rd Quartile	4th Quartile			
Number of subjects	106	122	118	114			
Anthropometric variables							
BMI (kg/m^2)	30.59 (4.06)	30.14 (4.82)	30.17 (4.70)	29.16 (3.77)	0.023	0.030	0.914
Waist circumference (cm)	102.0 (11.6)	100.6 (13.6)	99.3 (12.9)	96.8 (11.0)	0.001	0.002	0.685
Body fat percentage (%)	28.96 (5.64)	28.61 (6.38)	28.42 (7.06)	26.42 (6.75)	0.005	0.002	0.886
Blood pressure variables							
Resting SBP (mmHg)	125.7 (10.8)	124.7 (11.4)	126.6 (12.7)	125.1 (9.5)	0.980	0.836	0.515
Resting DBP (mmHg)	79.6 (7.2)	78.8 (6.7)	79.3 (6.3)	78.6 (7.1)	0.418	0.522	0.927
Biochemical variables							
Total Cholesterol (mg/dL)	200.2 (36.6)	193.1 (37.0)	198.2 (41.4)	197.5 (35.4)	0.894	0.876	0.742
HDL-Cholesterol (mg/dL)	45.6 (10.1)	48.6 (11.9)	48.7 (11.5)	50.9 (11.4)	0.001	0.002	0.022
LDL-Cholesterol (mg/dL)	127.3 (32.7)	119.5 (30.1)	124.4 (35.3)	123.6 (32.2)	0.703	0.690	0.587
Total Cholesterol/HDL ratio	4.60 (1.31)	4.19 (1.58)	4.27 (1.28)	4.03 (0.96)	0.004	0.007	0.020
Triglycerides (mg/dL)	140.8 (85.9)	118.4 (62.7)	129.2 (88.4)	116.9 (65.7)	0.071	0.107	0.364
Glucose (mg/dL)	99.9 (14.3)	100.9 (23.2)	98.6 (20.5)	98.6 (18.9)	0.450	0.594	0.770

* unadjusted; † adjusted for gender and age; ‡ adjusted for age, gender, race, physical activity, and smoking.

After further adjustment for subjects' ethnicity, physical activity, and smoking (Table 2), being in a higher mMDS quartile remained significantly inversely associated with the total cholesterol/HDL ratio ($p = 0.020$) and positively associated with HDL-cholesterol ($p = 0.022$).

3.4. Effects of a Unitary Increase in the Modified Mediteranean Score on Anthropometric Measures, Blood Pressure, and Biochemical Indices

The association of mMDS with subjects' anthropometric measures, blood pressure, and biochemical variables, as a continuous variable, was further analyzed using linear regression models (Table 3).

Table 3. Effect of a unitary increase in the mMDS on anthropometric measures, blood pressure, and biochemical variables.

| Risk Factor | Linear Regression Models | | | | | |
| | Adjusted by Gender and Age | | | Adjusted by Age, Gender, Race, Physical Activity, and Smoking | | |
	B Coefficient	SE	p Value	B Coefficient	SE	p Value
Anthropometric variables						
BMI (kg/m^2)	−0.080	0.030	0.008	−0.026	0.038	0.490
Waist circumference (in)	−0.114	0.031	<0.001	−0.045	0.039	0.241
Body fat percentage (%)	−0.141	0.043	0.001	−0.028	0.057	0.627
Blood pressure variables						
Resting SBP (mmHg)	−0.041	0.076	0.590	0.004	0.107	0.969
Resting DBP (mmHg)	−0.056	0.046	0.223	−0.037	0.062	0.552
Biochemical variables						
Total Cholesterol (mg/dL)	−0.160	0.264	0.546	−0.289	0.332	0.385
HDL Cholesterol (mg/dL)	0.254	0.075	<0.001	0.286	0.100	0.004
LDL Cholesterol (mg/dL)	−0.193	0.230	0.402	−0.341	0.300	0.256
Total cholesterol-HDL ratio	−0.028	0.009	0.002	−0.030	0.010	0.002
Triglycerides (mg/dL)	−1.010	0.532	0.058	−0.909	0.644	0.159
Glucose (mg/dL)	−0.137	0.135	0.313	−0.155	0.186	0.404

SD, standard deviation; B, unstandardized Beta coefficient; SE, standard error.

Multivariate linear regression analysis, adjusting for subjects' age and gender, revealed that a unitary increase in the mMDS was significantly inversely associated with BMI (β-coefficient −0.080, $p = 0.008$), waist circumference (β-coefficient −0.114, $p < 0.001$), body fat percentage (β-coefficient −0.141, $p = 0.001$), and total cholesterol/HDL ratio (β-coefficient −0.028, $p = 0.002$), whereas it was positively associated with HDL-cholesterol (β-coefficient 0.254, $p < 0.001$). After further adjustment for subjects' ethnicity, physical activity, and smoking, mMDS was significantly associated with a lower total cholesterol/HDL ratio (β-coefficient −0.030, $p = 0.002$), whereas there was a positive association of mMDS with HDL-cholesterol (β-coefficient 0.286, $p = 0.004$).

3.5. Effects of Single Components of the Modified Mediteranean Score on Anthropometric Measures, Blood Pressure, and Biochemical Indices

Examining component food items of the mMDS and total cholesterol/HDL ratio, total cholesterol-HDL ratio, and blood glucose, fast-food consumption was positively associated with a total cholesterol/HDL ratio >6 ($p = 0.003$) and with triglycerides levels ≥150 mg/dL ($p < 0.001$). Sweet desserts consumption was associated with a total cholesterol/HDL ratio >6 ($p = 0.004$) and with triglycerides levels ≥150 mg/dL ($p = 0.002$), while lower consumption of fruits and vegetables was associated with a total cholesterol/HDL ratio >6 ($p = 0.049$). Fried food consumption was associated with a total cholesterol/HDL ratio >6 ($p = 0.004$) and with triglycerides levels ≥150 mg/dL ($p = 0.037$), and consumption of non-alcoholic beverages at home was associated with glucose levels ≥100 mg/dL ($p = 0.036$). No other statistically significant associations were observed (Appendix A Table A1).

4. Discussion

Our study shows that greater adherence to a Mediterranean diet, as measured by higher mMDS, was favorably associated, as expected, with various anthropometric and biochemical parameters after adjustment by age and gender. After further adjustment for ethnicity, physical activity, and smoking, a higher mMDS remained associated with a lower total cholesterol/HDL ratio and increased HDL-cholesterol. These results are generally in agreement with those of our previous larger study in a different Midwest firefighter cohort of 780 career male firefighters. The study sample was representative, as the participants had similar demographics, anthropometrics, and dietary habits to those of their entire fire departments and other mid-Western firefighters [39]. In our former cross-sectional study, the results indicated that a higher mMDS was associated with HDL-cholesterol and with lower LDL-cholesterol when adjusted for age, BMI, and physical activity and that the firefighters who adhere the most to the Mediterranean diet had a 35% lower risk of prevalent metabolic syndrome [39]. Taken together, our findings are biologically plausible based on previous research and lend additional credibility and validity to the mMDS. The PREDIMED study also found similar results for the Mediterranean diet arms of the intervention, where a reduction of carbohydrates and the increase of monounsaturated dietary fatty acids (MUFA) resulted in lower cholesterol levels and increased HDL cholesterol levels [46]. Similar results were reported from another recent randomized control trial from Italy [47]. In summary, the present study is consistent with past research demonstrating that the Mediterranean diet has cardioprotective effects by improving HDL-cholesterol levels and the total cholesterol/HDL ratio [19,23,48].

Regarding anthropometrics, our results adjusted for age and gender were consistent with previous findings associating the Mediterranean diet with BMI, waist circumference, and weight loss [19,34,49–52]. However, we found no statistically significant associations, after further adjusting for ethnicity, physical activity, and smoking status. Similarly, several other scores such as the Mediterranean Diet Scale (MDScale), Mediterranean Food Pattern (MFP), MD Score (MDS), Short Mediterranean Diet Questionnaire (SMDQ), and MedDiet score were also not significantly associated with BMI [51,52]. The difference between our unadjusted and adjusted models may indicate an insufficient sample size in the current study.

In our study, there was no statistically significant association between the mMDS and glucose levels, consistent with previous research and the most recent RCT meta-analysis studies [23,24,53], although we did find that high consumption of non-alcoholic sugar-sweetened beverages at home was associated with higher glucose levels, as has been shown elsewhere [54,55]. Sweet desserts consumption was associated with a total cholesterol/HDL ratio >6 and with triglycerides levels ≥150 mg/dL. Firefighters with low fruit consumption were more likely to have a total cholesterol/HDL ratio >6. On average, the firefighters were consuming three servings of fruits and vegetables per day, in contrast with the recommendations of five or more daily servings of fruits and vegetables of the American Heart Association (AHA) [56]. Thus, our results highlight the need to increase the consumption of fruits and vegetables, because of their cardioprotective role, as an integral part of the Mediterranean diet [48,57,58]. In a recent study based on how the American population can adopt the Mediterranean diet, it was recommended that the American population should replace their usual desserts such us cookies, ice creams, pies, and sweet and creamy desserts with fresh fruits to optimize their health [59]. Increased fried food consumption was also associated with a total cholesterol/HDL ratio >6 and with triglycerides levels ≥150 mg/dL. It is well documented that the quality of fried food depends on the type of the oil used for frying [60]. Even though the scores for cooking with oils or fats at home and at work were not associated with any of the indices, these scores were below 4, indicating

The major limitation of this study is its cross-sectional nature, which does not allow us to infer causation. Another limitation of our study is that the firefighters were mainly men (94.4%). However, this reflects the current demographic of the US career fire service. Our study was also subject to a that the consumed fat or oils were mostly oils and spreads other than olive oil (e.g., margarine, corn or vegetable oil, and other spreads). Because at baseline the firefighters were unlikely to use olive oil for cooking, their olive oil consumption was reduced, and they were missing a basic component of the Mediterranean diet which is very important for its anti-inflammatory and antioxidant benefits [61–63]. degree of non-response bias, as the lifestyle questionnaires were completed online by firefighters and not during the face-to-face study visits.

One of our study's strengths is that the firefighters' anthropometrics included their body fat percentage and waist circumference, not only their BMI. In fact, BMI may cause some false positives due to the increased muscle mass of some firefighters [64]. Another strength is that all our data were collected using standardized procedures, which limits bias. Also, the mMDS was created so to cover the eating habits of the firefighters at work and at home for better accuracy [39]. Finally, one of the strengths of our study is that the previously validated instrument [43] we used to examine Mediterranean diet adherence was created for the American firefighters, based on their lifestyle, eating habits, nature of work (meals at home and at work), type of drinks, and alcohol consumption and therefore is a good-quality validated instrument for this population, as it is known that the quality of Mediterranean diet scores has been questioned in different populations [38].

5. Conclusions

In conclusion, greater adherence to a Mediterranean diet, as measured by a higher mMDS, was favorably associated with lower measures of cardiometabolic risk. In fully adjusted models including physical activity level and smoking, the associations of a higher mMDS with a lower total cholesterol/HDL ratio and increased HDL-cholesterol remained robust. The mMDS has now evidence of validity with respect to more established questionnaires and has been determined in relation to additional biologically plausible associations from two different and independent mid-western (US) firefighter cohorts. Therefore, the mMDS should be a valid tool for assessing the outcome of cluster-randomized controlled trials of Mediterranean lifestyle interventions in this population and similar ones. It may also have further utility not only in research but also in clinical practice.

Author Contributions: Conceptualization, M.R., G.T., T.C.C., and S.N.K.; methodology, M.R., M.S.H., M.S.-P., S.N.K., G.T., C.C., formal analysis, M.R. and G.T.; resources and analysis of the samples S.M., M.R., G.T.,M.S.-P.; data curation, G.T., C.C.; writing—original draft preparation, M.R.; writing—review and editing, M.R., M.S.-P., C.C., S.N.K., G.T., M.S.H., T.C.C.; supervision, S.N.K., G.T., T.C.C.; project administration, S.M. and S.N.K.; funding acquisition, S.N.K and M.S.-P. All authors contributed to the interpretation of data and critical revision of the manuscript and approved the final version. All authors have read and agreed to the published version of the manuscript.

Acknowledgments: We want to acknowledge the participation of the Indianapolis Fire Departments, the firefighters, and their spouses. We also thank Indiana Clinical and Translational Science Institute for the help with sample processing, Kroger Company (coupons and customer loyalty discounts), Barilla America (Barilla Plus Products), Arianna Trading Company, Innoliva and Molino de Zafra, Spain (extra virgin olive oil samples and discounts), and the Almond Board of California (free samples of roasted unsalted almonds). The sponsors have had no involvement in the overall study design; collection, analysis and interpretation of data; writing of the report; or the decision to submit the report for publication.

Appendix A

Table A1. Comparison of the single items of the modified Mediterranean diet scores (mMDS) according to biochemical indices.

	Total Cholesterol-HDL Ratio > 6					Triglycerides ≥ 150 mg/dL					Glucose ≥ 100 mg/dL				
	No (N = 374)		Yes (N = 27)		p Value	No (N = 300)		Yes (N = 100)		p Value	No (N = 243)		Yes (N = 158)		p Value
	Mean	SD	Mean	SD		Mean	SD	Mean	SD		Mean	SD	Mean	SD	
Total mMDS	22.23	6.80	18.19	6.63	0.003	22.47	6.80	20.44	6.86	0.010	22.12	6.67	21.70	7.15	0.549
Single item mMDS															
Fast food consumption *	1.57	0.95	1.00	0.83	0.003	1.66	0.93	1.14	0.92	<.001	1.51	0.97	1.56	0.93	0.634
Fruit consumption	1.57	0.90	1.22	0.70	0.049	1.58	0.91	1.44	0.82	0.163	1.58	0.94	1.49	0.80	0.270
Vegetable consumption	2.56	1.06	2.44	0.93	0.586	2.53	1.05	2.63	1.08	0.396	2.56	1.07	2.54	1.03	0.841
Sweet desserts consumption	1.85	1.57	0.96	1.22	0.004	1.93	1.57	1.37	1.50	0.002	1.76	1.57	1.84	1.56	0.625
Cooking oil or fat use at home	2.12	1.85	1.63	1.74	0.185	2.12	1.86	1.99	1.84	0.554	2.22	1.83	1.88	1.86	0.073
Fried food consumption	1.56	1.18	0.89	0.93	0.004	1.58	1.19	1.30	1.10	0.037	1.47	1.18	1.58	1.17	0.374
Breads or starches consumed at home	1.75	1.48	1.67	1.52	0.782	1.82	1.47	1.50	1.51	0.062	1.73	1.49	1.77	1.48	0.805
Ocean fish consumption	1.64	1.14	1.70	0.99	0.765	1.67	1.13	1.57	1.12	0.459	1.66	1.07	1.61	1.21	0.700
Non-alcoholic beverages at home	2.66	1.13	2.44	1.37	0.339	2.69	1.14	2.50	1.17	0.144	2.74	1.12	2.50	1.18	0.036
Alcoholic beverages	2.09	1.57	1.78	1.48	0.317	2.02	1.60	2.24	1.44	0.224	2.03	1.59	2.13	1.54	0.516
Wine consumption	0.81	0.98	0.89	1.01	0.679	0.81	0.98	0.82	0.99	0.953	0.83	0.99	0.78	0.98	0.645
Legumes consumption	0.67	1.26	0.74	1.29	0.791	0.66	1.26	0.74	1.29	0.585	0.71	1.29	0.63	1.23	0.510
Nuts consumption	1.39	1.62	0.81	1.44	0.073	1.40	1.62	1.20	1.61	0.277	1.32	1.59	1.41	1.66	0.612

* Fast-food consumption per week (score 0–4), i.e., frequency of choosing options such as McDonalds, Burger King, Kentucky Fried Chicken, etc.

References

1. Soares, E.M.K.V.K.; Smith, D.; Porto, L.G.G. Worldwide prevalence of obesity among firefighters: A systematic review protocol. *BMJ Open* **2020**, *10*, e031282. [CrossRef] [PubMed]
2. Tsismenakis, A.J.; Christophi, C.A.; Burress, J.W.; Kinney, A.M.; Kim, M.; Kales, S.N. The obesity epidemic and future emergency responders. *Obesity* **2009**, *17*, 1648–1650. [CrossRef] [PubMed]
3. Lavie, C.J.; Milani, R.V.; Ventura, H.O. Obesity and cardiovascular disease. risk factor, paradox, and impact of weight loss. *J. Am. Coll. Cardiol.* **2009**, *53*, 1925–1932. [CrossRef] [PubMed]
4. Dunlay, S.M.; Givertz, M.M.; Aguilar, D.; Allen, L.A.; Chan, M.; Desai, A.S.; Deswal, A.; Dickson, V.V.; Kosiborod, M.N.; Lekavich, C.L.; et al. Type 2 diabetes mellitus and heart failure, a scientific statement from the American Heart Association and Heart Failure Society of America. *J. Card. Fail.* **2019**, *25*, 584–619. [CrossRef] [PubMed]
5. Donovan, R.; Nelson, T.; Peel, J.; Lipsey, T.; Voyles, W.; Israel, R.G. Cardiorespiratory fitness and the metabolic syndrome in firefighters. *Occup. Med.* **2009**, *59*, 487–492. [CrossRef]
6. Soteriades, E.S.; Hauser, R.; Kawachi, I.; Liarokapis, D.; Christiani, D.C.; Kales, S.N. Obesity and cardiovascular disease risk factors in firefighters: A prospective cohort study. *Obes. Res.* **2005**, *13*, 1756–1763. [CrossRef]
7. Navarro, K.M.; Kleinman, M.T.; Mackay, C.E.; Reinhardt, T.E.; Balmes, J.R.; Broyles, G.A.; Ottmar, R.D.; Naher, L.P.; Domitrovich, J.W. Wildland firefighter smoke exposure and risk of lung cancer and cardiovascular disease mortality. *Environ. Res.* **2019**, *173*, 462–468. [CrossRef]
8. Kales, S.; Smith, D.L. Firefighting and the heart. *Circulation* **2017**, *135*, 1296–1299. [CrossRef]
9. Smith, D.L.; Haller, J.M.; Korre, M.; Fehling, P.C.; Sampani, K.; Porto, L.G.G.; Christophi, C.A.; Kales, S.N. Pathoanatomic findings associated with duty-related cardiac death in US firefighters: A case-control study. *J. Am. Heart Assoc.* **2018**, *7*, e009446. [CrossRef]
10. Smith, D.L.; Haller, J.M.; Korre, M.; Sampani, K.; Porto, L.G.G.; Fehling, P.C.; Christophi, C.A.; Kales, S.N. The relation of emergency duties to cardiac death among US firefighters. *Am. J. Cardiol.* **2019**, *123*, 736–741. [CrossRef]
11. Kahn, S.A.; Leonard, C.; Siordia, C. Firefighter fatalities: Crude mortality rates and risk factors for line of duty injury and death. *J. Burn Care Res.* **2018**, *40*, 196–201. [CrossRef] [PubMed]
12. Gao, X.; Deming, N.J.; Moore, K.; Alam, T. Cardiorespiratory fitness decline in aging firefighters. *Am. J. Public Health* **2020**, *110*, E1. [CrossRef] [PubMed]
13. Neovius, M.; Kark, M.; Rasmussen, F. Association between obesity status in young adulthood and disability pension. *Int. J. Obes.* **2008**, *32*, 1319–1326. [CrossRef] [PubMed]
14. Linde, J.A.; Andrade, K.; MacLehose, R.F.; Mitchell, N.R.; Harnack, L.; Cousins, J.M.; Graham, D.J.; Jeffery, R.W. HealthWorks: Results of a multi-component group-randomized worksite environmental intervention trial for weight gain prevention. *Int. J. Behav. Nutr. Phys. Act.* **2012**, *9*, 14. [CrossRef]
15. Baur, D.M.; Christophi, C.A.; Cook, E.F.; Kales, S. Age-Related decline in cardiorespiratory fitness among career firefighters: Modification by physical activity and adiposity. *J. Obes.* **2012**, *2012*, 1–6. [CrossRef]
16. Eleftheriou, D.; Benetou, V.; Trichopoulou, A.; La Vecchia, C.; Bamia, C. Mediterranean diet and its components in relation to all-cause mortality: Meta-analysis. *Br. J. Nutr.* **2018**, *120*, 1081–1097. [CrossRef]
17. Barbagallo, M.; Barbagallo, M. Mediterranean diet and longevity. *Eur. J. Cancer Prev.* **2004**, *13*, 453–456. [CrossRef]
18. Bo, S.; Ponzo, V.; Goitre, I.; Fadda, M.; Pezzana, A.; Beccuti, G.; Gambino, R.; Cassader, M.; Soldati, L.; Broglio, F. Predictive role of the Mediterranean diet on mortality in individuals at low cardiovascular risk: A 12-year follow-up population-based cohort study. *J. Transl. Med.* **2016**, *14*, 91. [CrossRef]
19. Korre, M.; Tsoukas, M.A.; Frantzeskou, E.; Yang, J.; Kales, S. Mediterranean diet and workplace health promotion. *Curr. Cardiovasc. Risk Rep.* **2014**, *8*, 1–7. [CrossRef]
20. Nissensohn, M.; Román-Viñas, B.; Sánchez-Villegas, A.; Piscopo, S.; Serra-Majem, L. The Effect of the Mediterranean diet on hypertension: A systematic review and meta-analysis. *J. Nutr. Educ. Behav.* **2016**, *48*, 42–53.e1. [CrossRef]
21. Korre, M.; Sotos-Prieto, M.; Kales, S. Survival Mediterranean style: Lifestyle changes to improve the health of the US fire service. *Front. Public Health* **2017**, *5*, 7–13. [CrossRef]

22. Benhammou, S.; Heras-González, L.; Ibáñez-Peinado, D.; Barceló, C.; Hamdan, M.; Rivas, A.; Mariscal-Arcas, M.; Olea-Serrano, F.; Monteagudo, C. Comparison of Mediterranean diet compliance between European and non-European populations in the Mediterranean basin. *Appetite* **2016**, *107*, 521–526. [CrossRef] [PubMed]

23. Dinu, M.; Pagliai, G.; Casini, A.; Sofi, F. Mediterranean diet and multiple health outcomes: An umbrella review of meta-analyses of observational studies and randomised trials. *Eur. J. Clin. Nutr.* **2018**, *72*, 30–43. [CrossRef]

24. Malakou, E.; Linardakis, M.; Armstrong, M.E.; Zannidi, D.; Foster, C.; Johnson, L.; Papadaki, A. The combined effect of promoting the Mediterranean diet and physical activity on metabolic risk factors in adults: A systematic review and meta-analysis of randomised controlled trials. *Nutrients* **2018**, *10*, 1577. [CrossRef] [PubMed]

25. Sotos-Prieto, M.; Moreno-Franco, B.; Ordovás, J.M.; León, M.; Casasnovas, J.A.; Peñalvo, J.L. Design and development of an instrument to measure overall lifestyle habits for epidemiological research: The Mediterranean Lifestyle (MEDLIFE) index. *Public Health Nutr.* **2015**, *18*, 959–967. [CrossRef] [PubMed]

26. Della Corte, C.; Mosca, A.; Vania, A.; Alterio, A.; Iasevoli, S.; Nobili, V. Good adherence to the Mediterranean diet reduces the risk for NASH and diabetes in pediatric patients with obesity: The results of an Italian Study. *Nutrition* **2017**, *39–40*, 8–14. [CrossRef] [PubMed]

27. Serra-Majem, L.; Román-Viñas, B.; Sanchez-Villegas, A.; Guasch-Ferré, M.; Corella, D.; La Vecchia, C. Benefits of the Mediterranean diet: Epidemiological and molecular aspects. *Mol. Asp. Med.* **2019**, *67*, 1–55. [CrossRef]

28. Foscolou, A.; Magriplis, E.; Tyrovolas, S.; Soulis, G.; Bountziouka, V.; Mariolis, A.; Piscopo, S.; Valacchi, G.; Anastasiou, F.; Gotsis, E.; et al. Lifestyle determinants of healthy ageing in a Mediterranean population: The multinational MEDIS study. *Exp. Gerontol.* **2018**, *110*, 35–41. [CrossRef]

29. Izadi, V.; Tehrani, H.; Haghighatdoost, F.; Dehghan, A.; Surkan, P.J.; Azadbakht, L. Adherence to the DASH and Mediterranean diets is associated with decreased risk for gestational diabetes mellitus. *Nutrition* **2016**, *32*, 1092–1096. [CrossRef]

30. Panagiotakos, D.B.; Georgousopoulou, E.N.; Pitsavos, C.; Chrysohoou, C.; Metaxa, V.; Georgiopoulos, G.; Kalogeropoulou, K.; Tousoulis, D.; Stefanadis, C. Ten-Year (2002–2012) cardiovascular disease incidence and all-cause mortality, in urban Greek population: The ATTICA Study. *Int. J. Cardiol.* **2015**, *180*, 178–184. [CrossRef]

31. Panagiotakos, D.B.; Pitsavos, C.; Stefanadis, C. Dietary patterns: A Mediterranean diet score and its relation to clinical and biological markers of cardiovascular disease risk. *Nutr. Metab. Cardiovasc. Dis.* **2006**, *16*, 559–568. [CrossRef] [PubMed]

32. Trichopoulos, D. Adherence to a Mediterranean diet and survival in a Greek population. *N. Engl. J. Med.* **2003**, 2599–2608. [CrossRef] [PubMed]

33. Naska, A.; Trichopoulou, A. Back to the future: The Mediterranean diet paradigm. *Nutr. Metab. Cardiovasc. Dis.* **2014**, *24*, 216–219. [CrossRef] [PubMed]

34. Gnagnarella, P.; Dragà, D.; Misotti, A.M.; Sieri, S.; Spaggiari, L.; Cassano, E.; Baldini, F.; Soldati, L.; Maisonneuve, P. Validation of a short questionnaire to record adherence to the Mediterranean diet: An Italian experience. *Nutr. Metab. Cardiovasc. Dis.* **2018**, *28*, 1140–1147. [CrossRef] [PubMed]

35. Abu-Saad, K.; Endevelt, R.; Goldsmith, R.; Shimony, T.; Nitsan, L.; Shahar, D.R.; Keinan-Boker, L.; Ziv, A.; Kalter-Leibovici, O. Adaptation and predictive utility of a Mediterranean diet screener score. *Clin. Nutr.* **2019**, *38*, 2928–2935. [CrossRef] [PubMed]

36. Guasch-Ferré, M.; Salas-Salvadó, J.; Ros, E.; Estruch, R.; Corella, D.; Fitó, M.; Martinez-Gonzalez, M.; Arós Borau, F.; Gómez-Gracia, E.; Fiol, M.; et al. The PREDIMED trial, Mediterranean diet and health outcomes: How strong is the evidence? *Nutr. Metab. Cardiovasc. Dis.* **2017**, *27*, 624–632. [CrossRef]

37. Martínez-González, M.Á.; García-Arellano, A.; Toledo, E.; Salas-Salvadó, J.; Buil-Cosiales, P.; Corella, D.; Covas, M.I.; Schröder, H.; Arós, F.; Gómez-Gracia, E.; et al. A 14-Item Mediterranean diet assessment tool and obesity indexes among high-risk subjects: The PREDIMED Trial. *PLoS ONE* **2012**, *7*, e43134. [CrossRef]

38. Zaragoza-Martí, A.; Cabañero-Martínez, M.J.; Hurtado-Sánchez, J.A.; Laguna-Pérez, A.; Ferrer-Cascales, R. Evaluation of Mediterranean diet adherence scores: A systematic review. *BMJ Open* **2018**, *8*, 1–8. [CrossRef]

39. Yang, J.; Farioli, A.; Korre, M.; Kales, S.N. Modified Mediterranean Diet score and cardiovascular risk in a north American working population. *PLoS ONE* **2014**, *9*, e87539. [CrossRef]

40. Sotos-Prieto, M.; Cash, S.B.; Christophi, C.; Folta, S.C.; Moffatt, S.; Muegge, C.M.; Korre, M.; Mozaffarian, D.; Kales, S.N. Rationale and design of feeding America's bravest: Mediterranean diet-based intervention to change firefighters' eating habits and improve cardiovascular risk profiles. *Contemp. Clin. Trials* **2017**, *61*, 101–107. [CrossRef]

41. Willett, W.C.; Sampson, L.; Stampfer, M.J.; Rosner, B.; Bain, C.; Witschi, J.; Hennekens, C.H.; Speizer, F.E. Reproducibility and validity of a semiquantitative food frequency questionnaire. *Am. J. Epidemiol.* **1985**, *122*, 51–65. [CrossRef] [PubMed]

42. Salvini, S.; Hunter, D.J.; Sampson, L.; Stampfer, M.J.; Colditz, G.A.; Rosner, B.; Willett, W.C. Food-Based validation of a dietary questionnaire: The effects of week-to-week variation in food consumption. *Int. J. Epidemiol.* **1989**, *18*, 858–867. [CrossRef] [PubMed]

43. Sotos-Prieto, M.; Christophi, C.; Black, A.; Furtado, J.D.; Song, Y.; Magiatis, P.; Papakonstantinou, A.; Melliou, E.; Moffatt, S.; Kales, S.N. Assessing validity of self-reported dietary intake within a Mediterranean diet cluster randomized controlled trial among US firefighters. *Nutrients* **2019**, *11*, 2250. [CrossRef]

44. Jackson, A.S.; Blair, S.N.; Mahar, M.T.; Wier, L.T.; Ross, R.M.; Stuteville, J.E. Prediction of functional aerobic capacity without exercise testing. *Med. Sci. Sports Exerc.* **1990**, *22*, 863–870. [CrossRef] [PubMed]

45. Hershey, M.S.; Sotos-Prieto, M.; Ruiz-Canela, M.; Martínez-González, M.Á.; Cassidy, A.; Moffatt, S.; Kales, S. Anthocyanin intake and physical activity: Associations with the lipid profile of a US working population. *Molecules* **2020**, *25*, 4398. [CrossRef] [PubMed]

46. Estruch, R. Anti-Inflammatory effects of the Mediterranean diet: The experience of the PREDIMED study. *Proc. Nutr. Soc.* **2010**, *69*, 333–340. [CrossRef] [PubMed]

47. Amato, M.; Bonomi, A.; Laguzzi, F.; Veglia, F.; Tremoli, E.; Werba, J.P.; Giroli, M.G. Overall dietary variety and adherence to the Mediterranean diet show additive protective effects against coronary heart disease. *Nutr. Metab. Cardiovasc. Dis.* **2020**, *30*, 1315–1321. [CrossRef]

48. Merino, J.; Kones, R.; Ros, E. Effects of Mediterranean diet on endothelial function. In *Endothelium and Cardiovascular Diseases*; Academic Press: Cambridge, MA, USA, 2018; pp. 363–389.

49. Romaguera, D.; Norat, T.; Mouw, T.; May, A.M.; Bamia, C.; Slimani, N.; Travier, N.; Besson, H.; Luan, J.; Wareham, N.; et al. Adherence to the Mediterranean Diet is associated with lower abdominal adiposity in European men and women. *J. Nutr.* **2009**, *139*, 1728–1737. [CrossRef]

50. Mattei, J.; Sotos-Prieto, M.; Bigornia, S.J.; Noel, S.E.; Tucker, K.L. The Mediterranean diet score is more strongly associated with favorable cardiometabolic risk factors over 2 years than other diet quality indexes in puerto rican adults. *J. Nutr.* **2017**, *147*, 661–669. [CrossRef]

51. Aoun, C.; Papazian, T.; Helou, K.; El Osta, N.; Khabbaz, L.R. Comparison of five international indices of adherence to the Mediterranean diet among healthy adults: Similarities and differences. *Nutr. Res. Pract.* **2019**, *13*, 333–343. [CrossRef]

52. Trichopoulou, A.; Naska, A.; Orfanos, P.; Trichopoulos, D. Mediterranean diet in relation to body mass index and waist-to-hip ratio: The Greek European prospective investigation into cancer and nutrition study. *Am. J. Clin. Nutr.* **2005**, *82*, 935–940. [CrossRef] [PubMed]

53. Estruch, R.; Martínez-González, M.A.; Corella, D.; Salas-Salvadó, J.; Ruiz-Gutiérrez, V.; Covas, M.I.; Fiol, M.; Gómez-Gracia, E.; López-Sabater, M.C.; Vinyoles, E.; et al. Effects of a Mediterranean-style diet on cardiovascular risk factors a randomized trial. *Ann. Intern. Med.* **2006**, *145*, 1–11. [CrossRef] [PubMed]

54. Estruch, R.; Ros, E.; Salas-Salvadó, J.; Covas, M.-I.; Corella, D.; Arós, F.; Gómez-Gracia, E.; Ruiz-Gutiérrez, V.; Fiol, M.; Lapetra, J.; et al. Primary prevention of cardiovascular disease with a Mediterranean diet. *N. Engl. J. Med.* **2013**, *368*, 1279–1290. [CrossRef] [PubMed]

55. Sahingoz, S.A.; Sanlier, N. Compliance with Mediterranean Diet Quality Index (KIDMED) and nutrition knowledge levels in adolescents. A case study from Turkey. *Appetite* **2011**, *57*, 272–277. [CrossRef] [PubMed]

56. Krauss, R.M.; Eckel, R.H.; Howard, B.; Appel, L.J.; Daniels, S.R.; Deckelbaum, R.J.; Erdman, J.W.; Kris-Etherton, P.; Goldberg, I.J.; Kotchen, T.A.; et al. AHA Dietary Guidelines: Revision 2000: A statement for healthcare professionals from the Nutrition Committee of the American Heart Association. *Circulation* **2000**, *102*, 2284–2299. [CrossRef]

57. Willett, W.C. The Mediterranean diet: Science and practice. *Public Health Nutr.* **2006**, *9*, 105–110. [CrossRef]

58. Mozaffarian, D. Dietary and policy priorities for cardiovascular disease, diabetes, and obesity. *Circulation* **2016**, *133*, 187–225. [CrossRef]

59. Martínez-González, M.A.; Hershey, M.S.; Zazpe, I.; Trichopoulou, A. Transferability of the Mediterranean diet to non-mediterranean countries. What is and what is not the Mediterranean diet. *Nutrients* **2017**, *9*, 1226. [CrossRef]

60. Soriguer, F.; Rojo-Martínez, G.; Dobarganes, M.C.; Almeida, J.M.G.; Esteva, I.; Beltrán, M.; De Adana, M.S.R.; Tinahones, F.; Gómez-Zumaquero, J.M.; García-Fuentes, E.; et al. Hypertension is related to the degradation of dietary frying oils. *Am. J. Clin. Nutr.* **2003**, *78*, 1092–1097. [CrossRef]

61. Godos, J.; Rapisarda, G.; Marventano, S.; Galvano, F.; Mistretta, A.; Grosso, G. Association between polyphenol intake and adherence to the Mediterranean diet in Sicily, southern Italy. *NFS J.* **2017**, *8*, 1–7. [CrossRef]

62. Pérez-Martínez, P.; Mikhailidis, D.P.; Athyros, V.G.; Bullo, M.; Couture, P.; Covas, M.I.; De Koning, L.; Delgado-Lista, J.; Díaz-López, A.; Drevon, C.A.; et al. Lifestyle recommendations for the prevention and management of metabolic syndrome: An international panel recommendation. *Nutr. Rev.* **2017**, *75*, 307–326. [CrossRef] [PubMed]

63. Morin, S.J.; Gaziano, J.M.; Djoussé, L. Relation between plasma phospholipid oleic acid and risk of heart failure. *Eur. J. Nutr.* **2017**, *57*, 2937–2942. [CrossRef] [PubMed]

64. Gurevich, K.; Poston, W.S.C.; Anders, B.; Ivkina, M.A.; Archangelskaya, A.; Jitnarin, N.; Starodubov, V.I. Obesity prevalence and accuracy of BMI-defined obesity in Russian firefighters. *Occup. Med.* **2016**, *67*, 61–63. [CrossRef] [PubMed]

8

Ethnicity and Metabolic Syndrome: Implications for Assessment, Management and Prevention

Scott A. Lear [1,2,*] and Danijela Gasevic [3,4]

[1]   Faculty of Health Sciences, Simon Fraser University, Burnaby, BC V5A 1S6, Canada
[2]   Division of Cardiology, Providence Health Care, Vancouver, BC V6Z 1Y6, Canada
[3]   School of Public Health and Preventive Medicine, Monash University, Melbourne, VIC 3004, Australia;
      danijela.gasevic@monash.edu
[4]   Usher Institute, University of Edinburgh, Edinburgh EH8 9AG, UK
[*]   Correspondence: slear@providencehealth.bc.ca

Abstract: The metabolic syndrome (MetS) is a constellation of cardiometabolic risk factors that identifies people at increased risk for type 2 diabetes and cardiovascular disease. While the global prevalence is 20%–25% of the adult population, the prevalence varies across different racial/ethnic populations. In this narrative review, evidence is reviewed regarding the assessment, management and prevention of MetS among people of different racial/ethnic groups. The most popular definition of MetS considers race/ethnicity for assessing waist circumference given differences in visceral adipose tissue and cardiometabolic risk. However, defining race/ethnicity may pose challenges in the clinical setting. Despite 80% of the world's population being of non-European descent, the majority of research on management and prevention has focused on European-derived populations. In these studies, lifestyle management has proven an effective therapy for reversal of MetS, and randomised studies are underway in specific racial/ethnic groups. Given the large number of people at risk for MetS, prevention efforts need to focus at community and population levels. Community-based interventions have begun to show promise, and efforts to improve lifestyle behaviours through alterations in the built environment may be another avenue. However, careful consideration needs to be given to take into account the unique cultural context of the target race/ethnic group.

Keywords: metabolic syndrome; ethnicity; prevention; lifestyle; cardiometabolic

1. Introduction

The metabolic syndrome (MetS) is a constellation of cardiometabolic risk factors that results in an increased risk for type 2 diabetes (T2D), cardiovascular disease and premature mortality [1]. At its foundation is insulin resistance, in which the actions of insulin decrease, resulting in hyperinsulinemia. Left unchecked, insulin resistance can progress to MetS and prediabetes, and further to T2D. MetS is defined as the presence of at least three of the following five common clinical measures, which occur in people with insulin resistance: elevated triglycerides (TG), low high-density lipoprotein cholesterol (HDL-C), elevated blood sugar, elevated blood pressure (BP) and elevated waist circumference (WC) (Table 1, Table 2) [2].Within primary care and other front-line care environments, the MetS is a simple tool with which to identify people with insulin resistance and prediabetes, and therefore, at early risk for T2D and cardiovascular disease. As a result, it provides an opportune time for primary care providers to intervene and prevent progression to overt disease.

Table 1. Criteria of the metabolic syndrome defined as three of more of the five measures.

Measure	Threshold
Elevated triglycerides	≥1.70 mmol/L *
Reduced HDL-C	≤1.00 mmol/L (males) * ≤1.30 mmol/L (females) *
Elevated blood pressure	Systolic ≥ 130 mmHg and/or Diastolic ≥ 85 mmHg *
Elevated fasting glucose	≥5.6 mmol/L *
Elevated waist circumference	See population-specific thresholds in Table 2

* Or appropriate drug treatment. HDL-C = high-density lipoprotein cholesterol.

Table 2. Population-specific waist circumference thresholds [2].

Population	Men	Women
Central/South American, Chinese, Japanese, South Asian	≥90 cm	≥80 cm
Mediterranean, Middle East, Sub-Saharan African	≥94 cm	≥80 cm
Europid (includes Canada, Europe and United States) *	≥102 cm (≥94 cm)	≥88 cm (≥88 cm)

* While thresholds of ≥94 cm for men and ≥80 cm for women are more common in research, the thresholds of ≥102 for men and ≥88 for women are used more commonly in clinical practice.

Despite the ease of assessment, the worldwide prevalence of MetS is not known [3,4], in part due to MetS not being a common clinical indicator, such as T2D, and thus not widely assessed. Further complicating estimates is the variation in definitions used in countries before, and even since [5], the MetS definition was harmonised in 2009 [2]. However, estimates suggest the worldwide prevalence of MetS to be 20%–25% of the population, based on a presumed prevalence threefold higher than T2D [4]. As the prevalence of obesity and T2D is expected to rise, so too is the prevalence of MetS. In countries where prevalence data do exist, it is clear that it differs by country. For example, the estimated prevalence of MetS in the United States is 33.4% [6], while in China, it is 14.4% [7].

The difference in MetS prevalence across countries is likely the result of different governmental, institutional and sociocultural factors at the population level, which can affect a range of upstream determinants including, but not limited to, the type of available foods and access, health care policies, education, employment and the physical environment. This is in addition to individual factors such as biology/genetics and sociocultural aspects, which are also likely relevant to the different prevalence of MetS between countries. These latter aspects may be collectively referred to as ethnic or racial differences, as many of these characteristics often cluster in specific and identifiable populations. Even within the same country, in the same local environment, the prevalence of MetS differs along certain predefined racial/ethnic groups. For example, in the United States, the prevalence of MetS is highest in Hispanics and lowest in African-Americans, with the prevalence of MetS in whites in between the two [8]. (It is important to recognise that the term "white" does not describe an ethnicity or ethnic group. The use of the term "white" in this article is only used when the authors of the original article that has been cited have used this term to describe one of their study populations without providing additional information on that group's ethnic origins.) While recent national level data in Canada have not been reported, an earlier study reported MetS to be highest in people of Indigenous ancestry, followed by South Asians, Europeans and East Asians [9]. In Singapore, MetS is highest in South Asians, followed by Malays and then people of Chinese background [10]. Understanding the influence race/ethnicity has with respect to MetS is important for its proper assessment, treatment and prevention.

Ethnicity and race are fluid constructs that have no clear-cut definition, which are often (and incorrectly) used interchangeably. Despite these challenges, ethnicity and race are still used in medical literature as a means to differentiate between populations and recognise such differences in health management and disease prevention. Furthernore, ethnic and racial groupings often differ across the medical literature based on the research purpose, methods of data collection and even the lens of the researchers themselves. While individuals may ascribe their ethnicity within sociocultural aspects, medical guidelines such as those for the MetS attempt to define ethnicity primarily on common biomedical (whether biological or genetic) and/or geographical aspects. These are generally broad classifications, which often group multiple ethnic and racial groups into one. Sometimes this is based exclusively on geographical origins (for example, "Asian" or "European") without recognising the ethnic or racial heterogeneity within these groupings and thus incorrectly inferring that the populations are homogeneous. While some biomedical characteristics align with certain ethnic and racial groups, this should not be interpreted that ethnicity and race are biomedical constructs, nor should ethnic and racial classifications be interpreted to reflect genetic variation.

It should also be noted that ethnicity and race are not the same. Race infers some biological foundations for differences among groups, while ethnicity views populations from a more social/cultural lens. However, these terms may be used in medical literature as if they are the same. Across the many papers cited in this review, some authors grouped study participants into categories they termed "race", while others used groupings termed "ethnicity", commonly without defining the terms or the categories. This lack of consistency makes it challenging to compare and contrast across the various studies. As a result, for the sake of this review, the terms are combined (albeit not ideally) into one called "race/ethnicity", and when citing research, we have used the same race/ethnicity group names as the original authors.

2. Assessment

Of the five cardiometabolic risk factors, four of the definition thresholds apply to all race/ethnic groups. The fifth, WC, entails different threshold values based on race/ethnic background (Table 2). These differing thresholds are based on evidence that the association between WC, an indicator of abdominal obesity, and risk of cardiometabolic diseases differs by race/ethnicity. For example, at a similar WC, people of Chinese and South Asian background have higher values of total cholesterol and other cardiometabolic risk factors compared with people of European background [11–13]. If the goal is to identify people at the same level of cardiometabolic risk, lower WC thresholds for people of Asian background were created.

The requirement for lower WC thresholds in some racial/ethnic groups has its foundation in the differences in visceral adipose tissue (VAT). In particular, people of Asian backgrounds (South Asian, East Asian, Southeast Asian) have higher amounts of VAT at a given body size and WC [14]. For South Asians, this higher amount of VAT accounts for much of their elevated cardiometabolic risk compared with European-derived populations [15]. In African-Americans, VAT tends to be lower than whites at a similar body size [16]. Despite a higher prevalence of obesity and T2D [17,18], levels of VAT in North American Indigenous populations appear to be similar to that of Europeans of the same size [14,19].

While the use of race/ethnic-specific WC thresholds is reflective of the differing risk in different racial/ethnic groups, it can pose a challenge during assessment of MetS. This is reflected in the above biological foundations for having different WC thresholds for MetS. It must be acknowledged that the MetS uses a broad definition of race/ethnicity and population grouping based on geographical location, which does not reflect the many varying races and ethnicities within those groupings. There is even limited agreement in how race/ethnicity is defined [20]; however, it is probably best defined by self-report, meaning, each individual is likely to provide the most "accurate" identification of their own race/ethnicity.

In predominantly homogeneous populations found in many parts of Asia, the use of race/ethnic-specific WC thresholds should not pose a challenge [21]. However, in diverse populations such as in Europe and the Americas, determining the race/ethnicity of a patient can be challenging [22]. While self-identification may be the best indicator of race/ethnicity, this may be a conversation in which health care professionals may feel uncomfortable engaging. In addition, people who descend from a different geographical or race/ethnic region from where they currently live may identify more with the local context than their ancestral one. This may result in a conflict between how an individual identifies his/herself and how race/ethnicity is defined in the health system. In many locations, people may also identify with more than one race/ethnicity. Guessing on the part of the health care professional may be no better. The increasingly common prevalence of offspring from mixed ethnic partnerships can further complicate the matter [23], as there are no studies on how to apply the race/ethnic-specific WC thresholds to these individuals.

3. Treatment

As MetS allows for the presence of overt risk factors such as hypercholesterolemia, hypertension and T2D, when present, these should be treated as per local clinical guidelines. For patients with MetS but without overt risk factors, treatment through lifestyle therapy is effective at reversing MetS. In the Diabetes Prevention Program (55% white, 20% African-American, 16% Hispanic, 5% Native American and 4% Asian in the original trial [24], no analysis by race/ethnicity), the combined intervention of physical activity and diet resulted in a more than twofold reversal of the MetS compared with the placebo group and a 65% greater reversal rate than the metformin group [25]. A subsequent meta-analysis of combined physical activity and diet interventions found a twofold greater rate of MetS reversal compared with control interventions [26].

In isolation, regular aerobic physical activity of low-to-moderate intensity has resulted in reversal of the MetS in postmenopausal women (65% white, 30% African-American and 6% other in original trial [27], no analysis by race/ethnicity) [28] and reduction in MetS severity in a workplace setting using a wrist-worn activity monitor and smartphone app designed to enhance physical activity (conducted in Germany, race/ethnicity not reported) [29]. In addition to aerobic exercise interventions, a 12-week resistance training program was effective in reversing MetS in older women (race/ethnicity not reported) [30]. However, aerobic physical activity alone in men and women (56% white, 44% African-American) or a combination of aerobic and resistance physical activity may be superior to resistance training alone [31]. A randomised trial in Norwegian men and women focused on differing intensities of exercise on reversing the MetS is currently underway [32].

A secondary analysis in the PREDIMED randomised trial of participants with the MetS (approximately 97% European) at the study's onset reported the Mediterranean diet resulted in an approximately 28%–35% reversal of MetS compared with the control diet [33]. However, due to later concerns with the PREDIMED methods [34] and republication with a smaller sample attesting to similar conclusions [35], the exact effect of the intervention may not be accurately reflected in this analysis.

Despite more than 80% of the world's population being of non-European descent, the overwhelming majority of research on MetS is limited by the predominant focus on European-derived populations and a lack of race/ethnic-specific analyses. In terms of the benefits of interventions aimed at reducing or reversing MetS in other race/ethnic groups, few studies exist. Short-term diet studies have reported reversal of MetS in Iranians [36], South Asians [37] and people of Asian descent living in the United States [38]. A combined lifestyle intervention in Arabs living in Saudi Arabia reported a greater reduction in MetS compared with the group receiving general advice [39]. One randomised trial currently underway is investigating a combined lifestyle intervention of physical activity, nutrition improvement and weight loss in a diverse population in the United Kingdom [40], while another exercise-focused trial in African-American women with MetS is also in progress [41].

3.1. Comprehensive Lifestyle Interventions

Much information on reversing MetS may also be gleaned from randomised intervention studies that target individual components of the MetS or prevention/treatment of T2D. A small randomised study of Japanese men with MetS reported that a three-month intervention of diet and physical activity reduced WC and glycated haemoglobin, along with a nonsignificant reduction in MetS prevalence compared to control [42]. In African-Americans with T2D, a lifestyle weight loss intervention of 12 weeks resulted in lower weight, improved BP and glycaemic control compared with usual care after six months [43]. Similarly, a six-month weight loss program in African-Americans in the Southern United States resulted in reduction of WC and BP [44]. The Da Qing Diabetes Prevention Study in China reported reduced incidence of T2D by 45% following six years of a diet and physical activity intervention in people with glucose intolerance [45]. In Hispanic obese women, a community implementation of the Diabetes Prevention Program resulted in a greater decrease in WC and improved glycaemic control compared with metformin or standard care after 12 months [46]. In Brazil, a randomised intervention of lifestyle counselling resulted in improvements in WC and BP [47]. A nonrandomised study of translation of the Diabetes Prevention Program in Aboriginal people in the United States showed promise in reducing risk for T2D [48]. In Jewish and Bedouin women with post-gestational diabetes, a lifestyle counselling intervention resulted in reduction in glucose [49]. In South Asians living in the United Kingdom, compared with control, a diet and physical activity intervention resulted in improved WC but not glucose and BP after two years [50].

3.2. Nutritional Interventions

A wide variety of nutritional interventions ranging from macronutrient comparisons to supplementation with single foods or supplements have been carried out in a number of racial/ethnic groups. The most common dietary interventions are those focused on energy restriction in order to target weight loss, which generally improves cardiometabolic risk factors [51–53]. More recent attention has focused on the macronutrient combinations, and in particular, low-carbohydrate diets. A number of small randomised studies have indicated low-carbohydrate diets to result in more favourable improvements to glucose, insulin sensitivity, triglycerides and HDL-C [54], which may be independent of weight loss, suggesting a specific mechanism by which carbohydrates may promote cardiometabolic risk [55]. However, not all studies are in agreement and a meta-analysis of 23 randomised trials reported no difference in cardiometabolic risk factors between low-carbohydrate and low-fat diets [56].

In non-European-derived populations, diets with an emphasis on fruits and vegetables, healthy proteins and sodium reduction (such as the DASH diet) have demonstrated reductions in BP among African-Americans [57,58], East Asians [59,60] and South Asians [61,62]. For people with T2D, dietary interventions consisting of nutrition counselling following local guidelines for T2D care have resulted in improved glycaemic control, lipids and anthropometric measures in Arabs [63] and African-Americans [64]. Overweight and obese Malaysian adults undergoing a six-month trial of a high-protein, high-fibre diet had improvements to WC and glucose metabolism compared with control [65]. Studies in South Asians focusing on healthy protein, whether through meal replacement or nut supplementation, have reported reductions in glucose and WC, along with increases in HDL-C [61,62,66]. In Chinese men and women, a number of different randomised dietary interventions (high-protein, low-carbohydrate diets) have resulted in reductions in WC and lipid measures [67,68]. Diet supplemented with whole grain oats over six months reduced WC in Chinese men and women compared with control [69]. Very few studies have investigated interventions in Indigenous populations. A randomised study of flaxseed supplementation in Native Americans resulted in lowering low-density lipoprotein cholesterol (LDL-C) but did not affect HDL-C or TG [70], while a high-protein diet in Maori in New Zealand resulted in a greater decrease in WC compared with a low-fat or control diet [71].

3.3. Physical Activity Interventions

Numerous studies of various forms of physical activity have been conducted in a range of populations. In randomised trials, exercise interventions have demonstrated improvements in one or more of the components of MetS in South Asians [72–74] and East Asians [75,76]. In Chinese men, an intervention of Tai Chi was effective at reducing BP and TG [77]. Less is known about how similar interventions may be effective in African-American, Hispanic and Aboriginal/Indigenous populations. However, higher levels of physical activity and fitness have been reported to be associated with a lower prevalence of MetS in African-Americans [78], Hispanics [79] and Aboriginals [80].

To complement physical activity interventions, consideration should be given to interventions to limit sedentary behaviour such as sitting. Prospective studies have reported extended sedentary time to be positively associated with increased risk for type 2 diabetes, cardiovascular disease and premature mortality [81]. These associations occur even independently of physical activity levels. Cross-sectional studies in Americans [82], Brazilians [83] and Koreans [84] have reported positive associations between sedentary time and MetS. Randomised interventions aimed at reducing sedentary time have proven successful in increasing physical activity [85,86].

4. Prevention

Given the overall numbers of people with, and at risk for, MetS in most countries, individual-based prevention approaches are unlikely to be efficient and feasible. Instead, prevention strategies should be targeted to populations at the community level [87] and must be culturally tailored, as what works in one race/ethnic group may not necessarily work in another. These can vary from upstream, high-level policy initiatives to downstream, on the ground programs targeted at high-risk groups.

Policies such as the introduction of a sugar tax show promise. A high consumption of sugar, and sugar-sweetened beverages in particular, has been associated with a higher prevalence of MetS in a number of countries [88,89]. Countries and regions that have implemented a sugar tax have reported reductions in the consumption of sugar-sweetened beverages [90–92]. However, at present, there is no evidence to indicate this translates into a reduction in the incidence of MetS or its components, most likely because these policies are relatively new and may need more time for a downstream effect to be realised.

Another area influenced by policy at the local level is the built environment, which comprises the human-made infrastructure in which we live. This consists of such things as the street network, the placement of stores, community centres and residential areas, as well as the presence of sidewalks. Aspects of the built environment are associated with both physical activity and diet [93] and may be an upstream determinant for MetS.

People living in areas that are considered walkable (such as those with high street connectivity, mixed land use, and sidewalks) have higher physical activity levels and are at lower risk for T2D compared with those living in nonwalkable areas [94]. Similarly, living in an area with a high proportion of fast food restaurants and limited opportunities to buy healthy foods is associated with a greater prevalence of obesity [95]. These findings are consistent with a systematic review, which found cross-sectional associations of the built environment with obesity, hypertension and MetS, such that areas considered more walkable had a lower prevalence of these conditions [96]. Being cross-sectional, these studies cannot provide insight into causal relations or address the possible numerous confounders such as socioeconomic status (SES) and that some people are able to choose their neighbourhood based on their preferred lifestyle, while others may be limited in opportunities of residential movement as a result of their SES and race/ethnic minority status due to historical segregation. A limited number of longitudinal studies have reported that changes in the built environment associated with more walkability have corresponded with increased walking [97,98].

While some studies have indicated that the local food environment is associated with diets of nearby residents [99,100], not all studies have [101]. Similarly, the association of the food environment with risk factors is less clear. Some studies reported a positive association between fast food restaurants and obesity [95,102], a negative association between supermarkets and obesity [103], while others observed no association between food stores and obesity [104]. However, it appears these associations may depend on socioeconomic strata, which in heterogeneous populations often aligns along race/ethnicity, as the positive relationship between fast food restaurants and obesity was strongest in those with the lowest income [100,105]. Whether interventions to change the local food environment affect risk for the MetS is not known. Introduction of a supermarket in an area previously absent of any had a modest effect on diet quality, such as reduced sugar consumption in nearby residents compared with a control neighbourhood [106]. However, dietary assessment was conducted less than a year after the supermarket opened, and it may take a longer time, and more supermarkets, to change food purchasing behaviours.

Of importance is that many people in high- and middle-income countries who are at high risk for MetS are also among those with the lowest SES [107,108]. In addition, in countries with a diverse population, racial/ethnic minorities tend to be the most marginalised in that society. In lower SES communities, there are fewer opportunities for physical activity (such as green areas and community centres), less access to grocery stores and supermarkets (which sell healthy foods) and a higher proportion of fast food restaurants [109,110]. Targeted built environment interventions in these high-risk communities may be worthwhile to improve lifestyle behaviours known to protect against MetS.

While built environment initiatives affect the whole population, targeting interventions in high-risk communities by bringing prevention strategies to places where people gather have demonstrated substantial promise. These types of programs are needed, as access to health services for prevention and treatment (whether physical or cultural) is often worse for those of lower SES and/or of a minority racial/ethnic status [111]. In African-American communities in the United States, this has taken on the form of BP interventions at local barbershops. Both encouragement of lifestyle modification by their barber and integration with onsite pharmacists resulted in significant BP reductions, with the latter intervention being significantly better than barber encouragement alone [112]. Similar intervention studies are ongoing in faith-based communities and places of worship [113].

Success has also been reported using workplace interventions, which have resulted in improvements in activity and nutrition compared with control [114]. In Delhi, a multifactorial six-month worksite intervention focusing on education resulted in improvements in HDL-C, TG and WC compared with control groups [115]. Others have looked at translating successful interventions in European-derived populations to different racial/ethnic groups and delivering them in local communities. These studies have demonstrated significant reduction in MetS risk factors in African-Americans, [116] Hispanics [117,118] and South Asians living in India, Pakistan and the United Kingdom [119–121]. Community initiatives have also worked in increasing physical activity through walking programs in Hispanic neighbourhoods [122] and improving nutrition through local dietary counselling in African-American neighbourhoods [123]. Other community-based interventions have reported improvements in HDL-C, BP and WC compared with control in Taiwan [124]. A cluster-randomised study of communes in Vietnam found a six-month physical activity and nutrition intervention also improved cardiometabolic risk factors and a slightly better reduction in prevalence of MetS compared with an educational intervention [125]. In Iran, community-based educational programs have been successful in reducing the incidence of MetS compared with nonintervention controls [126,127].

Another area of promise for individual interventions but on a population scale is the use of consumer technology devices such as tablets, smartphones and wearables. A number of randomised studies have reported on experimental interventions that have improved lifestyle behaviours and/or cardiometabolic risk factors related to MetS, whether through wearable technology, smartphone apps or simple text messaging [29,128,129]. With the increasing ubiquity of global ownership of these devices, the opportunity to leverage these technologies to intervene on a population level has grown.

Recent studies have demonstrated the possible effectiveness of large-scale interventions [130] and the feasibility of reach in pragmatic trials [131].

5. Other Considerations

While both physical activity and dietary interventions are likely to be efficacious treatments for MetS, the intervention that is effective in one racial/ethnic group may not be effective in a different racial/ethnic group. This can be due to not only different cultural contexts of physical activity and diet but also due to structural barriers and policies, which cater to the majority population and may pose barriers to maintaining health and disease prevention for minority populations. Various cultures also view physical activity in different lights. For example, South Asians have lower physical activity levels compared with other populations [132,133], which may be rooted in cultural context [134]. In addition, adherence to and enjoyment of exercise may be based on the physical activity type, which also may have cultural relevance, such as Bhangra dance in South Asians [73] or Tai Chi in East Asians [135].

Similarly, food is strongly rooted in culture, and availability and cost may differ from place to place. Therefore, interventions need to consider what foods target groups have access to, the cultural meaning of food and the financial opportunity of the individuals. If interventions are not designed taking cultural preferences into account, they are unlikely to be engaged by the population and be successful [136]. In addition to cultural differences, in many high-income countries, many racial/ethnic groups comprise a minority population and are commonly marginalised in society, creating further barriers for treatment. To be effective, interventions must also address real and perceived structural barriers and policies present within each racial/ethnic group. For example, as a result of residential schools in Canada, there is distrust between people of Aboriginal background and government-funded health care [137]. Therefore, trust in the health care system and health care professionals, who may not be from the same community, is needed before effective prevention and intervention can begin [138].

6. Future Directions and Conclusions

Despite more than 80% of the world's population being of non-European descent, the overwhelming majority of research on MetS, from prevalence to treatment, is in predominantly European-derived populations. This is a critical gap in knowledge given that cardiometabolic risk may differ along racial/ethnic lines. Indeed, the recognised different WC thresholds reflect the nuances of race/ethnicity when assessing MetS. Current evidence in prevention and treatment of MetS suggests lifestyle interventions proved in European-derived populations can be effective at treating and reversing MetS; however, they need to be translated into the local cultural context to ensure success. For widespread prevention of MetS, interventions targeted at the population level are likely to be most successful. In order to grow our knowledge of MetS in different populations around the world, we need to conduct more rigorous cohort and randomised trials in populations beyond those of European descent. In addition, studies in countries with significant diversity should include unrepresented racial/ethnic groups as well as analyses stratified by race/ethnicity.

Author Contributions: S.A.L. conceptualised and wrote the manuscript. D.G. reviewed and revised the manuscript. All authors have read and agreed to the published version of the manuscript.

Acknowledgments: S.A.L. holds the Pfizer/Heart and Stroke Foundation Chair in Cardiovascular Prevention Research at St. Paul's Hospital.

References

1. Ballantyne, C.M.; Hoogeveen, R.C.; McNeill, A.M.; Heiss, G.; Schmidt, M.I.; Duncan, B.B.; Pankow, J.S. Metabolic syndrome risk for cardiovascular disease and diabetes in the ARIC study. *Int. J. Obes. (Lond.)* **2008**, *32* (Suppl. S2), S21–S24. [CrossRef] [PubMed]

2. Alberti, K.G.; Eckel, R.H.; Grundy, S.M.; Zimmet, P.Z.; Cleeman, J.I.; Donato, K.A.; Fruchart, J.C.; James, W.P.; Loria, C.M.; Smith, S.C., Jr. Harmonizing the metabolic syndrome: A joint interim statement of the International Diabetes Federation Task Force on Epidemiology and Prevention; National Heart, Lung, and Blood Institute; American Heart Association; World Heart Federation; International Atherosclerosis Society; and International Association for the Study of Obesity. *Circulation* **2009**, *120*, 1640–1645. [CrossRef] [PubMed]

3. Nolan, P.B.; Carrick-Ranson, G.; Stinear, J.W.; Reading, S.A.; Dalleck, L.C. Prevalence of metabolic syndrome and metabolic syndrome components in young adults: A pooled analysis. *Prev. Med. Rep.* **2017**, *7*, 211–215. [CrossRef] [PubMed]

4. Saklayen, M.G. The Global Epidemic of the Metabolic Syndrome. *Curr. Hypertens. Rep.* **2018**, *20*, 12. [CrossRef]

5. O'Neill, S.; O'Driscoll, L. Metabolic syndrome: A closer look at the growing epidemic and its associated pathologies. *Obes. Rev.* **2015**, *16*, 1–12. [CrossRef]

6. Moore, J.X.; Chaudhary, N.; Akinyemiju, T. Metabolic Syndrome Prevalence by Race/Ethnicity and Sex in the United States, National Health and Nutrition Examination Survey, 1988–2012. *Prev. Chronic Dis.* **2017**, *14*, E24. [CrossRef]

7. Lan, Y.; Mai, Z.; Zhou, S.; Liu, Y.; Li, S.; Zhao, Z.; Duan, X.; Cai, C.; Deng, T.; Zhu, W.; et al. Prevalence of metabolic syndrome in China: An up-dated cross-sectional study. *PLoS ONE* **2018**, *13*, e0196012. [CrossRef]

8. Aguilar, M.; Bhuket, T.; Torres, S.; Liu, B.; Wong, R.J. Prevalence of the metabolic syndrome in the United States, 2003–2012. *JAMA* **2015**, *313*, 1973–1974. [CrossRef]

9. Anand, S.S.; Yi, Q.; Gerstein, H.; Lonn, E.; Jacobs, R.; Vuksan, V.; Teo, K.; Davis, B.; Montague, P.; Yusuf, S. Relationship of metabolic syndrome and fibrinolytic dysfunction to cardiovascular disease. *Circulation* **2003**, *108*, 420–425. [CrossRef]

10. Tan, C.E.; Ma, S.; Wai, D.; Chew, S.K.; Tai, E.S. Can we apply the National Cholesterol Education Program Adult Treatment Panel definition of the metabolic syndrome to Asians? *Diabetes Care* **2004**, *27*, 1182–1186. [CrossRef]

11. Lear, S.A.; Chen, M.M.; Birmingham, C.L.; Frohlich, J.J. The relationship between simple anthropometric indices and c-reactive protein: Ethnic and gender differences. *Metabolism* **2003**, *52*, 1542–1546. [CrossRef] [PubMed]

12. Lear, S.A.; Chen, M.M.; Frohlich, J.J.; Birmingham, C.L. The relationship between waist circumference and metabolic risk factors: Cohorts of European and Chinese descent. *Metabolism* **2002**, *51*, 1427–1432. [CrossRef] [PubMed]

13. Lear, S.A.; Toma, M.; Birmingham, C.L.; Frohlich, J.J. Modification of the relationship between simple anthropometric indices and risk factors by ethnic background. *Metabolism* **2003**, *52*, 1295–1301. [CrossRef]

14. Lear, S.A.; Humphries, K.H.; Kohli, S.; Chockalingam, A.; Frohlich, J.J.; Birmingham, C.L. Visceral adipose tissue accumulation differs according to ethnic background: Results of the Multicultural Community Health Assessment Trial (M-CHAT). *Am. J. Clin. Nutr.* **2007**, *86*, 353–359. [CrossRef] [PubMed]

15. Lear, S.A.; Chockalingam, A.; Kohli, S.; Richardson, C.G.; Humphries, K.H. Elevation in cardiovascular disease risk in South Asians is mediated by differences in visceral adipose tissue. *Obesity (Silver Spring)* **2012**, *20*, 1293–1300. [CrossRef] [PubMed]

16. Hoffman, D.J.; Wang, Z.; Gallagher, D.; Heymsfield, S.B. Comparison of visceral adipose tissue mass in adult African Americans and whites. *Obes. Res.* **2005**, *13*, 66–74. [CrossRef]

17. Katzmarzyk, P.T. Obesity and physical activity among Aboriginal Canadians. *Obesity (Silver Spring)* **2008**, *16*, 184–190. [CrossRef]

18. Turin, T.C.; Saad, N.; Jun, M.; Tonelli, M.; Ma, Z.; Barnabe, C.C.M.; Manns, B.; Hemmelgarn, B. Lifetime risk of diabetes among First Nations and non-First Nations people. *CMAJ* **2016**, *188*, 1147–1153. [CrossRef]

19. Gautier, J.F.; Milner, M.R.; Elam, E.; Chen, K.; Ravussin, E.; Pratley, R.E. Visceral adipose tissue is not increased in Pima Indians compared with equally obese Caucasians and is not related to insulin action or secretion. *Diabetologia* **1999**, *42*, 28–34. [CrossRef]

20. Gasevic, D.; Kohli, S.; Khan, N.; Lear, S.A. Abdominal Adipose Tissue and Insulin Resistance: The Role of Ethnicity. In *Nutrition in the Prevention and Treatment of Abdominal Obesity*; Academic Press; Elsivier, Inc.: Waltham, MA, USA, 2014; pp. 125–140.

21. Lear, S.A.; James, P.T.; Ko, G.T.; Kumanyika, S. Appropriateness of waist circumference and waist-to-hip ratio cutoffs for different ethnic groups. *Eur. J. Clin. Nutr.* **2010**, *64*, 42–61. [CrossRef]

22. Kaneshiro, B.; Geling, O.; Gellert, K.; Millar, L. The challenges of collecting data on race and ethnicity in a diverse, multiethnic state. *Hawaii Med. J.* **2011**, *70*, 168–171. [PubMed]

23. Aspinall, P.J. Concepts, terminology and classifications for the "mixed" ethnic or racial group in the United Kingdom. *J. Epidemiol. Community Health* **2010**, *64*, 557–560. [CrossRef] [PubMed]

24. Knowler, W.C.; Barrett-Connor, E.; Fowler, S.E.; Hamman, R.F.; Lachin, J.M.; Walker, E.A.; Nathan, D.M. Reduction in the incidence of type 2 diabetes with lifestyle intervention or metformin. *N. Engl. J. Med.* **2002**, *346*, 393–403. [CrossRef] [PubMed]

25. Orchard, T.J.; Temprosa, M.; Goldberg, R.; Haffner, S.; Ratner, R.; Marcovina, S.; Fowler, S. The effect of metformin and intensive lifestyle intervention on the metabolic syndrome: The Diabetes Prevention Program randomized trial. *Ann. Intern. Med.* **2005**, *142*, 611–619. [CrossRef]

26. Yamaoka, K.; Tango, T. Effects of lifestyle modification on metabolic syndrome: A systematic review and meta-analysis. *BMC Med.* **2012**, *10*, 138. [CrossRef]

27. Church, T.S.; Earnest, C.P.; Skinner, J.S.; Blair, S.N. Effects of different doses of physical activity on cardiorespiratory fitness among sedentary, overweight or obese postmenopausal women with elevated blood pressure: A randomized controlled trial. *JAMA* **2007**, *297*, 2081–2091. [CrossRef]

28. Earnest, C.P.; Johannsen, N.M.; Swift, D.L.; Lavie, C.J.; Blair, S.N.; Church, T.S. Dose effect of cardiorespiratory exercise on metabolic syndrome in postmenopausal women. *Am. J. Cardiol.* **2013**, *111*, 1805–1811. [CrossRef]

29. Haufe, S.; Kerling, A.; Protte, G.; Bayerle, P.; Stenner, H.T.; Rolff, S.; Sundermeier, T.; Kuck, M.; Ensslen, R.; Nachbar, L.; et al. Telemonitoring-supported exercise training, metabolic syndrome severity, and work ability in company employees: A randomised controlled trial. *Lancet Public Health* **2019**, *4*, e343–e352. [CrossRef]

30. Tomeleri, C.M.; Souza, M.F.; Burini, R.C.; Cavaglieri, C.R.; Ribeiro, A.S.; Antunes, M.; Nunes, J.P.; Venturini, D.; Barbosa, D.S.; Sardinha, L.B.; et al. Resistance training reduces metabolic syndrome and inflammatory markers in older women: A randomized controlled trial. *J. Diabetes* **2018**, *10*, 328–337. [CrossRef]

31. Earnest, C.P.; Johannsen, N.M.; Swift, D.L.; Gillison, F.B.; Mikus, C.R.; Lucia, A.; Kramer, K.; Lavie, C.J.; Church, T.S. Aerobic and strength training in concomitant metabolic syndrome and type 2 diabetes. *Med. Sci. Sports Exerc.* **2014**, *46*, 1293–1301. [CrossRef]

32. Tjonna, A.E.; Ramos, J.S.; Pressler, A.; Halle, M.; Jungbluth, K.; Ermacora, E.; Salvesen, O.; Rodrigues, J.; Bueno, C.R., Jr.; Munk, P.S.; et al. EX-MET study: Exercise in prevention on of metabolic syndrome—A randomized multicenter trial: Rational and design. *BMC Public Health* **2018**, *18*, 437. [CrossRef] [PubMed]

33. Babio, N.; Toledo, E.; Estruch, R.; Ros, E.; Martinez-Gonzalez, M.A.; Castaner, O.; Bullo, M.; Corella, D.; Aros, F.; Gomez-Gracia, E.; et al. Mediterranean diets and metabolic syndrome status in the PREDIMED randomized trial. *CMAJ* **2014**, *186*, E649–E657. [CrossRef] [PubMed]

34. Agarwal, A.; Ioannidis, J.P.A. PREDIMED trial of Mediterranean diet: Retracted, republished, still trusted? *BMJ* **2019**, *364*, l341. [CrossRef] [PubMed]

35. Estruch, R.; Ros, E.; Salas-Salvado, J.; Covas, M.I.; Corella, D.; Aros, F.; Gomez-Gracia, E.; Ruiz-Gutierrez, V.; Fiol, M.; Lapetra, J.; et al. Retraction and Republication: Primary Prevention of Cardiovascular Disease with a Mediterranean Diet. *N. Engl. J. Med.* **2018**, *378*, 2441–2442. [CrossRef] [PubMed]

36. Ehteshami, M.; Shakerhosseini, R.; Sedaghat, F.; Hedayati, M.; Eini-Zinab, H.; Hekmatdoost, A. The Effect of Gluten Free Diet on Components of Metabolic Syndrome: A Randomized Clinical Trial. *Asian Pac. J. Cancer Prev. APJCP* **2018**, *19*, 2979–2984. [CrossRef] [PubMed]

37. Gupta Jain, S.; Puri, S.; Misra, A.; Gulati, S.; Mani, K. Effect of oral cinnamon intervention on metabolic profile and body composition of Asian Indians with metabolic syndrome: A randomized double -blind control trial. *Lipids Health Dis.* **2017**, *16*, 113. [CrossRef]

38. Wu, H.; Pan, A.; Yu, Z.; Qi, Q.; Lu, L.; Zhang, G.; Yu, D.; Zong, G.; Zhou, Y.; Chen, X.; et al. Lifestyle counseling and supplementation with flaxseed or walnuts influence the management of metabolic syndrome. *J. Nutr.* **2010**, *140*, 1937–1942. [CrossRef]

39. Alfawaz, H.A.; Wani, K.; Alnaami, A.M.; Al-Saleh, Y.; Aljohani, N.J.; Al-Attas, O.S.; Alokail, M.S.; Kumar, S.; Al-Daghri, N.M. Effects of Different Dietary and Lifestyle Modification Therapies on Metabolic Syndrome in Prediabetic Arab Patients: A 12-Month Longitudinal Study. *Nutrients* **2018**, *10*, 383. [CrossRef]

40. Dunkley, A.J.; Davies, M.J.; Stone, M.A.; Taub, N.A.; Troughton, J.; Yates, T.; Khunti, K. The Reversal Intervention for Metabolic Syndrome (TRIMS) study: Rationale, design, and baseline data. *Trials* **2011**, *12*, 107. [CrossRef]

41. Dash, C.; Makambi, K.; Wallington, S.F.; Sheppard, V.; Taylor, T.R.; Hicks, J.S.; Adams-Campbell, L.L. An exercise trial targeting African-American women with metabolic syndrome and at high risk for breast cancer: Rationale, design, and methods. *Contemp. Clin. Trials* **2015**, *43*, 33–38. [CrossRef]

42. Nanri, A.; Tomita, K.; Matsushita, Y.; Ichikawa, F.; Yamamoto, M.; Nagafuchi, Y.; Kakumoto, Y.; Mizoue, T. Effect of six months lifestyle intervention in Japanese men with metabolic syndrome: Randomized controlled trial. *J. Occup. Health* **2012**, *54*, 215–222. [CrossRef] [PubMed]

43. Agurs-Collins, T.D.; Kumanyika, S.K.; Ten Have, T.R.; Adams-Campbell, L.L. A randomized controlled trial of weight reduction and exercise for diabetes management in older African-American subjects. *Diabetes Care* **1997**, *20*, 1503–1511. [CrossRef] [PubMed]

44. Ard, J.D.; Carson, T.L.; Shikany, J.M.; Li, Y.; Hardy, C.M.; Robinson, J.C.; Williams, A.G.; Baskin, M.L. Weight loss and improved metabolic outcomes amongst rural African American women in the Deep South: Six-month outcomes from a community-based randomized trial. *J. Intern. Med.* **2017**, *282*, 102–113. [CrossRef] [PubMed]

45. Li, G.; Zhang, P.; Wang, J.; An, Y.; Gong, Q.; Gregg, E.W.; Yang, W.; Zhang, B.; Shuai, Y.; Hong, J.; et al. Cardiovascular mortality, all-cause mortality, and diabetes incidence after lifestyle intervention for people with impaired glucose tolerance in the Da Qing Diabetes Prevention Study: A 23-year follow-up study. *Lancet Diabetes Endocrinol.* **2014**, *2*, 474–480. [CrossRef]

46. O'Brien, M.J.; Perez, A.; Scanlan, A.B.; Alos, V.A.; Whitaker, R.C.; Foster, G.D.; Ackermann, R.T.; Ciolino, J.D.; Homko, C. PREVENT-DM Comparative Effectiveness Trial of Lifestyle Intervention and Metformin. *Am. J. Prev. Med.* **2017**, *52*, 788–797. [CrossRef]

47. Saboya, P.P.; Bodanese, L.C.; Zimmermann, P.R.; Gustavo, A.D.; Macagnan, F.E.; Feoli, A.P.; Oliveira, M.D. Lifestyle Intervention on Metabolic Syndrome and its Impact on Quality of Life: A Randomized Controlled Trial. *Arq. Bras. Cardiol.* **2017**, *108*, 60–69. [CrossRef]

48. Jiang, L.; Manson, S.M.; Beals, J.; Henderson, W.G.; Huang, H.; Acton, K.J.; Roubideaux, Y. Translating the Diabetes Prevention Program into American Indian and Alaska Native communities: Results from the Special Diabetes Program for Indians Diabetes Prevention demonstration project. *Diabetes Care* **2013**, *36*, 2027–2034. [CrossRef]

49. Zilberman-Kravits, D.; Meyerstein, N.; Abu-Rabia, Y.; Wiznitzer, A.; Harman-Boehm, I. The Impact of a Cultural Lifestyle Intervention on Metabolic Parameters After Gestational Diabetes Mellitus A Randomized Controlled Trial. *Matern. Child Health J.* **2018**, *22*, 803–811. [CrossRef]

50. Bhopal, R.S.; Douglas, A.; Wallia, S.; Forbes, J.F.; Lean, M.E.; Gill, J.M.; McKnight, J.A.; Sattar, N.; Sheikh, A.; Wild, S.H.; et al. Effect of a lifestyle intervention on weight change in south Asian individuals in the UK at high risk of type 2 diabetes: A family-cluster randomised controlled trial. *Lancet Diabetes Endocrinol.* **2014**, *2*, 218–227. [CrossRef]

51. Bajerska, J.; Chmurzynska, A.; Muzsik, A.; Krzyzanowska, P.; Madry, E.; Malinowska, A.M.; Walkowiak, J. Weight loss and metabolic health effects from energy-restricted Mediterranean and Central-European diets in postmenopausal women: A randomized controlled trial. *Sci. Rep.* **2018**, *8*, 11170. [CrossRef]

52. Harvie, M.N.; Pegington, M.; Mattson, M.P.; Frystyk, J.; Dillon, B.; Evans, G.; Cuzick, J.; Jebb, S.A.; Martin, B.; Cutler, R.G.; et al. The effects of intermittent or continuous energy restriction on weight loss and metabolic disease risk markers: A randomized trial in young overweight women. *Int. J. Obes. (Lond.)* **2011**, *35*, 714–727. [CrossRef] [PubMed]

53. Sundfor, T.M.; Svendsen, M.; Tonstad, S. Effect of intermittent versus continuous energy restriction on weight loss, maintenance and cardiometabolic risk: A randomized 1-year trial. *Nutr. Metab. Cardiovasc. Dis.* **2018**, *28*, 698–706. [CrossRef] [PubMed]

54. Volek, J.S.; Phinney, S.D.; Forsythe, C.E.; Quann, E.E.; Wood, R.J.; Puglisi, M.J.; Kraemer, W.J.; Bibus, D.M.; Fernandez, M.L.; Feinman, R.D. Carbohydrate restriction has a more favorable impact on the metabolic syndrome than a low fat diet. *Lipids* **2009**, *44*, 297–309. [CrossRef] [PubMed]

55. Hyde, P.N.; Sapper, T.N.; Crabtree, C.D.; LaFountain, R.A.; Bowling, M.L.; Buga, A.; Fell, B.; McSwiney, F.T.; Dickerson, R.M.; Miller, V.J.; et al. Dietary carbohydrate restriction improves metabolic syndrome independent of weight loss. *JCI Insight* **2019**, *4*. [CrossRef]

56. Hu, T.; Mills, K.T.; Yao, L.; Demanelis, K.; Eloustaz, M.; Yancy, W.S., Jr.; Kelly, T.N.; He, J.; Bazzano, L.A. Effects of low-carbohydrate diets versus low-fat diets on metabolic risk factors: A meta-analysis of randomized controlled clinical trials. *Am. J. Epidemiol.* **2012**, *176* (Suppl. S7), S44–S54. [CrossRef]

57. Svetkey, L.P.; Erlinger, T.P.; Vollmer, W.M.; Feldstein, A.; Cooper, L.S.; Appel, L.J.; Ard, J.D.; Elmer, P.J.; Harsha, D.; Stevens, V.J. Effect of lifestyle modifications on blood pressure by race, sex, hypertension status, and age. *J. Hum. Hypertens.* **2005**, *19*, 21–31. [CrossRef]

58. Svetkey, L.P.; Simons-Morton, D.; Vollmer, W.M.; Appel, L.J.; Conlin, P.R.; Ryan, D.H.; Ard, J.; Kennedy, B.M. Effects of dietary patterns on blood pressure: Subgroup analysis of the Dietary Approaches to Stop Hypertension (DASH) randomized clinical trial. *Arch. Intern. Med.* **1999**, *159*, 285–293. [CrossRef]

59. Schroeder, N.; Park, Y.H.; Kang, M.S.; Kim, Y.; Ha, G.K.; Kim, H.R.; Yates, A.A.; Caballero, B. A randomized trial on the effects of 2010 Dietary Guidelines for Americans and Korean diet patterns on cardiovascular risk factors in overweight and obese adults. *J. Acad. Nutr. Diet.* **2015**, *115*, 1083–1092. [CrossRef]

60. Zhao, X.; Yin, X.; Li, X.; Yan, L.L.; Lam, C.T.; Li, S.; He, F.; Xie, W.; Sang, B.; Luobu, G.; et al. Using a low-sodium, high-potassium salt substitute to reduce blood pressure among Tibetans with high blood pressure: A patient-blinded randomized controlled trial. *PLoS ONE* **2014**, *9*, e110131. [CrossRef]

61. Gulati, S.; Misra, A.; Pandey, R.M.; Bhatt, S.P.; Saluja, S. Effects of pistachio nuts on body composition, metabolic, inflammatory and oxidative stress parameters in Asian Indians with metabolic syndrome: A 24-wk, randomized control trial. *Nutrition* **2014**, *30*, 192–197. [CrossRef]

62. Mohan, V.; Gayathri, R.; Jaacks, L.M.; Lakshmipriya, N.; Anjana, R.M.; Spiegelman, D.; Jeevan, R.G.; Balasubramaniam, K.K.; Shobana, S.; Jayanthan, M.; et al. Cashew Nut Consumption Increases HDL Cholesterol and Reduces Systolic Blood Pressure in Asian Indians with Type 2 Diabetes: A 12-Week Randomized Controlled Trial. *J. Nutr.* **2018**, *148*, 63–69. [CrossRef] [PubMed]

63. Al-Shookri, A.; Khor, G.L.; Chan, Y.M.; Loke, S.C.; Al-Maskari, M. Effectiveness of medical nutrition treatment delivered by dietitians on glycaemic outcomes and lipid profiles of Arab, Omani patients with Type 2 diabetes. *Diabet Med.* **2012**, *29*, 236–244. [CrossRef] [PubMed]

64. Ziemer, D.C.; Berkowitz, K.J.; Panayioto, R.M.; El-Kebbi, I.M.; Musey, V.C.; Anderson, L.A.; Wanko, N.S.; Fowke, M.L.; Brazier, C.W.; Dunbar, V.G.; et al. A simple meal plan emphasizing healthy food choices is as effective as an exchange-based meal plan for urban African Americans with type 2 diabetes. *Diabetes Care* **2003**, *26*, 1719–1724. [CrossRef] [PubMed]

65. Mitra, S.R.; Tan, P.Y. Effect of an individualised high-protein, energy-restricted diet on anthropometric and cardio-metabolic parameters in overweight and obese Malaysian adults: A 6-month randomised controlled study. *Br. J. Nutr.* **2019**, *121*, 1002–1017. [CrossRef]

66. Gulati, S.; Misra, A.; Tiwari, R.; Sharma, M.; Pandey, R.M.; Yadav, C.P. Effect of high-protein meal replacement on weight and cardiometabolic profile in overweight/obese Asian Indians in North India. *Br. J. Nutr.* **2017**, *117*, 1531–1540. [CrossRef]

67. Chen, W.; Liu, Y.; Yang, Q.; Li, X.; Yang, J.; Wang, J.; Shi, L.; Chen, Y.; Zhu, S. The Effect of Protein-Enriched Meal Replacement on Waist Circumference Reduction among Overweight and Obese Chinese with Hyperlipidemia. *J. Am. Coll. Nutr.* **2016**, *35*, 236–244. [CrossRef]

68. Liu, X.; Zhang, G.; Ye, X.; Li, H.; Chen, X.; Tang, L.; Feng, Y.; Shai, I.; Stampfer, M.J.; Hu, F.B.; et al. Effects of a low-carbohydrate diet on weight loss and cardiometabolic profile in Chinese women: A randomised controlled feeding trial. *Br. J. Nutr.* **2013**, *110*, 1444–1453. [CrossRef]

69. Zhang, J.; Li, L.; Song, P.; Wang, C.; Man, Q.; Meng, L.; Cai, J.; Kurilich, A. Randomized controlled trial of oatmeal consumption versus noodle consumption on blood lipids of urban Chinese adults with hypercholesterolemia. *Nutr. J.* **2012**, *11*, 54. [CrossRef]

70. Patade, A.; Devareddy, L.; Lucas, E.A.; Korlagunta, K.; Daggy, B.P.; Arjmandi, B.H. Flaxseed reduces total and LDL cholesterol concentrations in Native American postmenopausal women. *J. Womens Health (2002)* **2008**, *17*, 355–366. [CrossRef]

71. Brooking, L.A.; Williams, S.M.; Mann, J.I. Effects of macronutrient composition of the diet on body fat in indigenous people at high risk of type 2 diabetes. *Diabetes Res. Clin. Pract.* **2012**, *96*, 40–46. [CrossRef]

72. Andersen, E.; Hostmark, A.T.; Anderssen, S.A. Effect of a physical activity intervention on the metabolic syndrome in Pakistani immigrant men: A randomized controlled trial. *J. Immigr. Minor. Health* **2012**, *14*, 738–746. [CrossRef] [PubMed]

73. Lesser, I.A.; Singer, J.; Hoogbruin, A.; Mackey, D.C.; Katzmarzyk, P.T.; Sohal, P.; Leipsic, J.; Lear, S.A. Effectiveness of Exercise on Visceral Adipose Tissue in Older South Asian Women. *Med. Sci. Sports Exerc.* **2016**, *48*, 1371–1378. [CrossRef] [PubMed]

74. Martin, C.A.; Gowda, U.; Smith, B.J.; Renzaho, A.M.N. Systematic Review of the Effect of Lifestyle Interventions on the Components of the Metabolic Syndrome in South Asian Migrants. *J. Immigr. Minor. Health* **2018**, *20*, 231–244. [CrossRef] [PubMed]

75. Igarashi, Y.; Akazawa, N.; Maeda, S. Regular aerobic exercise and blood pressure in East Asians: A meta-analysis of randomized controlled trials. *Clin. Exp. Hypertens. (NY 1993)* **2018**, *40*, 378–389. [CrossRef]

76. Matsuo, T.; So, R.; Shimojo, N.; Tanaka, K. Effect of aerobic exercise training followed by a low-calorie diet on metabolic syndrome risk factors in men. *Nutr. Metab. Cardiovasc. Dis.* **2015**, *25*, 832–838. [CrossRef]

77. Choi, Y.S.; Song, R.; Ku, B.J. Effects of a T'ai Chi-Based Health Promotion Program on Metabolic Syndrome Markers, Health Behaviors, and Quality of Life in Middle-Aged Male Office Workers: A Randomized Trial. *J. Altern. Complement. Med.* **2017**, *23*, 949–956. [CrossRef]

78. Adams-Campbell, L.L.; Dash, C.; Kim, B.H.; Hicks, J.; Makambi, K.; Hagberg, J. Cardiorespiratory Fitness and Metabolic Syndrome in Postmenopausal African-American Women. *Int. J. Sports Med.* **2016**, *37*, 261–266. [CrossRef]

79. Vella, C.A.; Zubia, R.Y.; Ontiveros, D.; Cruz, M.L. Physical activity, cardiorespiratory fitness, and metabolic syndrome in young Mexican and Mexican-American women. *Appl. Physiol. Nutr. Metab.* **2009**, *34*, 10–17. [CrossRef]

80. Liu, J.; Young, T.K.; Zinman, B.; Harris, S.B.; Connelly, P.W.; Hanley, A.J. Lifestyle variables, non-traditional cardiovascular risk factors, and the metabolic syndrome in an Aboriginal Canadian population. *Obesity (Silver Spring)* **2006**, *14*, 500–508. [CrossRef]

81. Biswas, A.; Oh, P.I.; Faulkner, G.E.; Bajaj, R.R.; Silver, M.A.; Mitchell, M.S.; Alter, D.A. Sedentary time and its association with risk for disease incidence, mortality, and hospitalization in adults: A systematic review and meta-analysis. *Ann. Intern. Med.* **2015**, *162*, 123–132. [CrossRef]

82. Bankoski, A.; Harris, T.B.; McClain, J.J.; Brychta, R.J.; Caserotti, P.; Chen, K.Y.; Berrigan, D.; Troiano, R.P.; Koster, A. Sedentary activity associated with metabolic syndrome independent of physical activity. *Diabetes Care* **2011**, *34*, 497–503. [CrossRef] [PubMed]

83. Lemes, I.R.; Sui, X.; Fernandes, R.A.; Blair, S.N.; Turi-Lynch, B.C.; Codogno, J.S.; Monteiro, H.L. Association of sedentary behavior and metabolic syndrome. *Public Health* **2019**, *167*, 96–102. [CrossRef] [PubMed]

84. Nam, J.Y.; Kim, J.; Cho, K.H.; Choi, Y.; Choi, J.; Shin, J.; Park, E.C. Associations of sitting time and occupation with metabolic syndrome in South Korean adults: A cross-sectional study. *BMC Public Health* **2016**, *16*, 943. [CrossRef] [PubMed]

85. Compernolle, S.; DeSmet, A.; Poppe, L.; Crombez, G.; De Bourdeaudhuij, I.; Cardon, G.; van der Ploeg, H.P.; Van Dyck, D. Effectiveness of interventions using self-monitoring to reduce sedentary behavior in adults: A systematic review and meta-analysis. *Int. J. Behav. Nutr. Phys. Act.* **2019**, *16*, 63. [CrossRef]

86. Balducci, S.; D'Errico, V.; Haxhi, J.; Sacchetti, M.; Orlando, G.; Cardelli, P.; Vitale, M.; Bollanti, L.; Conti, F.; Zanuso, S.; et al. Effect of a Behavioral Intervention Strategy on Sustained Change in Physical Activity and Sedentary Behavior in Patients With Type 2 Diabetes: The IDES_2 Randomized Clinical Trial. *JAMA* **2019**, *321*, 880–890. [CrossRef]

87. Pandit, K.; Goswami, S.; Ghosh, S.; Mukhopadhyay, P.; Chowdhury, S. Metabolic syndrome in South Asians. *Indian J. Endocrinol. Metab.* **2012**, *16*, 44–55. [CrossRef]

88. Malik, V.S.; Popkin, B.M.; Bray, G.A.; Despres, J.P.; Willett, W.C.; Hu, F.B. Sugar-sweetened beverages and risk of metabolic syndrome and type 2 diabetes: A meta-analysis. *Diabetes Care* **2010**, *33*, 2477–2483. [CrossRef]

89. Seo, E.H.; Kim, H.; Kwon, O. Association between Total Sugar Intake and Metabolic Syndrome in Middle-Aged Korean Men and Women. *Nutrients* **2019**, *11*, 2042. [CrossRef]

90. Colchero, M.A.; Rivera-Dommarco, J.; Popkin, B.M.; Ng, S.W. In Mexico, Evidence Of Sustained Consumer Response Two Years After Implementing A Sugar-Sweetened Beverage Tax. *Health Aff. (Proj. Hope)* **2017**, *36*, 564–571. [CrossRef]

91. Lee, M.M.; Falbe, J.; Schillinger, D.; Basu, S.; McCulloch, C.E.; Madsen, K.A. Sugar-Sweetened Beverage Consumption 3 Years After the Berkeley, California, Sugar-Sweetened Beverage Tax. *Am. J. Public Health* **2019**, *109*, 637–639. [CrossRef]

92. Nakamura, R.; Mirelman, A.J.; Cuadrado, C.; Silva-Illanes, N.; Dunstan, J.; Suhrcke, M. Evaluating the 2014 sugar-sweetened beverage tax in Chile: An observational study in urban areas. *PLoS Med.* **2018**, *15*, e1002596. [CrossRef] [PubMed]

93. Papas, M.A.; Alberg, A.J.; Ewing, R.; Helzlsouer, K.J.; Gary, T.L.; Klassen, A.C. The built environment and obesity. *Epidemiol. Rev.* **2007**, *29*, 129–143. [CrossRef] [PubMed]

94. Booth, G.L.; Creatore, M.I.; Luo, J.; Fazli, G.S.; Johns, A.; Rosella, L.C.; Glazier, R.H.; Moineddin, R.; Gozdyra, P.; Austin, P.C. Neighbourhood walkability and the incidence of diabetes: An inverse probability of treatment weighting analysis. *J. Epidemiol. Community Health* **2019**, *73*, 287–294. [CrossRef]

95. Li, F.; Harmer, P.; Cardinal, B.J.; Bosworth, M.; Johnson-Shelton, D. Obesity and the built environment: Does the density of neighborhood fast-food outlets matter? *Am. J. Health Promot.* **2009**, *23*, 203–209. [CrossRef] [PubMed]

96. Malambo, P.; Kengne, A.P.; De Villiers, A.; Lambert, E.V.; Puoane, T. Built Environment, Selected Risk Factors and Major Cardiovascular Disease Outcomes: A Systematic Review. *PLoS ONE* **2016**, *11*, e0166846. [CrossRef] [PubMed]

97. Hirsch, J.A.; Moore, K.A.; Clarke, P.J.; Rodriguez, D.A.; Evenson, K.R.; Brines, S.J.; Zagorski, M.A.; Diez Roux, A.V. Changes in the built environment and changes in the amount of walking over time: Longitudinal results from the multi-ethnic study of atherosclerosis. *Am. J. Epidemiol.* **2014**, *180*, 799–809. [CrossRef]

98. Sun, G.; Oreskovic, N.M.; Lin, H. How do changes to the built environment influence walking behaviors? A longitudinal study within a university campus in Hong Kong. *Int. J. Health Geogr.* **2014**, *13*, 28. [CrossRef]

99. Morland, K.; Wing, S.; Diez Roux, A. The contextual effect of the local food environment on residents' diets: The atherosclerosis risk in communities study. *Am. J. Public Health* **2002**, *92*, 1761–1767. [CrossRef]

100. Mackenbach, J.D.; Burgoine, T.; Lakerveld, J.; Forouhi, N.G.; Griffin, S.J.; Wareham, N.J.; Monsivais, P. Accessibility and Affordability of Supermarkets: Associations With the DASH Diet. *Am. J. Prev. Med.* **2017**, *53*, 55–62. [CrossRef]

101. Jiao, J.; Moudon, A.V.; Kim, S.Y.; Hurvitz, P.M.; Drewnowski, A. Health Implications of Adults' Eating at and Living near Fast Food or Quick Service Restaurants. *Nutr. Diabetes* **2015**, *5*, e171. [CrossRef]

102. Inagami, S.; Cohen, D.A.; Brown, A.F.; Asch, S.M. Body mass index, neighborhood fast food and restaurant concentration, and car ownership. *J. Urban Health* **2009**, *86*, 683–695. [CrossRef] [PubMed]

103. Drewnowski, A.; Aggarwal, A.; Hurvitz, P.M.; Monsivais, P.; Moudon, A.V. Obesity and supermarket access: Proximity or price? *Am. J. Public Health* **2012**, *102*, e74–e80. [CrossRef] [PubMed]

104. Mazidi, M.; Speakman, J.R. Higher densities of fast-food and full-service restaurants are not associated with obesity prevalence. *Am. J. Clin. Nutr.* **2017**, *106*, 603–613. [CrossRef] [PubMed]

105. Burgoine, T.; Forouhi, N.G.; Griffin, S.J.; Brage, S.; Wareham, N.J.; Monsivais, P. Does neighborhood fast-food outlet exposure amplify inequalities in diet and obesity? A cross-sectional study. *Am. J. Clin. Nutr.* **2016**, *103*, 1540–1547. [CrossRef] [PubMed]

106. Dubowitz, T.; Ghosh-Dastidar, M.; Cohen, D.A.; Beckman, R.; Steiner, E.D.; Hunter, G.P.; Florez, K.R.; Huang, C.; Vaughan, C.A.; Sloan, J.C.; et al. Diet And Perceptions Change With Supermarket Introduction In A Food Desert, But Not Because Of Supermarket Use. *Health Aff. (Proj. Hope)* **2015**, *34*, 1858–1868. [CrossRef]

107. Karlamangla, A.S.; Merkin, S.S.; Crimmins, E.M.; Seeman, T.E. Socioeconomic and ethnic disparities in cardiovascular risk in the United States, 2001–2006. *Ann. Epidemiol.* **2010**, *20*, 617–628. [CrossRef]

108. Zhan, Y.; Yu, J.; Chen, R.; Gao, J.; Ding, R.; Fu, Y.; Zhang, L.; Hu, D. Socioeconomic status and metabolic syndrome in the general population of China: A cross-sectional study. *BMC Public Health* **2012**, *12*, 921. [CrossRef]

109. Block, J.P.; Scribner, R.A.; DeSalvo, K.B. Fast food, race/ethnicity, and income: A geographic analysis. *Am. J. Prev. Med.* **2004**, *27*, 211–217.

110. Burgoine, T.; Sarkar, C.; Webster, C.J.; Monsivais, P. Examining the interaction of fast-food outlet exposure and income on diet and obesity: Evidence from 51,361 UK Biobank participants. *Int. J. Behav. Nutr. Phys. Act.* **2018**, *15*, 71. [CrossRef]

111. Palafox, B.; McKee, M.; Balabanova, D.; AlHabib, K.F.; Avezum, A.J.; Bahonar, A.; Ismail, N.; Chifamba, J.; Chow, C.K.; Corsi, D.J.; et al. Wealth and cardiovascular health: A cross-sectional study of wealth-related

inequalities in the awareness, treatment and control of hypertension in high-, middle- and low-income countries. *Int. J. Equity Health* **2016**, *15*, 199. [CrossRef]

112. Victor, R.G.; Lynch, K.; Li, N.; Blyler, C.; Muhammad, E.; Handler, J.; Brettler, J.; Rashid, M.; Hsu, B.; Foxx-Drew, D.; et al. A Cluster-Randomized Trial of Blood-Pressure Reduction in Black Barbershops. *N. Engl. J. Med.* **2018**, *378*, 1291–1301. [CrossRef] [PubMed]

113. Carter-Edwards, L.; Lindquist, R.; Redmond, N.; Turner, C.M.; Harding, C.; Oliver, J.; West, L.B.; Ravenell, J.; Shikany, J.M. Designing Faith-Based Blood Pressure Interventions to Reach Young Black Men. *Am. J. Prev. Med.* **2018**, *55*, S49–S58. [CrossRef] [PubMed]

114. Smith, M.L.; Wilson, M.G.; Robertson, M.M.; Padilla, H.M.; Zuercher, H.; Vandenberg, R.; Corso, P.; Lorig, K.; Laurent, D.D.; DeJoy, D.M. Impact of a Translated Disease Self-Management Program on Employee Health and Productivity: Six-Month Findings from a Randomized Controlled Trial. *Int. J. Environ. Res. Public Health* **2018**, *15*, 851. [CrossRef] [PubMed]

115. Shrivastava, U.; Fatma, M.; Mohan, S.; Singh, P.; Misra, A. Randomized Control Trial for Reduction of Body Weight, Body Fat Patterning, and Cardiometabolic Risk Factors in Overweight Worksite Employees in Delhi, India. *J. Diabetes Res.* **2017**, *2017*, 7254174. [CrossRef]

116. Parra-Medina, D.; Wilcox, S.; Salinas, J.; Addy, C.; Fore, E.; Poston, M.; Wilson, D.K. Results of the Heart Healthy and Ethnically Relevant Lifestyle trial: A cardiovascular risk reduction intervention for African American women attending community health centers. *Am. J. Public Health* **2011**, *101*, 1914–1921. [CrossRef]

117. McCurley, J.L.; Gutierrez, A.P.; Gallo, L.C. Diabetes Prevention in U.S. Hispanic Adults: A Systematic Review of Culturally Tailored Interventions. *Am. J. Prev. Med.* **2017**, *52*, 519–529. [CrossRef]

118. Vincent, D.; McEwen, M.M.; Hepworth, J.T.; Stump, C.S. The effects of a community-based, culturally tailored diabetes prevention intervention for high-risk adults of Mexican descent. *Diabetes Educ.* **2014**, *40*, 202–213. [CrossRef]

119. Kandula, N.R.; Dave, S.; De Chavez, P.J.; Bharucha, H.; Patel, Y.; Seguil, P.; Kumar, S.; Baker, D.W.; Spring, B.; Siddique, J. Translating a heart disease lifestyle intervention into the community: The South Asian Heart Lifestyle Intervention (SAHELI) study; a randomized control trial. *BMC Public Health* **2015**, *15*, 1064. [CrossRef]

120. Telle-Hjellset, V.; Raberg Kjollesdal, M.K.; Bjorge, B.; Holmboe-Ottesen, G.; Wandel, M.; Birkeland, K.I.; Eriksen, H.R.; Hostmark, A.T. The InnvaDiab-DE-PLAN study: A randomised controlled trial with a culturally adapted education programme improved the risk profile for type 2 diabetes in Pakistani immigrant women. *Br. J. Nutr.* **2013**, *109*, 529–538. [CrossRef]

121. Wijesuriya, M.; Fountoulakis, N.; Guess, N.; Banneheka, S.; Vasantharajah, L.; Gulliford, M.; Viberti, G.; Gnudi, L.; Karalliedde, J. A pragmatic lifestyle modification programme reduces the incidence of predictors of cardio-metabolic disease and dysglycaemia in a young healthy urban South Asian population: A randomised controlled trial. *BMC Med.* **2017**, *15*, 146. [CrossRef]

122. Schulz, A.J.; Israel, B.A.; Mentz, G.B.; Bernal, C.; Caver, D.; DeMajo, R.; Diaz, G.; Gamboa, C.; Gaines, C.; Hoston, B.; et al. Effectiveness of a walking group intervention to promote physical activity and cardiovascular health in predominantly non-Hispanic black and Hispanic urban neighborhoods: Findings from the walk your heart to health intervention. *Health Educ. Behav.* **2015**, *42*, 380–392. [CrossRef] [PubMed]

123. Miller, E.R., 3rd; Cooper, L.A.; Carson, K.A.; Wang, N.Y.; Appel, L.J.; Gayles, D.; Charleston, J.; White, K.; You, N.; Weng, Y.; et al. A Dietary Intervention in Urban African Americans: Results of the "Five Plus Nuts and Beans" Randomized Trial. *Am. J. Prev. Med.* **2016**, *50*, 87–95. [CrossRef] [PubMed]

124. Chang, S.H.; Chen, M.C.; Chien, N.H.; Lin, H.F. Effectiveness of community-based exercise intervention programme in obese adults with metabolic syndrome. *J. Clin. Nurs.* **2016**, *25*, 2579–2589. [CrossRef] [PubMed]

125. Tran, V.D.; James, A.P.; Lee, A.H.; Jancey, J.; Howat, P.A.; Thi Phuong Mai, L. Effectiveness of a Community-Based Physical Activity and Nutrition Behavior Intervention on Features of the Metabolic Syndrome: A Cluster-Randomized Controlled Trial. *Metab. Syndr. Relat. Disord.* **2017**, *15*, 63–71. [CrossRef] [PubMed]

126. Azizi, F.; Mirmiran, P.; Momenan, A.A.; Hadaegh, F.; Habibi Moeini, A.; Hosseini, F.; Zahediasl, S.; Ghanbarian, A.; Hosseinpanah, F. The effect of community-based education for lifestyle intervention on the prevalence of metabolic syndrome and its components: Tehran lipid and glucose study. *Int. J. Endocrinol. Metab.* **2013**, *11*, 145–153. [CrossRef] [PubMed]

127. Khalili, D.; Asgari, S.; Lotfaliany, M.; Zafari, N.; Hadaegh, F.; Momenan, A.A.; Nowroozpoor, A.; Hosseini-Esfahani, F.; Mirmiran, P.; Amiri, P.; et al. Long-Term Effectiveness of a Lifestyle Intervention: A Pragmatic Community Trial to Prevent Metabolic Syndrome. *Am. J. Prev. Med.* **2019**, *56*, 437–446. [CrossRef]

128. Shariful Islam, S.M.; Farmer, A.J.; Bobrow, K.; Maddison, R.; Whittaker, R.; Pfaeffli Dale, L.A.; Lechner, A.; Lear, S.; Eapen, Z.; Niessen, L.W.; et al. Mobile phone text-messaging interventions aimed to prevent cardiovascular diseases (Text2PreventCVD): Systematic review and individual patient data meta-analysis. *Open Heart* **2019**, *6*, e001017. [CrossRef]

129. Kim, E.K.; Kwak, S.H.; Jung, H.S.; Koo, B.K.; Moon, M.K.; Lim, S.; Jang, H.C.; Park, K.S.; Cho, Y.M. The Effect of a Smartphone-Based, Patient-Centered Diabetes Care System in Patients With Type 2 Diabetes: A Randomized, Controlled Trial for 24 Weeks. *Diabetes Care* **2019**, *42*, 3–9. [CrossRef]

130. Ganesan, A.N.; Louise, J.; Horsfall, M.; Bilsborough, S.A.; Hendriks, J.; McGavigan, A.D.; Selvanayagam, J.B.; Chew, D.P. International Mobile-Health Intervention on Physical Activity, Sitting, and Weight: The Stepathlon Cardiovascular Health Study. *J. Am. Coll. Cardiol.* **2016**, *67*, 2453–2463. [CrossRef]

131. Perez, M.V.; Mahaffey, K.W.; Hedlin, H.; Rumsfeld, J.S.; Garcia, A.; Ferris, T.; Balasubramanian, V.; Russo, A.M.; Rajmane, A.; Cheung, L.; et al. Large-Scale Assessment of a Smartwatch to Identify Atrial Fibrillation. *N. Engl. J. Med.* **2019**, *381*, 1909–1917. [CrossRef]

132. Liu, R.; So, L.; Mohan, S.; Khan, N.; King, K.; Quan, H. Cardiovascular risk factors in ethnic populations within Canada: Results from national cross-sectional surveys. *Open Med.* **2010**, *4*, e143–e153. [PubMed]

133. Williams, E.D.; Stamatakis, E.; Chandola, T.; Hamer, M. Physical activity behaviour and coronary heart disease mortality among South Asian people in the UK: An observational longitudinal study. *Heart* **2011**, *97*, 655–659. [CrossRef] [PubMed]

134. Lucas, A.; Murray, E.; Kinra, S. Heath beliefs of UK South Asians related to lifestyle diseases: A review of qualitative literature. *J. Obes.* **2013**, *2013*, 827674. [CrossRef] [PubMed]

135. Huston, P.; McFarlane, B. Health benefits of tai chi: What is the evidence? *Can. Fam. Physician* **2016**, *62*, 881–890. [PubMed]

136. Vlaar, E.M.A.; Nierkens, V.; Nicolaou, M.; Middelkoop, B.J.C.; Busschers, W.B.; Stronks, K.; van Valkengoed, I.G.M. Effectiveness of a targeted lifestyle intervention in primary care on diet and physical activity among South Asians at risk for diabetes: 2-year results of a randomised controlled trial in the Netherlands. *BMJ Open* **2017**, *7*, e012221. [CrossRef] [PubMed]

137. Vogel, L. Broken trust drives native health disparities. *CMAJ* **2015**, *187*, E9–E10. [CrossRef]

138. Kirkendoll, K.; Clark, P.C.; Grossniklaus, D.; Igho-Pemu, P.; Mullis, R.; Dunbar, S.B. Metabolic syndrome in African Americans: Views on making lifestyle changes. *J. Transcult. Nurs.* **2010**, *21*, 104–113. [CrossRef]

9

Linseed Components Are More Effective Than Whole Linseed in Reversing Diet-Induced Metabolic Syndrome in Rats

Siti Raihanah Shafie [1,†], Stephen Wanyonyi [1], Sunil K. Panchal [1] and Lindsay Brown [1,2,*]

1   Functional Foods Research Group, University of Southern Queensland, Toowoomba, QLD 4350, Australia
2   School of Health and Wellbeing, University of Southern Queensland, Toowoomba, QLD 4350, Australia
*   Correspondence: Lindsay.Brown@usq.edu.au
†   Current Address: Department of Nutrition and Dietetics, Faculty of Medicine and Health Sciences, Universiti Putra Malaysia, 43000 UPM Serdang, Selangor, Malaysia.

Abstract: Linseed is a dietary source of plant-based ω–3 fatty acids along with fiber as well as lignans including secoisolariciresinol diglucoside (SDG). We investigated the reversal of signs of metabolic syndrome following addition of whole linseed (5%), defatted linseed (3%), or SDG (0.03%) to either a high-carbohydrate, high-fat or corn starch diet for rats for the final eight weeks of a 16–week protocol. All interventions reduced plasma insulin, systolic blood pressure, inflammatory cell infiltration in heart, ventricular collagen deposition, and diastolic stiffness but had no effect on plasma total cholesterol, nonesterified fatty acids, or triglycerides. Whole linseed did not change the body weight or abdominal fat in obese rats while SDG and defatted linseed decreased abdominal fat and defatted linseed increased lean mass. Defatted linseed and SDG, but not whole linseed, improved heart and liver structure, decreased fat vacuoles in liver, and decreased plasma leptin concentrations. These results show that the individual components of linseed produce greater potential therapeutic responses in rats with metabolic syndrome than whole linseed. We suggest that the reduced responses indicate reduced oral bioavailability of the whole seeds compared to the components.

Keywords: linseed; secoisolariciresinol diglucoside; obesity; blood pressure; high-carbohydrate; high-fat diet

---

1. Introduction

Linseed or flax (*Linum usitatissimum* L.) has widely reported health benefits from studies with many forms including whole or ground seeds, oil, defatted meal, and mucilage extracts [1,2]. Linseed and its components, especially α–linolenic acid (ALA, C18:3n–3) and the lignan, secoisolariciresinol diglucoside (SDG), may protect against metabolic syndrome and cardiovascular disease by lowering blood pressure, reducing blood glucose concentrations, delaying postprandial glucose absorption, and decreasing oxidative stress and inflammation [3–5]. However, the health benefits of introducing linseed into the diet have not been fully defined [6]. In addition, processing including dehusking, crushing, milling, and defatting may increase bioavailability of individual components such as lignans and ALA [7–9]. Furthermore, no studies have compared physiological responses to whole linseed or linseed components using the same animal model or humans.

Linseed has a hard outer layer which may allow the seeds to pass unchanged through the gut and reduce absorption of useful nutrients by the body [10]. Thus, it may be more beneficial to consume ground linseeds over whole linseeds. This implied difference in oral bioavailability could markedly alter the choice of linseed preparations as functional foods, since both whole linseeds and ground linseed flour are readily available. In humans fed muffins with either 30 g whole or ground linseed, or flaxseed oil with 6 g ALA, plasma ALA concentrations were 0.024 mg/mL with whole linseed (not significantly different from control) but increased to 0.031 mg/mL with ground linseed and 0.055 mg/mL with linseed oil, suggesting reduced absorption from whole linseeds [11]. In a randomized, crossover study involving 12 healthy subjects, the bioavailability of enterolignans formed as lignan metabolites in the liver more than tripled after feeding on crushed linseed relative to whole linseed and further increased with milled linseed [8]. In rats following oral administration, SDG was metabolized in the gastrointestinal tract and not absorbed while the oral bioavailability of secoisolariciresinol was about 25% with a half–life within the body following intravenous administration of 4 h [12].

In this study, we evaluated the cardiovascular, liver, and metabolic responses of whole linseed, and two of its components, defatted ground linseed, and SDG–enriched fraction, by using an established model of high-carbohydrate, high-fat diet-fed rats mimicking the human metabolic syndrome [13]. We have compared these results with our earlier study on 3% linseed oil containing ALA, which normalized systolic blood pressure, and improved heart function and glucose tolerance [14]. Measurements included body weight, systolic blood pressure, oral glucose tolerance test, left ventricular diastolic stiffness, histology of the heart and liver, and plasma biochemistry. Doses of the linseed components were chosen so as to be similar to the proportion in whole linseed. Our hypothesis was that whole linseeds and the isolated components would improve cardiovascular, metabolic, and liver changes in diet-induced metabolic syndrome in rats.

2. Materials and Methods

2.1. Rats and Diet

All experimental protocols were approved by the University of Southern Queensland Animal Ethics Committee under the guidelines of the National Health and Medical Research Council of Australia. Male Wistar rats were purchased from Animal Resource Centre, Murdoch, WA, Australia. Rats were housed individually in temperature-controlled, 12 h light/dark conditions in the animal house facility of the University of Southern Queensland. The rats were acclimatized and given free access to water and standard rat powdered food prior to initiation of the protocol diets.

Rats (8–9 weeks old, weighing 330–340 g, $n = 96$) were randomly divided into 8 experimental groups: corn starch diet-fed rats (C; $n = 12$), corn starch diet-fed rats treated with 5% whole linseed in food (CW; $n = 12$), corn starch diet-fed rats treated with 3% defatted ground linseed in food (CD; $n = 12$), corn starch diet-fed rats treated with 0.03% SDG in food (CS; $n = 12$), high-carbohydrate, high-fat diet-fed rats (H; $n = 12$), high-carbohydrate, high-fat diet-fed rats treated with 5% whole linseed in food (HW; $n = 12$), high-carbohydrate, high-fat diet-fed rats treated with 3% defatted ground linseed in food (HD; $n = 12$), and high-carbohydrate, high-fat diet-fed rats treated with 0.03% SDG in food (HS; $n = 12$). Preparation of C and H diets has been described previously [13]. The energy densities of C and H diets were 11.23 kJ/g and 17.83 kJ/g, respectively, with an additional 3.85 kJ/mL in drinking water for fructose intake in high-carbohydrate, high-fat diet-fed rats [13].

Whole linseed- and defatted linseed–supplemented diets were prepared by replacing 5% water with 5% whole linseed (not ground) and 3% water with 3% defatted linseed, respectively, in C and H diets. The whole linseed dose replicated our previous study which used 5% chia seeds in food [15], as the oil composition of chia seed and linseed are similar. Since the oil content of linseed is about 40% [16], the non-oil component, defined here as defatted linseed, is 60% so defatted linseed flour was added at 3% in the food. The SDG-supplemented diets were prepared by adding 0.03% SDG (0.3 g of SDG/kg food) in C and H diets.

The whole linseed, defatted linseed, and SDG diets were administered for 8 weeks starting 8 weeks after the initiation of C or H diet. H, HW, HD, and HS groups were given 25% fructose in drinking water along with the diets for the 16-week duration of the study. Normal drinking water without any supplementation was given to C, CW, CD, and CS rats. Rats were monitored daily for body weight and food and water intakes. Energy intake and food conversion efficiency were calculated based on the food intake and body weight gain [14,15].

Whole linseed was a gift from AustGrains (Moree, NSW, Australia) and was also ground and extracted with n-hexane to produce defatted linseed. SDG (40% purity) was a gift from the Archer Daniels Midland Company (Chicago, IL, USA). The analysis of SDG content was conducted by St. Boniface Hospital Research, Winnipeg, MB, Canada. Total gross energy content of whole linseed, defatted linseed, and SDG samples were measured by bomb calorimetry (XRY-1A Oxygen Bomb calorimeter, Shanghai Changji Geological Instrument Co. Ltd., Shanghai, China) in triplicate. One gram of whole linseed, defatted linseed, or SDG were burnt in compressed oxygen (25 kg/cm^2) in the calorimetric bomb immersed in water. The energy densities for whole linseed, defatted linseed, and SDG were 23.76 kJ/g, 16.98 kJ/g, and 17.48 kJ/g, respectively.

2.2. Measurements in Live Rats

Systolic blood pressure was measured at the end of the protocol under light sedation by intraperitoneal injection with Zoletil (tiletamine 10 mg/kg, zolazepam 10 mg/kg; Virbac, Peakhurst, NSW, Australia). Measurements were performed using an MLT1010 Piezo-Electric Pulse Transducer (ADInstruments, Sydney, NSW, Australia) and an inflatable tail-cuff connected to an MLT844 Physiological Pressure Transducer (ADInstruments) connected to a PowerLab data acquisition unit (ADInstruments) [13].

Oral glucose tolerance tests were performed at the end of the protocol on rats after overnight (12 h) food deprivation. During this time, fructose-supplemented drinking water in H, HW, HD, and HS rats was replaced with tap water. Basal blood glucose concentrations were determined in tail vein blood using Medisense Precision Q.I.D. glucometer (Abbott Laboratories, Bedford, MA, USA). The rats were given 2 g/kg body weight of glucose as a 40% (w/v) aqueous glucose solution via oral gavage. Tail vein blood samples were taken at 30, 60, 90, and 120 min following glucose administration [13].

Dual-energy X-ray absorptiometry (DXA) was performed on all rats after 16 weeks of feeding using a Norland XR36 DXA instrument (Norland Corp., Fort Atkinson, WI, USA). Rats were anesthetized using intraperitoneal injection of Zoletil (tiletamine 10 mg/kg and zolazepam 10 mg/kg) and Ilium Xylazil (xylazine 6 mg/kg; Troy Laboratories, Smithfield, NSW, Australia). Scans were analyzed using the manufacturer's recommended software for use in laboratory animals (Small Subject Analysis Software, version 2.5.3/1.3.1; Norland Corp.) [13]. Visceral adiposity index (%) was calculated based on the abdominal fat content obtained during terminal experiments [15].

2.3. Measurements after Euthanasia

Terminal euthanasia was induced by intraperitoneal injection of Lethabarb (pentobarbitone sodium, 100 mg/kg; Virbac) and ~6 mL blood was immediately drawn from the abdominal aorta, collected into heparinized tubes, and centrifuged for plasma [13]. Hearts ($n = 8$–10) were separated into right ventricle and left ventricle with septum for weighing. Liver and abdominal fat pads (retroperitoneal, epididymal, and omental) were isolated and weighed ($n = 8$–10). Organ weights were normalized to the tibial length and presented in mg of tissue/mm of tibial length [13].

A portion of the heart, liver, small intestine, and large intestine was collected and fixed in 10% neutral buffered formalin for 3 days. Standard histological procedures were followed to process tissues for staining with hematoxylin and eosin or picrosirius red staining [13]. Two slides were prepared per tissue specimen and two random, non-overlapping fields per slide were taken to avoid biased analysis. To examine collagen distribution in the heart, the tissue was stained with picrosirius red stain and imaged using EVOS FL Color Imaging System (version 1.4 (Rev 26059); Advanced Microscopy Group, Bothwell, WA, USA) [14]. Small and large intestine sections were stained with periodic acid-Schiff stain to identify goblet cells [17]. Left ventricular collagen deposition was estimated by analysis with NIH ImageJ software (https://imagej.nih.gov/ij/).

Plasma samples collected during terminal experiments were used to test plasma activities of alanine transaminase and aspartate transaminase, and plasma concentrations of total cholesterol, triglycerides, and nonesterified fatty acids [13].

2.4. Statistical Analysis

All data are presented as mean ± standard error of the mean (SEM). Group data were tested for variance using Bartlett's test. Variables that were not normally distributed were transformed (using log 10 function) prior to statistical analysis. Groups were tested for effects of diet, treatment, and their interactions using two-way analysis of variance. When interaction and/or the main effects were significant, means were compared using Newman-Keuls multiple-comparison post hoc test. All statistical analyses were performed using Prism version 6.00 for Windows (GraphPad Software, San Diego, CA, USA). p-value of < 0.05 was considered as statistically significant.

3. Results

3.1. Dietary Intakes

Food and water intakes were lower in H rats than in C rats but energy intakes were higher in H rats than in C rats (Table 1). There were no differences between food intakes of C, CW, CD, and CS or between H, HW, HD, and HS groups (Table 1). Water intake was unchanged among C, CW, CD, and CS groups and there was no difference in water intake among H, HW, HD, and HS rats (Table 1). Doses of SDG were 31.9 ± 1.3 mg/kg/day and 15.9 ± 0.3 mg/kg/day for CS and HS rats, respectively. Intakes of whole linseed were 4.36 ± 0.14 g/kg/day and 2.51 ± 0.16 g/kg/day for CW and HW rats, respectively, while intakes of defatted linseed were 2.64 ± 0.09 g/kg/day and 1.57 ± 0.04 g/kg/day for CD and HD rats, respectively.

3.2. Body Composition and Organ Weights

Body weight was higher in H rats than in C rats and whole linseed, defatted linseed and SDG did not change body weight in HW, HD, and HS rats, whereas the body weight was higher in CW rats than in C rats, and CS and CD rats had intermediate body weights to C and CW rats (Figure 1A and Table 1). Body weight gain was lower in HS rats compared to H, HW, and HD rats, whereas body weight gain was in the order C=CS>CD>CW among the C diet groups (Table 1). Feed conversion efficiency was higher in H rats than in C rats. Interventions did not change feed conversion efficiency in H diet-fed rats (HW, HD, and HS rats), whereas whole linseed increased the feed conversion efficiency in CW rats with no change in CS and CD rats (Table 1). Bone mineral content was higher in H rats than in C rats. None of the interventions changed bone mineral content in C diet groups (CW, CD, and CS), whereas HD rats showed reduction in this parameter compared to H, HW, and HS rats (Table 1). Lean mass did not differ between C and H rats. CW, CD, and HD rats had higher lean mass; CS, H, and HS rats had lower lean mass, whereas C and HW had intermediate lean mass (Table 1). H rats had higher fat mass compared to all C diet groups (C, CW, CD, and CS rats). HD rats had lower fat mass compared to H and HW rats, whereas HS rats had fat mass intermediate to H and HD rats (Table 1). Abdominal circumference and visceral adiposity index were unchanged in CW, CD, and CS rats compared to C rats, whereas these parameters were increased in H rats compared to C rats (Table 1). HD rats had lower abdominal circumference compared to H and HW rats, whereas visceral adiposity index was higher in HW rats compared to HS and HD rats (Table 1).

Table 1. Dietary intakes, body composition, and organ wet weights.

Variables	C	CW	CD	CS	H	HW	HD	HS	Diet	Treatment	Interaction
										p Value	
Food intake, g/day	35.0 ± 0.6 a	34.6 ± 1.2 a	33.9 ± 1.2 a	35.5 ± 0.8 a	25.2 ± 0.6 b	23.4 ± 0.6 b	24.4 ± 0.4 b	26.3 ± 0.4 b	<0.0001	0.06	0.59
Water intake, mL/day	28.7 ± 1.8 a	30.7 ± 2.1 a	32.7 ± 0.9 a	30.4 ± 2.7 a	25.6 ± 1.0 b	26.9 ± 0.4 ab	25.7 ± 1.1 b	25.2 ± 1.0 b	<0.0001	0.54	0.61
Energy intake, kJ/day	392 ± 7 b	433 ± 14 b	397 ± 14 b	420 ± 13 b	552 ± 13 a	561 ± 14 a	542 ± 9 a	555 ± 8 a	<0.0001	0.11	0.37
Body weight gained (week 8–16), %	7.4 ± 1.0 d	18.2 ± 0.8 b	13.2 ± 1.6 c	9.1 ± 1.7 d	23.3 ± 0.9 a	23.4 ± 0.6 a	22.7 ± 1.4 a	18.9 ± 1.3 b	<0.0001	<0.0001	0.0006
Final body weight (week 16)	375 ± 4 a	432 ± 6 b	400 ± 5 a	392 ± 10 a	526 ± 10 c	539 ± 10 c	521 ± 8 c	519 ± 11 c	< 0.0001	0.0004	0.06
Feed conversion efficiency, %	1.8 ± 0.2 c	4.9 ± 0.3 b	3.2 ± 0.4 c	2.6 ± 0.5 c	9.6 ± 0.6 a	9.2 ± 0.6 a	9.0 ± 0.6 a	8.1 ± 0.7 a	<0.0001	0.004	0.005
Bone mineral content, g	12.0 ± 0.4 c	12.1 ± 0.2 c	11.9 ± 0.2 c	13.2 ± 0.6 c	16.5 ± 0.4 a	17.3 ± 0.7 a	15.3 ± 0.6 b	16.8 ± 0.4 a	<0.0001	0.024	0.20
Total fat mass, g	98 ± 16 c	103 ± 7 c	77 ± 6 c	122 ± 16 c	256 ± 21 a	253 ± 21 a	189 ± 22 b	227 ± 7 ab	<0.0001	0.014	0.25
Total lean mass, g	276 ± 14 ab	317 ± 7 a	309 ± 5 a	267 ± 9 b	268 ± 14 b	277 ± 11 ab	312 ± 15 a	246 ± 7 b	0.035	<0.0001	0.24
Abdominal circumference, cm	18.4 ± 0.2 c	19.1 ± 0.2 c	19.1 ± 0.1 c	18.9 ± 0.2 c	23.0 ± 0.2 a	23.6 ± 0.4 a	21.2 ± 0.2 b	22.7 ± 0.2 a	<0.0001	0.016	0.19
Visceral adiposity index, %	4.9 ± 0.4 d	4.7 ± 0.3 d	4.2 ± 0.1 d	4.8 ± 0.6 d	9.6 ± 0.7 ab	10.4 ± 0.9 a	7.3 ± 0.5 c	8.5 ± 0.4 bc	<0.0001	0.007	0.09
Retroperitoneal fat, mg/mm *	189 ± 18 c	179 ± 18 c	151 ± 20 c	194 ± 31 c	531 ± 41 a	554 ± 59 a	407 ± 31 ab	469 ± 31 ab	<0.0001	0.55	0.34
Epididymal fat, mg/mm *	89 ± 10 d	98 ± 8 d	74 ± 5 d	112 ± 20 cd	259 ± 17 a	278 ± 28 a	154 ± 16 c	211 ± 11 b	<0.0001	0.29	0.037
Omental fat, mg/mm *	114 ± 15 c	124 ± 9 c	102 ± 7 c	102 ± 13 c	240 ± 25 ab	280 ± 18 a	198 ± 14 b	207 ± 8 b	<0.0001	0.013	0.26
Total abdominal fat, mg/mm *	392 ± 39 d	401 ± 35 d	308 ± 36 d	408 ± 63 d	1031 ± 79 ab	1113 ± 105 a	683 ± 92 c	887 ± 45 b	<0.0001	0.23	0.18
Liver, mg/mm *	201 ± 5 b	213 ± 12 b	216 ± 7 b	213 ± 8 b	327 ± 12 a	337 ± 15 a	310 ± 8 a	306 ± 9 a	<0.0001	0.32	0.22

Values are expressed as mean ± SEM, n = 8–12. Means with different superscripts (a, b, c, or d) differ, $p < 0.05$. C, corn starch diet-fed rats; CW, corn starch diet-fed rats treated with whole linseed; CD, corn starch diet-fed rats treated with defatted linseed; CS, corn starch diet-fed rats treated with secoisolariciresinol diglucoside (SDG); H, high-carbohydrate, high-fat diet-fed rats; HW, high-carbohydrate, high-fat diet-fed rats treated with whole linseed; HD, high-carbohydrate, high-fat diet-fed rats treated with defatted linseed; and HS, high-carbohydrate, high-fat diet-fed rats treated with SDG. * Denotes the values that were normalized against tibial length and presented as tissue weight in mg/mm of tibial length.

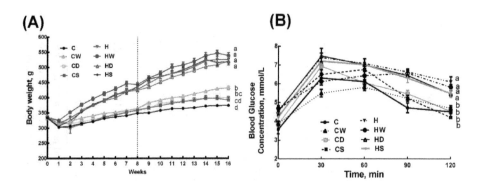

Figure 1. Effects of whole linseed, defatted linseed, and secoisolariciresinol diglucoside (SDG) on (**A**) body weight and (**B**) oral glucose tolerance test. The vertical dotted grid line in (**A**) at week 8 represents the start of treatment for rats. Data are presented as mean ± SEM, n = 10–12. End-point means with different letters (a, b, c, or d) are significantly different, $p < 0.05$. C, corn starch diet-fed rats; CW, corn starch diet-fed rats treated with whole linseed; CD, corn starch diet-fed rats treated with defatted linseed; CS, corn starch diet-fed rats treated with SDG; H, high-carbohydrate, high-fat diet-fed rats; HW, high-carbohydrate, high-fat diet-fed rats treated with whole linseed; HD, high-carbohydrate, high-fat diet-fed rats treated with defatted linseed; HS, high-carbohydrate, high-fat diet-fed rats treated with SDG.

Retroperitoneal, epididymal, and omental fat pads were higher in H rats than in C rats. CW, CD, and CS rats had no difference in these fat pads and total abdominal fat compared to C rats. SDG decreased epididymal fat in HS rats, whereas retroperitoneal, omental, and total abdominal fats were unchanged compared to H rats. Whole linseed did not change the individual fat pads in HW rats compared to H rats, whereas defatted linseed lowered retroperitoneal, epididymal, and total abdominal fat in HD rats compared to H rats (Table 1). Liver wet weights were higher in H rats than in C rats. Whole linseed, defatted linseed, and SDG treatment did not change liver wet weight compared to C or H rats (Table 1).

3.3. Metabolic Parameters

During oral glucose tolerance test, H rats showed higher basal blood glucose concentrations than C rats. Similarly, H rats showed higher 120 min glucose concentration (Figure 1B). Area under the curve for glucose tolerance test was higher in H rats compared to C, CW, CD, and CS rats. HW, HD, and HS rats were similar to H rats in area under the curve for glucose tolerance test (Table 2). Plasma total cholesterol concentrations were not different among all groups (Table 2). Plasma nonesterified fatty acids and triglyceride concentrations were higher in H rats compared to C rats, and these were unchanged with whole linseed, defatted linseed, or SDG treatment in any of the groups compared to their diet respective controls (Table 2). Plasma insulin concentrations were higher in H rats compared to C rats. HW, HD, and HS rats had lower plasma insulin concentrations compared to H rats, whereas plasma insulin concentrations were higher in CW, CD, and CS rats compared to C rats (Table 2). Plasma leptin concentrations were higher in H rats compared to C rats. CW, CD, and CS rats had no change in plasma leptin concentrations compared to C rats. Whole linseed did not change plasma leptin concentrations, whereas both SDG and defatted linseed decreased plasma leptin concentrations (Table 2).

Table 2. Metabolic, cardiovascular, and liver parameters.

Variables	C	CW	CD	CS	H	HW	HD	HS	p Value Diet	p Value Treatment	p Value Interaction
Area under the curve, mmol/L×min	636 ± 19 bc	625 ± 14 c	680 ± 14 b	687 ± 20 b	794 ± 13 a	735 ± 17 ab	770 ± 17 a	765 ± 25 a	<0.0001	0.037	0.09
Plasma total cholesterol, mmol/L	1.5 ± 0.05 a	1.3 ± 0.10 a	1.4 ± 0.10 a	1.6 ± 0.06 a	1.6 ± 0.04 a	1.5 ± 0.10 a	1.6 ± 0.10 a	1.6 ± 0.06 a	0.09	0.023	0.39
Plasma nonesterified fatty acids, mmol/L	0.9 ± 0.2 b	1.5 ± 0.2 b	1.5 ± 0.2 b	1.4 ± 0.2 b	4.3 ± 0.6 a	4.0 ± 0.3 a	3.7 ± 0.4 a	3.7 ± 0.5 a	<0.0001	0.86	0.31
Plasma triglycerides, mmol/L	0.4 ± 0.06 b	0.4 ± 0.10 b	0.5 ± 0.01 b	0.4 ± 0.06 b	1.6 ± 0.30 a	1.5 ± 0.20 a	1.3 ± 0.20 a	1.3 ± 0.20 a	<0.0001	0.68	0.68
Plasma insulin, μmol/L	1.3 ± 0.01 e	2.9 ± 0.05 c	1.7 ± 0.05 d	1.7 ± 0.01 d	7.7 ± 0.09 a	5.9 ± 0.12 b	5.8 ± 0.04 b	6.0 ± 0.11 b	<0.0001	<0.0001	<0.0001
Plasma leptin, μmol/L	3.2 ± 0.40 d	4.2 ± 0.06 d	3.9 ± 0.03 d	2.1 ± 0.62 d	12.3 ± 1.54 a	13.1 ± 0.03 a	10.2 ± 0.08 b	6.3 ± 0.97 c	<0.0001	<0.0001	0.005
Heart, mg/mm *	22.0 ± 1.0 c	25.4 ± 0.7 bc	25.3 ± 0.9 bc	21.5 ± 0.4 c	26.8 ± 1.1 b	31.5 ± 2.1 a	26.9 ± 0.9 b	23.6 ± 0.9 bc	<0.0001	<0.0001	0.18
Left ventricle + septum, mg/mm *	18.1 ± 0.7 b	21.6 ± 0.6 b	20.8 ± 0.8 b	17.2 ± 0.3 b	20.8 ± 0.8 b	27.1 ± 1.8 a	22.3 ± 0.8 b	18.5 ± 0.8 b	0.0002	<0.0001	0.09
Right ventricle, mg/mm *	4.0 ± 0.4	4.5 ± 0.4	4.5 ± 0.3	4.4 ± 0.2	6.3 ± 1.7	5.8 ± 0.4	4.7 ± 0.2	5.0 ± 0.1	0.03	0.79	0.53
Systolic blood pressure, mmHg	128 ± 3 bc	129 ± 2 bc	120 ± 3 c	133 ± 2 b	148 ± 2 a	134 ± 2 b	129 ± 5 bc	133 ± 3 b	<0.0001	0.026	0.0004
Diastolic stiffness constant (κ)	23.0 ± 0.4 bc	24.2 ± 0.7 abc	21.9 ± 0.3 c	23.0 ± 0.8 bc	26.6 ± 0.9 a	25.1 ± 0.5 ab	23.7 ± 1.3 bc	22.0 ± 0.5 c	0.034	0.001	0.004
Plasma alanine transaminase, U/L	26.8 ± 2.5 b	30.9 ± 3.8 b	28.3 ± 2.0 b	23.2 ± 1.6 b	33.7 ± 1.5 a	27.8 ± 2.5 ab	33.8 ± 1.5 a	33.6 ± 1.7 a	0.017	0.74	0.017
Plasma aspartate transaminase, U/L	64.6 ± 4.6 a	66.4 ± 5.9 a	66.3 ± 2.8 a	61.6 ± 1.8 a	68.8 ± 2.6 a	61.6 ± 3.7 a	67.5 ± 2.9 a	69.6 ± 6.8 a	0.52	0.84	0.38
Left ventricle collagen deposition, %	6.51 ± 1.0 b	6.57 ± 1.1 b	5.29 ± 0.2 b	4.96 ± 0.5 b	16.1 ± 3.7 a	13.9 ± 1.3 a	8.2 ± 0.5 b	8.3 ± 1.0 b	<0.0001	<0.0001	<0.0001
Left ventricle inflammatory cells, n	9.0 ± 2.5 b	7.5 ± 1.2 b	10.5 ± 1.6 b	12.3 ± 1.1 b	60.0 ± 4.0 a	10.8 ± 1.4 b	12.3 ± 1.1 b	10.8 ± 1.1 b	<0.0001	<0.0001	<0.0001
Liver fat vacuoles, n	4.0 ± 0.6 c	10.8 ± 1.6 c	4.0 ± 1.2 c	3.5 ± 1.0 c	75.0 ± 4.6 a	39.7 ± 4.4 b	3.5 ± 1.0 c	1.5 ± 0.9 c	<0.0001	<0.0001	<0.0001
Ileum goblet cells, n	91.5 ± 6.0 c	82.3 ± 6.1 d	107.3 ± 2.1 abc	100.3 ± 2.5 cd	124.3 ± 3.4 ab	118.3 ± 8.6 ab	94.8 ± 3.4 bc	110.8 ± 4.4 ab	0.0005	0.3224	0.0004
Colon goblet cells, n	97.5 ± 2.9 c	42 ± 5.1 d	84.5 ± 2.6 c	90.8 ± 5.2 c	78.8 ± 3.9 c	135.3 ± 2.3 b	203.8 ± 14.5 a	131.3 ± 7.3 b	<0.0001	<0.0001	<0.0001

Values are expressed as mean ± SEM, n = 8–12. Means with different superscripts (a, b, c, d, or e) differ, $p < 0.05$. C, corn starch diet-fed rats; CW, corn starch diet-fed rats treated with whole linseed; CD, corn starch diet-fed rats treated with defatted linseed; CS, corn starch diet-fed rats treated with secoisolariciresinol diglucoside (SDG); H, high-carbohydrate, high-fat diet-fed rats; HW, high-carbohydrate, high-fat diet-fed rats treated with whole linseed; HD, high-carbohydrate, high-fat diet-fed rats treated with defatted linseed; and HS, high-carbohydrate, high-fat diet-fed rats treated with SDG. For histological scoring, values are expressed as mean ± SEM, n = 4. * Denotes the values that were normalized against tibial length and presented as tissue weight in mg/mm of tibial length.

3.4. Cardiovascular, Liver, and Gut Parameters

Heart wet weights were higher in H rats compared to C rats. CW, CD, and CS rats showed no difference in heart weight compared to C rats. HW rats had higher heart weight compared to H rats, whereas HS and HD rats had similar heart weight to H rats (Table 2). H rats had higher systolic blood pressure than C rats. Whole linseed, defatted linseed, and SDG reduced blood pressure in HW, HD, and HS rats, respectively, compared to H rats, whereas these interventions did not change systolic blood pressure in CW, CD, and CS rats compared to C rats (Table 2). H rats had higher ventricular diastolic stiffness than C rats. SDG and defatted linseed reduced diastolic stiffness in HS and HD rats, respectively, compared to H rats, whereas none of the interventions reduced diastolic stiffness in CW, CD, or CS rats compared to C rats (Table 2).

H rats showed increased infiltration of inflammatory cells (Figure 2E) and greater interstitial collagen deposition (Figure 3E) as compared to other groups (Figure 2; Figure 3; Table 2). HW, HD, and HS rats had reduced infiltration of inflammatory cells (Figure 2F–H) and ventricular collagen deposition (Figure 3F–H; Table 2) compared to H rats.

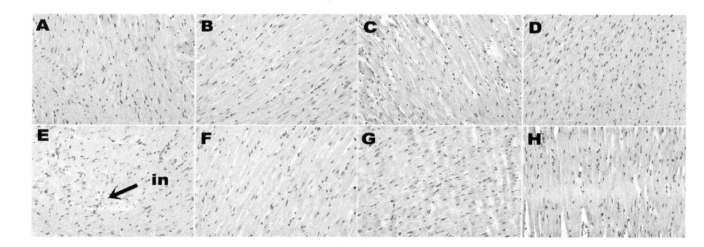

Figure 2. Hematoxylin and eosin staining of left ventricle showing infiltration of inflammatory cells (magnification ×20; shown by arrow) in rats fed corn starch diet-fed rats (**A**), corn starch diet-fed rats treated with whole linseed (**B**), corn starch diet-fed rats treated with defatted linseed (**C**), corn starch diet-fed rats treated with SDG (**D**), high-carbohydrate, high-fat diet-fed rats (**E**), high-carbohydrate, high-fat diet-fed rats treated with whole linseed (**F**), high-carbohydrate, high-fat diet-fed rats treated with defatted linseed (**G**), and high-carbohydrate, high-fat diet-fed rats treated with SDG (**H**). Inflammatory cells are marked as "in".

H rats had higher plasma alanine transaminase activity than C rats. None of the treatments in this study changed the plasma activities of alanine transaminase or aspartate transaminase (Table 2). Staining of liver sections showed increased lipid deposition and inflammatory cell infiltration in H rats (Figure 4E) compared to C rats (Figure 4A). HW (Figure 4F), HD (Figure 4G), and HS (Figure 4H) rats showed decreased inflammatory cell infiltration compared to H rats. HW rats showed some reduction in liver lipid deposition (Figure 4F), whereas HD (Figure 4G) and HS (Figure 4H) rats showed minimal lipid deposition (Table 2). CW (Figure 4B), CS (Figure 4C), and CD (Figure 4D) rats showed no changes in the liver in inflammatory cell infiltration and lipid deposition compared to C rats (Figure 4A; Table 2).

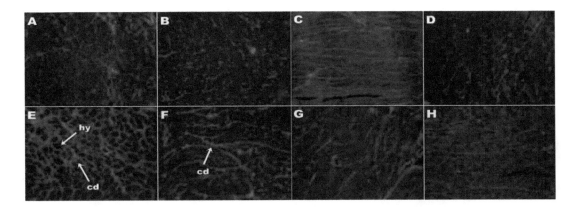

Figure 3. Picrosirius red staining of left ventricular interstitial collagen deposition (magnification ×20; shown by arrows) in rats fed corn starch diet-fed rats (**A**), corn starch diet-fed rats treated with whole linseed (**B**), corn starch diet-fed rats treated with defatted linseed (**C**), corn starch diet-fed rats treated with SDG (**D**), high-carbohydrate, high-fat diet-fed rats (**E**), high-carbohydrate, high-fat diet-fed rats treated with whole linseed (**F**), high-carbohydrate, high-fat diet-fed rats treated with defatted linseed (**G**), and high-carbohydrate, high-fat diet-fed rats treated with SDG (**H**). Collagen deposition is marked as "cd" and hypertrophied cardiomyocytes are marked as "hy".

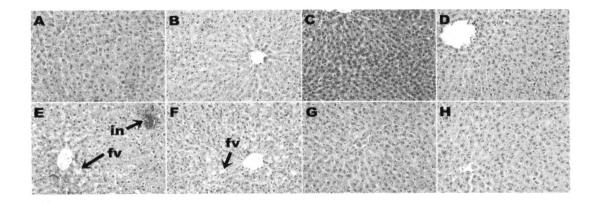

Figure 4. Hematoxylin and eosin staining of liver showing fat vacuoles and infiltration of inflammatory cells (magnification ×20; shown by arrows) in corn starch diet-fed rats (**A**), corn starch diet-fed rats treated with whole linseed (**B**), corn starch diet-fed rats treated with defatted linseed (**C**), corn starch diet-fed rats treated with SDG (**D**), high-carbohydrate, high-fat diet-fed rats (**E**), high-carbohydrate, high-fat diet-fed rats treated with whole linseed (**F**), high-carbohydrate, high-fat diet-fed rats treated with defatted linseed (**G**), and high-carbohydrate, high-fat diet-fed rats treated with SDG (**H**). Fat vacuoles are marked as "fv" and inflammatory cells are marked as "in".

Histological analyses of small intestine showed more goblet cells in H rats (Figure 5E) compared to C rats (Figure 5A; Table 2). HW (Figure 5F) and HS (Figure 5H) rats showed no change in the number of goblet cells in the small intestine, whereas HD rats (Figure 5G) showed reduction in the number of goblet cells (Table 2) compared to H rats (Figure 5E). Colon from C rats (Figure 6A) and H rats (Figure 6E) showed no difference in the number of goblet cells (Table 2). HW (Figure 6F), HD (Figure 6G), and HS (Figure 6H) rats showed an increase in the number of goblet cells in colons compared to H rats (Figure 6E; Table 2).

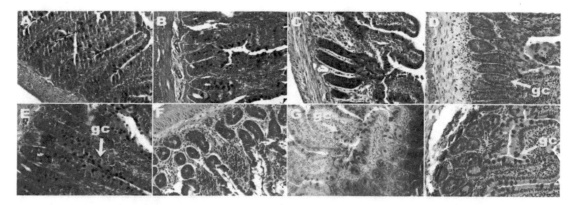

Figure 5. Periodic acid-Schiff staining of ileum showing goblet cells (magnification ×20; shown by arrows) in corn starch diet-fed rats (**A**), corn starch diet-fed rats treated with whole linseed (**B**), corn starch diet-fed rats treated with defatted linseed (**C**), corn starch diet-fed rats treated with SDG (**D**), high-carbohydrate, high-fat diet-fed rats (**E**), high-carbohydrate, high-fat diet-fed rats treated with whole linseed (**F**), high-carbohydrate, high-fat diet-fed rats treated with defatted linseed (**G**), and high-carbohydrate, high-fat diet-fed rats treated with SDG (**H**). Goblet cells are marked as "gc".

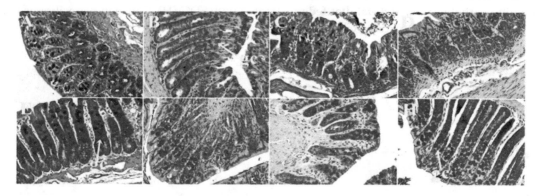

Figure 6. Periodic acid-Schiff staining of colon showing goblet cells (magnification ×20; shown by arrows) in corn starch diet-fed rats (**A**), corn starch diet-fed rats treated with whole linseed (**B**), corn starch diet-fed rats treated with defatted linseed (**C**), corn starch diet-fed rats treated with SDG (**D**), high-carbohydrate, high-fat diet-fed rats (**E**), high-carbohydrate, high-fat diet-fed rats treated with whole linseed (**F**), high-carbohydrate, high-fat diet-fed rats treated with defatted linseed (**G**), and high-carbohydrate, high-fat diet-fed rats treated with SDG (**H**). Goblet cells are marked as "gc".

4. Discussion

Metabolic syndrome, including obesity, hypertension, impaired glucose tolerance, insulin resistance, dyslipidemia, and fatty liver, is a major risk factor for cardiovascular disease and type 2 diabetes, and may be attenuated by functional foods [18]. Many trials have been conducted to determine the responses to linseed and its components in humans with obesity, hypertension, or diabetes [19,20]. However, few trials have compared responses to individual components of linseed in patients with metabolic syndrome or in appropriate rat models. Rats fed a diet with increased content of fructose, sucrose, and saturated and *trans* fatty acids developed signs of metabolic syndrome in humans, especially abdominal obesity, hypertension, impaired glucose and leptin, dyslipidemia, and diminished cardiac function [13–15]. Using this rat model of diet-induced metabolic syndrome, we have now compared responses to whole linseed, defatted linseed flour, and SDG and included comparison with an earlier study on ALA from linseed oil with the same rat model [14].

Our results show that addition of defatted linseed or SDG improved metabolic parameters and the structure and function of the heart and liver, as we previously showed with linseed oil [14]. In contrast, the only metabolic parameter to be improved by whole linseed was plasma insulin concentration, while body weight, abdominal fat pads, and liver parameters were unchanged. Although whole linseed decreased systolic blood pressure, left ventricular diastolic stiffness, infiltration of inflammatory cells, and collagen deposition in the heart, these changes were to a lesser extent than defatted linseed, showing reduced or absent responses in cardiovascular, hepatic structure and function, adiposity, lipid, and glucose parameters. We suggest that the reason for these reduced responses to whole linseed is that the oral bioavailability of ALA, fiber, and SDG when presented as whole linseed is reduced, leading to reduced responses to the whole seeds, even though the components are effective when given individually. This could be tested in further studies by measurement of the pharmacokinetics of linseed components such as ALA, fiber, or SDG in rats fed an obesogenic diet.

In this study with whole linseeds and their components in rats, we were unable to show decreases in body weight or abdominal circumference with whole linseed treatment in diet-induced obese rats. In contrast, we showed decreased total fat and abdominal fat in rats treated with defatted linseed or SDG. We have previously shown that ALA from linseed decreased obesity in the same diet-induced rat model of metabolic syndrome [14]. Other studies also showed decreased obesity with linseed products: young rats fed a linseed flour intervention for the first 90 days showed higher lean mass, lower fat mas, and a smaller adipocyte area [21] and linseed dietary fiber reduced apparent energy and fat digestibility leading to decreased abdominal fat and body weight [22]. Linseed contains 20 to 30% globulin-rich proteins with a high content of arginine [23,24] which has been associated with increases in lean mass [25,26] thereby providing a possible mechanism for lean mass increase as well as fat mass decrease [27]. In high-fat diet-fed mice, SDG decreased abdominal fat and body weight by inducing adiponectin expression at a much higher dose of 0.5 or 1% in diet [28] and inhibiting adipogenesis at a dose of 50 mg/kg/day [29]. Furthermore, the SDG metabolites, enterolactone and enterodiol, induced adiponectin expression, adipogenesis, and lipid uptake in 3T3-L1 adipocytes [28,30]. We are not aware of any studies with whole linseeds in obese rats, but freshly ground flaxseed did not change body weight or blood pressure in non-obese WKY or SHR rats and in cyclosporine-induced hypertensive rats [31,32].

These rodent results translate to some extent to humans. Linseed products reduced human obesity in randomized controlled trials, shown by a meta-analysis of 45 of these trials with 2561 subjects aged 25.6–67.0 years including 21 trials on milled or ground linseed, one on defatted linseed, 18 on linseed oil, and five on linseed lignan but none on whole linseeds [19]. This meta-analysis showed that supplementation of linseed products for more than 12 weeks in individuals with a body mass index higher than 27 kg/m^2 reduced body weight by an average of 0.99 kg, body mass index by an average of 0.30 kg/m^2, and waist circumference by an average of 0.80 cm [19]. These changes are relatively small, approximating 1% of these parameters in a 1.80 m tall person weighing 88 kg to give a body mass index of 27 kg/m^2 fitting the definition of obesity with waist circumference more than 94 cm. Differences of around 1% as in the above meta-analysis on human trials would not be statistically significant in our group of 12 rats treated for eight weeks. In addition, data from the US National Health and Nutrition Examination Survey 2001-10 provided epidemiological evidence that urinary enterolactone is inversely associated with obesity in adult males [33].

Linseed products also reduced blood pressure in rodents. Both linseed oil and SDG prevented the increase in systolic blood pressure in rats with metabolic syndrome induced by feeding with 30% fructose, likely due to decreased oxidative stress [34]. In deoxycorticosterone acetate (DOCA)-salt hypertensive rats, linseed lignan concentrate lowered blood pressure, and improved antioxidant status, serum electrolytes, and lipid profiles [35]. A lignan-enriched linseed powder reduced blood pressure, body weight, and fat accumulation, and improved lipid profiles in rats fed a high-fat and high-fructose diet [36]. In humans with peripheral artery disease, ground linseed (30 g/day) for 12 months decreased central systolic and diastolic blood pressure by 10 and 6 mmHg, respectively, with corresponding changes in plasma oxylipins [37]. Meta-analysis of 15 randomized controlled trials with linseed components on hypertension have shown reductions in both systolic and diastolic blood pressure of 3.10 and 2.62 mmHg, respectively, in a subset of trials of 12 weeks or longer, but there were no effects with linseed oil or SDG on systolic blood pressure [20].

Hyperlipidemia is a key component of metabolic syndrome. In rats fed a high-fat diet, a lignan-enriched linseed powder improved the plasma lipid profile as well as decreasing body weight, visceral fat accumulation, and blood pressure [36]. In rats fed with lard and cholic acid, treatment with powdered linseed or defatted linseed for eight weeks did not change plasma cholesterol, low-density lipoproteins (LDL) cholesterol, or triglyceride concentrations but decreased liver fat and cholesterol and increased bacterial glycolytic activity in the distal intestine [38]. Intervention with linseed powder (30 g/day for 40 days) produced small but significant decreases in body weight and decreased plasma cholesterol, LDL, and triglyceride concentrations in 35 hyperlipidemic subjects [39]. Furthermore, linseed may reduce plasma concentrations of the inflammatory marker, C-reactive protein, in subjects with a body mass index (BMI) > 30 kg/m^2 [40]; this meta-analysis included trials on ground linseed, flour, oil, and ALA-enriched products, but there were no studies on whole linseeds.

The combination of ALA, dietary fiber, and lignans in linseed may be useful in preventing and treating diabetes, especially in rodent models [41]. SDG and its enteric metabolite enterodiol affected glucose transport and adipogenesis by regulating the transcription of adiponectin, leptin, and peroxisome proliferator-activated receptor gamma (PPARγ) genes [28]. By altering the expression profile of adiponectin and leptin, SDG may increase rates of fatty acid oxidation and mediate an insulin-sensitizing effect [42]. Although these findings are consistent with the decrease in plasma insulin and leptin observed in our study, it is not clear why glucose tolerance was only improved in the whole linseed group.

Thus, our results are broadly consistent with both rodent and human studies on individual signs of metabolic syndrome and individual components of linseeds. However, these literature studies do not compare results in the range of signs in metabolic syndrome in the same subject groups or rodent models, nor allow comparison of linseed components. Furthermore, no study has administered whole linseeds, so the comparison between whole linseeds and components has not been previously made.

Gastrointestinal changes could play a role in the metabolic responses to ground or defatted linseed, but studies on whole linseeds have not been reported. Linseed is a rich source of dietary fiber (35–45%) consisting of soluble and insoluble fiber in ratios that vary between 1:4 and 2:3 [43]. Rats on a control diet fed 10% dietary fiber from linseeds showed decreased body weight with decreased fat digestibility, which was greater when the proportion of viscous dietary fiber was increased [22]. In obese rats fed a high-fat diet with cholic acid, ground linseed prevented an increase in intestinal glucosidase activity while defatted ground linseed increased mucosal disaccharidase activities; both forms decreased fat absorption but only the defatted product decreased liver expression of PPARα, showing important differences between defatted and whole ground linseed [38]. Fermentation of dietary fiber by colonic microflora generates short-chain fatty acids such as acetate, propionate, and butyrate which decrease signs of metabolic syndrome and other gastrointestinal disorders [44]. High-fermentable fiber of milled whole linseed led to increased Enterobacteriaceae diversity in mice which was associated with an increased body weight compared to milled defatted linseed [45]. In healthy, non-obese adult men given 0.3 g/kg/day ground linseed for one week, enterolignan production was increased, but there were no changes in fecal metabolome or dominant bacterial communities [46]. Thus, the responses to defatted linseed in contrast to whole linseed could be produced by the increased bioavailable fiber content acting on the colonic microflora and liver, and possibly on goblet cell function. Goblet cells in the gastrointestinal tract are responsible for secretion of mucus, but the location of the goblet cells determines whether secretion is continuous or upon stimulation to form the protective inner colonic mucosal layer [47]. Mice fed a high-fat diet showed increased goblet cells in the duodenum [48]. Dietary intervention with whole ground linseed increased goblet cells, mucus secretion, and concentrations of short-chain fatty acids in healthy male mice which should be beneficial [49]. This increase could be due to an increase in fiber [50], consistent with our results in rats fed defatted linseed. However, the intervention with whole ground linseed worsened the damage by dextran sodium sulfate suggesting a role for context in interventions [49], but similar studies in high-fat diet-fed rats are not available. The different results in rats fed whole linseed, SDG, and defatted linseed suggest that these components of linseed produce different responses in goblet cells in the colon, possibly due to different types of goblet cells, requiring detailed research to define adequately.

The marked differences in responses between whole linseeds and the components of linseeds could be due to toxic compounds present in the whole linseed, such as the cyanogenic glycosides, leading to cyanide production by the activity of bacterial glucosidases in the large intestine [51]. However, ingestion of 30 g linseed by humans produced small and transient increases in plasma thiocyanate concentrations, indicating a low bioavailability of the cyanide from cyanogenic glycosides such as linustatin [52]. Thus, we suggest that a more likely explanation for the lower responses in whole linseeds is a markedly reduced oral bioavailability of the bioactive components when whole linseeds are given.

5. Conclusions

This study has highlighted the importance of using a single animal model to investigate the bioactivities of individual functional foods contained in linseed. We hypothesized that whole linseeds and the isolated components would improve cardiovascular, metabolic, and liver changes. We showed that the responses to the whole linseeds were reduced compared to defatted linseed, SDG, and ALA. We suggest that a markedly reduced bioavailability of these components from the whole linseeds underlies the reduced responses. Thus, our hypothesis was substantiated by measurements of physiological responses to the components of linseeds. However, ALA, defatted linseed, or SDG are likely to be better therapeutic agents in metabolic syndrome than whole linseeds.

Author Contributions: Conceptualization, S.K.P. and L.B.; Formal analysis, S.R.S. and S.W.; Investigation, S.R.S. and S.W.; Methodology, S.R.S., S.W., and S.K.P.; Project administration, S.K.P.; Resources, L.B.; Supervision, S.K.P. and L.B. All authors read and approved the final manuscript.

Acknowledgments: We thank Brian Bynon (School of Veterinary Science, The University of Queensland, Gatton, QLD, Australia) for helping with plasma analyses for this study. SDG (40% purity) was a gift from Archer Daniels Midland Company (Chicago, IL, USA). We thank St. Boniface Hospital Research (Winnipeg, MB, Canada) for providing SDG and its analysis. We also thank AustGrains (Moree, NSW, Australia) for providing linseed for this study.

References

1.   Goyal, A.; Sharma, V.; Upadhyay, N.; Gill, S.; Sihag, M. Flax and flaxseed oil: An ancient medicine & modern functional food. *J. Food Sci. Technol.* **2014**, *51*, 1633–1653. [CrossRef]
2.   Shim, Y.Y.; Gui, B.; Arnison, P.G.; Wang, Y.; Reaney, M.J.T. Flaxseed (*Linum usitatissimum* L.) bioactive compounds and peptide nomenclature: A review. *Trends Food Sci. Technol.* **2014**, *38*, 5–20. [CrossRef]
3.   Parikh, M.; Netticadan, T.; Pierce, G.N. Flaxseed: Its bioactive components and their cardiovascular benefits. *Am. J. Physiol. Heart Circ. Physiol.* **2018**, *314*, H146–H159. [CrossRef]
4.   Shafie, S.R.; Poudyal, H.; Panchal, S.K.; Brown, L. Linseed as a functional food for the management of obesity. In *Omega-3 Fatty Acids: Keys to Nutritional Health*; Hegde, M.V., Zanwar, A.A., Adekar, S.P., Eds.; Springer International Publishing: Cham, Switzerland, 2016; pp. 173–187.
5.   Imran, M.; Ahmad, N.; Anjum, F.M.; Khan, M.K.; Mushtaq, Z.; Nadeem, M.; Hussain, S. Potential protective properties of flax lignan secoisolariciresinol diglucoside. *Nutr. J.* **2015**, *14*, 71. [CrossRef]
6.   Parikh, M.; Pierce, G.N. Dietary flaxseed: What we know and don't know about its effects on cardiovascular disease. *Can. J. Physiol. Pharmacol.* **2018**, *97*, 75–81. [CrossRef]
7.   Oomah, B.D.; Mazza, G. Effect of dehulling on chemical composition and physical properties of flaxseed. *LWT—Food Sci. Technol.* **1997**, *30*, 135–140. [CrossRef]
8.   Kuijsten, A.; Arts, I.C.W.; van't Veer, P.; Hollman, P.C.H. The relative bioavailability of enterolignans in humans is enhanced by milling and crushing of flaxseed. *J. Nutr.* **2005**, *135*, 2812–2816. [CrossRef]

9.   Waszkowiak, K.; Gliszczynska-Swiglo, A.; Barthet, V.; Skrety, J. Effect of extraction method on the phenolic and cyanogenic glucoside profile of flaxseed extracts and their antioxidant capacity. *J. Am. Oil Chem. Soc.* **2015**, *92*, 1609–1619. [CrossRef]

10. Kajla, P.; Sharma, A.; Sood, D.R. Flaxseed-a potential functional food source. *J. Food Sci. Technol.* **2015**, *52*, 1857–1871. [CrossRef]

11. Austria, J.A.; Richard, M.N.; Chahine, M.N.; Edel, A.L.; Malcolmson, L.J.; Dupasquier, C.M.; Pierce, G.N. Bioavailability of a-linolenic acid in subjects after ingestion of three different forms of flaxseed. *J. Am. Coll. Nutr.* **2008**, *27*, 214–221. [CrossRef]

12. Mukker, J.K.; Singh, R.S.; Muir, A.D.; Krol, E.S.; Alcorn, J. Comparative pharmacokinetics of purified flaxseed and associated mammalian lignans in male Wistar rats. *Br. J. Nutr.* **2015**, *113*, 749–757. [CrossRef] [PubMed]

13. Panchal, S.K.; Poudyal, H.; Iyer, A.; Nazer, R.; Alam, M.A.; Diwan, V.; Kauter, K.; Sernia, C.; Campbell, F.; Ward, L.; et al. High-carbohydrate, high-fat diet-induced metabolic syndrome and cardiovascular remodeling in rats. *J. Cardiovasc. Pharmacol.* **2011**, *57*, 611–624. [CrossRef] [PubMed]

14. Poudyal, H.; Kumar, S.A.; Iyer, A.; Waanders, J.; Ward, L.C.; Brown, L. Responses to oleic, linoleic and a-linolenic acids in high-carbohydrate, high-fat diet-induced metabolic syndrome in rats. *J. Nutr. Biochem.* **2013**, *24*, 1381–1392. [CrossRef] [PubMed]

15. Poudyal, H.; Panchal, S.K.; Waanders, J.; Ward, L.; Brown, L. Lipid redistribution by a-linolenic acid-rich chia seed inhibits stearoyl-CoA desaturase-1 and induces cardiac and hepatic protection in diet-induced obese rats. *J. Nutr. Biochem.* **2012**, *23*, 153–162. [CrossRef] [PubMed]

16. Khattab, R.Y.; Zeitoun, M.A. Quality evaluation of flaxseed oil obtained by different extraction techniques. *LWT—Food Sci. Technol.* **2013**, *53*, 338–345. [CrossRef]

17. Ghattamaneni, N.K.R.; Panchal, S.K.; Brown, L. An improved rat model for chronic inflammatory bowel disease. *Pharmacol. Rep.* **2018**, *71*, 149–155. [CrossRef] [PubMed]

18. Brown, L.; Poudyal, H.; Panchal, S.K. Functional foods as potential therapeutic options for metabolic syndrome. *Obes. Rev.* **2015**, *16*, 914–941. [CrossRef] [PubMed]

19. Mohammadi-Sartang, M.; Mazloom, Z.; Raeisi-Dehkordi, H.; Barati-Boldaji, R.; Bellissimo, N.; Totosy de Zepetnek, J.O. The effect of flaxseed supplementation on body weight and body composition: A systematic review and meta-analysis of 45 randomized placebo-controlled trials. *Obes. Rev.* **2017**, *18*, 1096–1107. [CrossRef]

20. Ursoniu, S.; Sahebkar, A.; Andrica, F.; Serban, C.; Banach, M. Effects of flaxseed supplements on blood pressure: A systematic review and meta-analysis of controlled clinical trial. *Clin. Nutr.* **2016**, *35*, 615–625. [CrossRef]

21. Da Costa, C.A.; da Silva, P.C.; Ribeiro, D.C.; Pereira, A.D.; dos Santos Ade, S.; de Abreu, M.D.; Pessoa, L.R.; Boueri, B.F.; Pessanha, C.R.; do Nascimento-Saba, C.C.; et al. Effects of diet containing flaxseed flour (*Linum usitatissimum*) on body adiposity and bone health in young male rats. *Food Funct.* **2016**, *7*, 698–703. [CrossRef]

22. Kristensen, M.; Knudsen, K.E.; Jorgensen, H.; Oomah, D.; Bugel, S.; Toubro, S.; Tetens, I.; Astrup, A. Linseed dietary fibers reduce apparent digestibility of energy and fat and weight gain in growing rats. *Nutrients* **2013**, *5*, 3287–3298. [CrossRef] [PubMed]

23. Sammour, R.H. Proteins of linseed (*Linum usitatissimum* L.), extraction and characterization by electrophoresis. *Bot. Bull. Acad. Sin.* **1999**, *40*, 121–126.

24. Chung, M.W.Y.; Lei, B.; Li-Chan, E.C.Y. Isolation and structural characterization of the major protein fraction from NorMan flaxseed (*Linum usitatissimum* L.). *Food Chem.* **2005**, *90*, 271–279. [CrossRef]

25. Borsheim, E.; Bui, Q.U.; Tissier, S.; Kobayashi, H.; Ferrando, A.A.; Wolfe, R.R. Effect of amino acid supplementation on muscle mass, strength and physical function in elderly. *Clin. Nutr.* **2008**, *27*, 189–195. [CrossRef] [PubMed]

26. Pahlavani, N.; Entezari, M.H.; Nasiri, M.; Miri, A.; Rezaie, M.; Bagheri-Bidakhavidi, M.; Sadeghi, O. The effect of L-arginine supplementation on body composition and performance in male athletes: A double-blinded randomized clinical trial. *Eur. J. Clin. Nutr.* **2017**, *71*, 544–548. [CrossRef] [PubMed]

27. Alam, M.A.; Kauter, K.; Withers, K.; Sernia, C.; Brown, L. Chronic L-arginine treatment improves metabolic, cardiovascular and liver complications in diet-induced obesity in rats. *Food Funct.* **2013**, *4*, 83–91. [CrossRef] [PubMed]

28. Fukumitsu, S.; Aida, K.; Ueno, N.; Ozawa, S.; Takahashi, Y.; Kobori, M. Flaxseed lignan attenuates high-fat diet-induced fat accumulation and induces adiponectin expression in mice. *Br. J. Nutr.* **2008**, *100*, 669–676. [CrossRef] [PubMed]

29. Kang, J.; Park, J.; Kim, H.L.; Jung, Y.; Youn, D.H.; Lim, S.; Song, G.; Park, H.; Jin, J.S.; Kwak, H.J.; et al. Secoisolariciresinol diglucoside inhibits adipogenesis through the AMPK pathway. *Eur. J. Pharmacol.* **2018**, *820*, 235–244. [CrossRef] [PubMed]

30. Biasiotto, G.; Zanella, I.; Predolini, F.; Archetti, I.; Cadei, M.; Monti, E.; Luzzani, M.; Pacchetti, B.; Mozzoni, P.; Andreoli, R.; et al. 7-Hydroxymatairesinol improves body weight, fat and sugar metabolism in C57BJ/6 mice on a high-fat diet. *Br. J. Nutr.* **2018**, *120*, 751–762. [CrossRef] [PubMed]

31. Talom, R.T.; Judd, S.A.; McIntosh, D.D.; McNeill, J.R. High flaxseed (linseed) diet restores endothelial function in the mesenteric arterial bed of spontaneously hypertensive rats. *Life Sci.* **1999**, *64*, 1415–1425. [CrossRef]

32. Al-Bishri, W.M. Favorable effects of flaxseed supplemented diet on liver and kidney functions in hypertensive Wistar rats. *J. Oleo Sci.* **2013**, *62*, 709–715. [CrossRef] [PubMed]

33. Xu, C.; Liu, Q.; Zhang, Q.; Gu, A.; Jiang, Z.Y. Urinary enterolactone is associated with obesity and metabolic alteration in men in the US National Health and Nutrition Examination Survey 2001-10. *Br. J. Nutr.* **2015**, *113*, 683–690. [CrossRef] [PubMed]

34. Pilar, B.; Gullich, A.; Oliveira, P.; Stroher, D.; Piccoli, J.; Manfredini, V. Protective role of flaxseed oil and flaxseed lignan secoisolariciresinol diglucoside against oxidative stress in rats with metabolic syndrome. *J. Food Sci.* **2017**, *82*, 3029–3036. [CrossRef] [PubMed]

35. Sawant, S.H.; Bodhankar, S.L. Flax lignan concentrate reverses alterations in blood pressure, left ventricular functions, lipid profile and antioxidant status in DOCA-salt induced renal hypertension in rats. *Ren. Fail.* **2016**, *38*, 411–423. [CrossRef] [PubMed]

36. Park, J.B.; Velasquez, M.T. Potential effects of lignan-enriched flaxseed powder on bodyweight, visceral fat, lipid profile, and blood pressure in rats. *Fitoterapia* **2012**, *83*, 941–946. [CrossRef] [PubMed]

37. Caligiuri, S.P.; Rodriguez-Leyva, D.; Aukema, H.M.; Ravandi, A.; Weighell, W.; Guzman, R.; Pierce, G.N. Dietary flaxseed reduces central aortic blood pressure without cardiac involvement but through changes in plasma oxylipins. *Hypertension* **2016**, *68*, 1031–1038. [CrossRef] [PubMed]

38. Opyd, P.M.; Jurgonski, A.; Juskiewicz, J.; Fotschki, B.; Koza, J. Comparative effects of native and defatted flaxseeds on intestinal enzyme activity and lipid metabolism in rats fed a high-fat diet containing cholic acid. *Nutrients* **2018**, *10*, 1181. [CrossRef]

39. Torkan, M.; Entezari, M.H.; Siavash, M. Effect of flaxseed on blood lipid level in hyperlipidemic patients. *Rev. Recent Clin. Trials* **2015**, *10*, 61–67. [CrossRef]

40. Ren, G.Y.; Chen, C.Y.; Chen, G.C.; Chen, W.G.; Pan, A.; Pan, C.W.; Zhang, Y.H.; Qin, L.Q.; Chen, L.H. Effect of flaxseed intervention on inflammatory marker C-reactive protein: A systematic review and meta-analysis of randomized controlled trials. *Nutrients* **2016**, *8*, 136. [CrossRef]

41. Kailash, P.; Arti, D. Flaxseed and diabetes. *Curr. Pharm. Des.* **2016**, *22*, 141–144. [CrossRef]

42. Dyck, D.J.; Heigenhauser, G.J.; Bruce, C.R. The role of adipokines as regulators of skeletal muscle fatty acid metabolism and insulin sensitivity. *Acta Physiol.* **2006**, *186*, 5–16. [CrossRef] [PubMed]

43. Singh, K.K.; Mridula, D.; Rehal, J.; Barnwal, P. Flaxseed: A potential source of food, feed and fiber. *Crit. Rev. Food Sci. Nutr.* **2011**, *51*, 210–222. [CrossRef] [PubMed]

44. Requena, T.; Martínez-Cuesta, M.C.; Peláez, C. Diet and microbiota linked in health and disease. *Food Funct.* **2018**, *9*, 688–704. [CrossRef] [PubMed]

45. Pulkrabek, M.; Rhee, Y.; Gibbs, P.; Hall, C. Flaxseed- and buckwheat-supplemented diets altered *Enterobacteriaceae* diversity and prevalence in the cecum and feces of obese mice. *J. Diet. Suppl.* **2017**, *14*, 667–678. [CrossRef] [PubMed]

46. Lagkouvardos, I.; Kläring, K.; Heinzmann, S.S.; Platz, S.; Scholz, B.; Engel, K.-H.; Schmitt-Kopplin, P.; Haller, D.; Rohn, S.; Skurk, T.; et al. Gut metabolites and bacterial community networks during a pilot intervention study with flaxseeds in healthy adult men. *Mol. Nutr. Food Res.* **2015**, *59*, 1614–1628. [CrossRef] [PubMed]

47. Birchenough, G.M.; Johansson, M.E.; Gustafsson, J.K.; Bergstrom, J.H.; Hansson, G.C. New developments in goblet cell mucus secretion and function. *Mucosal Immunol.* **2015**, *8*, 712–719. [CrossRef] [PubMed]

48. Lecomte, M.; Couedelo, L.; Meugnier, E.; Plaisancie, P.; Letisse, M.; Benoit, B.; Gabert, L.; Penhoat, A.; Durand, A.; Pineau, G.; et al. Dietary emulsifiers from milk and soybean differently impact adiposity and inflammation in association with modulation of colonic goblet cells in high-fat fed mice. *Mol. Nutr. Food Res.* **2016**, *60*, 609–620. [CrossRef] [PubMed]

49. Power, K.A.; Lepp, D.; Zarepoor, L.; Monk, J.M.; Wu, W.; Tsao, R.; Liu, R. Dietary flaxseed modulates the colonic microenvironment in healthy C57Bl/6 male mice which may alter susceptibility to gut-associated diseases. *J. Nutr. Biochem.* **2016**, *28*, 61–69. [CrossRef] [PubMed]

50. Tanabe, H.; Ito, H.; Sugiyama, K.; Kiriyama, S.; Morita, T. Dietary indigestible components exert different regional effects on luminal mucin secretion through their bulk-forming property and fermentability. *Biosci. Biotechnol. Biochem.* **2006**, *70*, 1188–1194. [CrossRef]

51. Cressey, P.; Reeve, J. Metabolism of cyanogenic glycosides: A review. *Food Chem. Toxicol.* **2019**, *125*, 225–232. [CrossRef]

52. Schulz, V.; Loffler, A.; Gheorghiu, T. Resorption of hydrocyanic acid from linseed. *Leber Magen Darm* **1983**, *13*, 10–14.

10

Metabolic Syndrome in Arab Adults with Low Bone Mineral Density

Kaiser Wani [1], Sobhy M. Yakout [1], Mohammed Ghouse Ahmed Ansari [1], Shaun Sabico [1],
Syed Danish Hussain [1], Majed S. Alokail [1], Eman Sheshah [2], Naji J. Aljohani [3],
Yousef Al-Saleh [1,4,5,6], Jean-Yves Reginster [1,7] and Nasser M. Al-Daghri [1,*]

[1] Chair for Biomarkers of Chronic Diseases, Department of Biochemistry, College of Science, King Saud University, Riyadh 11451, Saudi Arabia; wani.kaiser@gmail.com (K.W.); sobhy.yakout@gmail.com (S.M.Y.); ansari.bio1@gmail.com (M.G.A.A.); eaglescout01@yahoo.com (S.S.); danishhussain121@gmail.com (S.D.H.); msa85@yahoo.co.uk (M.S.A.); alaslawi@hotmail.com (Y.A.-S.); jyr.ch@bluewin.ch (J.-Y.R.)
[2] Diabetes Care Center, King Salman Bin Abdulaziz Hospital, Riyadh 12769, Saudi Arabia; eman_shesha@hotmail.com
[3] Specialized Diabetes and Endocrine Center, King Fahad Medical City, Riyadh 12231, Saudi Arabia; najij@hotmail.com
[4] College of Medicine, King Saud bin Abdulaziz University for Health Sciences, Riyadh 22490, Saudi Arabia
[5] King Abdullah International Medical Research Center, Riyadh 11481, Saudi Arabia
[6] Department of Medicine, Ministry of the National Guard—Health Affairs, Riyadh 14611, Saudi Arabia
[7] Department of Public Health, Epidemiology and Health Economics, University of Liège, 4000 Liège, Belgium
* Correspondence: aldaghri2011@gmail.com

Abstract: There are discrepancies in the reports on the association of metabolic syndrome (MetS) and its components with bone mineral density (BMD) and hence more population-based studies on this subject are needed. In this context, this observational study was aimed to investigate the association between T-scores of BMD at lumbar L1–L4 and full MetS and its individual components. A total of 1587 participants (84.7% females), >35 years and with risk factors associated with bone loss were recruited from February 2013 to August 2016. BMD was done at L1–L4 using dual-energy X-ray absorptiometry (DXA). T-Scores were calculated. Fasting blood samples and anthropometrics were done at recruitment. Fasting lipid profile and glucose were measured. Screening for full MetS and its components was done according to the National Cholesterol Education Programme Adult Treatment Panel III (NCEP ATP III) criteria. Logistic regression analysis revealed that the odds of having full MetS increased significantly from the lowest T-score tertile to the highest one in both sexes (OR, odd ratio (95% CI, confidence interval) of tertile 2 and 3 at 1.49 (0.8 to 2.8) and 2.46 (1.3 to 4.7), $p = 0.02$ in males and 1.35 (1.0 to 1.7) and 1.45 (1.1 to 1.9), $p < 0.01$ in females). The odds remained significant even after adjustments with age, body mass index (BMI), and other risk factors associated with bone loss. Among the components of MetS, only central obesity showed a significant positive association with T-score. The study suggests a significant positive association of T-score (spine) with full MetS irrespective of sex, and among the components of MetS this positive association was seen specifically with central obesity.

Keywords: metabolic syndrome; bone mineral density; obesity; insulin resistance; bone health; osteoporosis

1. Introduction

Metabolic syndrome (MetS), a syndrome consisting of several disorders like abdominal obesity, dyslipidemia, increased blood pressure and impaired glucose regulation, represents characteristics such as low-grade inflammation and increased oxidative stress [1,2]. The increased prevalence of MetS in Saudi Arabia in recent years is blamed on rapid economic growth and Westernization of lifestyle [3,4]. The clinical impact of MetS is immense, considering its vascular harm and its predisposition to the progression of cardiovascular diseases and metabolic complications like type 2 diabetes mellitus (T2DM) [5,6].

The National Cholesterol Education Programme Adult Treatment Panel III (NCEP ATP III) [7] definition for full MetS requires the presence of at least three out of five components namely central obesity, hyperglycemia, low high-density cholesterol, hypertriglyceridemia and hypertension. The NCEP-ATPIII definition of MetS is the most commonly used definition for epidemiologic studies in the region since it does not require a pre-requisite risk factor (e.g., obesity for the International Diabetes Federation (IDF), hyperglycemia for the World Health Organization (WHO)) to reach a diagnosis. Interestingly, these components of MetS may also affect the bone mineral density (BMD) and bone metabolism through several mechanisms, one of which is the reduced blood flow to bone mass due to micro-vascular complications associated with impaired glucose regulation [8]. The other proposed mechanism is hypercalciuria induced by higher glucose levels and elevated blood pressure [9]. In spite of the associations, the overall relationship of MetS components, bone health and BMD remains blurred. For instance, although individuals with T2DM are at an increased risk for fractures [10], higher BMDs are seen in T2DM individuals [11,12]. However, a recent meta-analysis conducted on eight epidemiologic studies involving 39,938 participants suggested no explicit effect of MetS on bone fractures [13]. Apart from this, there are discrepancies in the reports on the association of MetS components and bone health in different sexes [14,15].

Clearly, more population-based studies are needed to decipher the relationship between MetS and its components on bone health. The authors' hypothesize a statistically significant association between different components of MetS and full MetS with the BMD at lumbar L1–L4 bone site. In this context, this observational study was aimed to investigate the association between T-scores of BMD at lumbar L1–L4 and full MetS and its individual components in Saudi Arab adults with risk factors associated with bone loss. Both sexes were included in this study to investigate the sexual disparity, if any, in these associations.

2. Materials and Methods

This observation study is part of a larger study dedicated to finding the biomarkers associated with bone health (titled: Osteoporosis Disease Registry); it was approved by the Ethics Committee at College of Science, King Saud University (KSU), Saudi Arabia (# H-01-R-012).

2.1. Study Design and Participants

The study was conducted in several hospitals around Riyadh city; the most prominent of them being King Fahad Medical City (KFMC), King Khalid University Hospital (KKUH) and King Salman Hospital (KSH), where the bulk of the recruitment was done. The study began in early 2013 and the recruitment ended in August 2016. The inclusion criteria were consenting males and females, >35 years old, who in their general physician visits had been advised of a bone mineral density (BMD) scan owing to their being at a risk associated with bone loss. There were no specific exclusion criteria except being ≤35 years of age or participants with malignancy, cardiac or lung diseases, etc. that required immediate medical attention. A total of 1587 participants (84.7% females and 15.3% males) were recruited during the period.

2.2. Bone Mineral Density (BMD) Scan and T-Score

A dual-energy X-ray absorptiometry (DXA) machine (Hologic Inc., Marlborough, MA, USA) was utilized to measure the bone mineral density (BMD) at lumbar vertebrae L1–L4 and the average scores were used to calculate sex-specific T-scores by the software installed in the machine which shows how much the measured bone density is higher or lower than the bone density of a healthy 30-year-old same sex individual. The machine was calibrated using a standard phantom provided by the manufacturer and the test was performed by a certified bone densitometry technologist. The results of the bone density scan were printed and transported to the Chair for Biomarkers in Chronic Diseases (CBCD) at KSU for data entry.

2.3. Anthropometry, Blood Collection and Sample Analysis

The study participants were invited for a fasting blood withdrawal procedure and administration of a standard questionnaire on the risk factors associated with the bone loss. Anthropometry measurements included height, weight, waist and hip circumference, and systolic/diastolic blood pressure, measured by trained nurses using standard procedures. Weight (Kg) was recorded using an international standard scale (Digital Pearson scale, ADAM Equipment Inc., Oxford, CT, USA). Height and waist and hip circumference (to the nearest 0.5 cm) were measured utilizing a standardized measuring tape. Body mass index (BMI) was calculated as weight in Kgs divided by height in square meters. Blood pressure (mmHG) was recorded by a trained nurse twice after 10 minutes rest using a conventional mercurial sphygmomanometer and the average was noted. A one-on-one interview was conducted by trained research associates where the participants were informed about the study and reported risk factors associated with bone loss through a 12-point questionnaire. The risk factors included whether or not the subject had T2DM, thyroid dysfunction, family history of diabetes, osteoporosis, arthritis, etc., whether they had a barium test, presence of scoliosis or kyphosis, loss of height in the last two years and history of fractures in the last five years.

Collected fasting blood samples were transported to CBCD laboratory for biochemical analysis which included lipid profile as well as glucose, calcium and albumin analysis quantified using an automated biochemical analyzer (Konelab 20, Thermo-Fischer Scientific, Espoo, Finland). The reagents were purchased from Thermo Fischer (catalogue# 981379 for glucose, 981812 for total cholesterol, 981823 for high density lipoprotein (HDL)-cholesterol, 981301 for triglyceride, 981367 for calcium and 981766 for albumin). Glucose kit employed the routine glucose-oxidase, peroxidase method; total cholesterol test employed cholesterol-esterase, oxidase method; HDL-cholesterol test employed the two-step polyethylene glycol modified cholesterol esterase and oxidase methodology; triglyceride kit employed enzymes like lipoprotein lipase and oxidase; calcium kit employed Arsenazo III methodology while albumin kit employed bromocresol purple method. The imprecision calculated as the total coefficient of variation (CV) was ≤5%, ≤3.5%, ≤4%, ≤4%, ≤4.5% and ≤3% for these tests, respectively. Insulin was also measured in these samples using Luminex multiplex (Luminexcorp, Austin, TX, USA) with fluorescent microbead technology.

2.4. T-Score Tertiles and MetS Components

Data for both males and females were divided into T-score tertiles with tertile 1 having the lowest T-score (spine) and tertile 3 having the highest T-score. The status of full MetS and its five components was assessed as present/absent (dichotomous data) using the criteria set in the National Cholesterol Education Programme Adult Treatment Panel III (NCEP-ATP III) [16] which states MetS being present if at least three of the following five components are present.

1. Central obesity: waist circumference >102 cm (males), >88 cm (females).
2. Hyperglycemia: fasting glucose >5.6 mmol/l or pharmacologic treatment for hyperglycemia (both sexes).
3. Hypertriglyceridemia: serum triglycerides ≥1.7 mmol/l (both sexes).
4. Low HDL-cholesterol: serum HDL-cholesterol <1.03 mmol/l (males), <1.30 mmol/l (females).
5. Hypertension: systolic blood pressure >130 mmHg and/or diastolic blood pressure >85 mmHg or current use of antihypertensive medications.

2.5. Data Analysis

SPSS (Version 23.0, SPSS Inc., Chicago, IL, USA) was used to analyze the data. Kolmogorov–Smirnov test was employed to assess the normal distribution of the preliminary data. Continuous normally distributed variables were presented as mean ± standard deviation while median (25th and 75th percentile) was used for continuous non-normal variables. Categorical variables like status of full MetS and its individual components; and data obtained from the bone loss risk factor questionnaires were presented as percentages. Chi-squared test (3 × 2 contingency table) was used for checking the differences in prevalence of MetS and its components in the three tertiles of T-scores. Multinomial logistic regression was performed using the T-score tertile as a dependent variable (with lowest tertile as reference) and full MetS or its individual components (present vs. absent) as independent variables. Data was presented as odds ratio 95% confidence interval (OR (95% CI)) and respective *p*-values represented odds of having different components of MetS at higher tertiles of T-score compared to the lowest. Different models were employed with model "a" as univariate, and all other models were adjusted accordingly for + age (model "b"), + BMI (model "c"), + other components of MetS (model "d") and + risk factors associated with bone loss like T2DM, thyroid dysfunction, etc.; family history of diabetes, osteoporosis, arthritis, etc.; barium test done previously; scoliosis or kyphosis of spine; loss of height reported; history of broken bones (model "e"). The analysis was conducted at 95% confidence level and a *p*-value < 0.05 was considered statistically significant. MS excel 2010 was used to prepare figures.

3. Results

3.1. General and Biochemical Characteristics of the Study Participants

Table 1 show the general and biochemical characteristics of the study participants. A total of 1587 participants were recruited for the study, out of which 84.7% (N = 1344) were females. Participants who were older than 35 years with risk factors associated with bone loss were recruited. The mean age for females and males were 56 and 58 years, respectively. It was determined that 87.3% of females and 79.4% of males were either overweight or obese (BMI >25 kg/m^2) with an average BMI in females at 32.93 kg/m^2 and males at 29.86 kg/m^2. Among the risk factors associated with bone loss, the most prominent in the participants were age greater than 50 years (77% in females and 79.8% in males); family history of diabetes (58.6% in females and 74.5% in males); and those diagnosed with T2DM (51.4% in females and 70.8% in males). The other risk factors like family history of osteoporosis and arthritis were moderately found in both males and females. The percentage of females who reported having thyroid disease, done a barium test (last two weeks of recruitment), and had scoliosis of the spine was 9.2%, 10.7% and 8.9%, respectively, while these risk factors were negligibly found in males. Additionally, 10% and 11.7% of the females reported loss of height in the last two years and a history of broken bones in the last five years of recruitment, respectively. The median (Q1, Q3) values for T-score at spine (L1–L4) for females and males were −1.70 (−2.5, −0.8) and −0.91 (−1.7, 0.1), respectively. The table also shows the biochemical characteristics of the participants, like lipid profile and fasting glucose, that were analyzed to assess different components of MetS.

3.2. Prevalence of Different MetS Components in T-Score Tertiles

Table 2 shows the prevalence of the five components of MetS and full MetS in participants with tertiles according to the T-score (L1-L4 spine). The lowest T-score (least BMD) in both groups represents the tertile 1 and the highest T-score represents the tertile 3. Among the five components of MetS, the prevalence of central obesity was significantly different in the three T-score tertiles in all participants as well as in males and females. It increased from 66.9% in tertile 1 to 82.7% in tertile 3 (*p* < 0.01). A similar trend was followed in males where it increased from 38.3% in tertile 1 to 71.6% in tertile 3 (*p* < 0.01), and in females where it increased from 72.1% in tertile 1 to 84.7% in tertile 3 (*p* < 0.01). The prevalence of other four components (hyperglycemia, low HDL-cholesterol, hypertriglyceridemia and hypertension) was more or less similar in different tertiles of T-score and this was seen in both males and females except for hypertriglyceridemia in all participants where it increased from 40.3% in tertile 1 to 47.7% in tertile 3 ($p = 0.04$). The prevalence of full MetS, however, increased significantly from the lowest T-score tertile to the highest and this was seen in all participants as well as when data was divided according to sexes (56.1% in tertile 1 to 67.7% in tertile 3, $p < 0.01$ in all participants as well as in males where full Mets was 50.6% in tertile 1 and 71.6% in tertile 3, $p = 0.02$; and females where it increased from 57.1% to 65.8%, $p = 0.003$).

Table 1. General and biochemical characteristics of participants.

	Overall	Males	Females
N	1587	243	1344
Anthropometrics			
Age (years)	56.7 ± 8.2	58.1 ± 9.4	56.4 ± 7.9
BMI (kg/m^2)	32.4 ± 6.4	29.9 ± 5.2	32.93 ± 6.4
Waist (cm)	100.3 ± 14.1	103.7 ± 14.2	99.7 ± 14
Hips (cm)	107.9 ± 12.9	104.4 ± 12	108.6 ± 13
Systolic BP (mmHg)	126.2 ± 16.4	131.1 ± 13.1	125.4 ± 16.8
Diastolic BP (mmHg)	76.8 ± 9.9	79.5 ± 8.2	76.3 ± 10.1
Risk Factors			
Age (>50 years) [$]	77.4	79.8	77.0
Family History			
Diabetes Mellitus [$]	61.0	74.5	58.6
Osteoporosis [$]	9.8	9.9	9.7
Arthritis [$]	6.2	4.9	6.5
Subject History			
Diabetes Mellitus [$]	54.4	70.8	51.4
Thyroid Disease [$]	8.1	2.5	9.2
Barium Test (last 2 weeks) [$]	9.4	2.1	10.7
Scoliosis of Spine [$]	7.8	1.6	8.9
Kyphosis [$]	3.5	0.8	4.0
Lost Height (2 years) [$]	8.8	1.6	10.0
Fracture (last 5 years) [$]	10.7	5.3	11.7
T-Score (L1–L4 Spine)	−1.49 ± 1.3	−0.84 ± 1.3	−1.60 ± 1.3
Biochemical Characteristics			
Glucose (mmol/l) [#]	6.7 (5.5, 9.9)	9.2 (6.5–14.1)	6.5 (5.4–9.3)
Insulin (μU/ml) [#]	10.4 (5.9, 18.4)	21.6 (10.7, 33.6)	9.4 (5.4, 15.6)
Total Cholesterol (mmol/l)	5.0 ± 1.1	4.9 ± 1.3	5.08 ± 1.1
Triglycerides (mmol/l) [#]	1.6 (1.2, 2.2)	1.9 (1.4, 2.8)	1.55 (1.1, 2.2)
HDL-Cholesterol (mol/l)	1.2 ± 0.4	1.1 ± 0.4	1.17 ± 0.4
Calcium (mmol/l)	2.3 ± 0.3	2.3 ± 0.2	2.3 ± 0.3
Albumin (g/l)	38.7 ± 6.7	40.2 ± 5.8	38.4 ± 6.8

Note: Data presented as mean ± standard deviation for normal variables; median (Q1, Q3) for non-normal variables (#) and as frequency (%) for categorical variables ($). BMI, body mass index; BP, blood pressure.

Table 2. Prevalence of metabolic syndrome (MetS) components in tertiles of T-score (spine) according to sex.

T-Score (L1–L4 Spine)	All (N = 1587)				Males (N = 243)				Females (N = 1344)			
	T1	T2	T3	p	T1	T2	T3	p	T1	T2	T3	p
Central Obesity	66.9	79.8	82.7	<0.01	38.3	60.5	71.6	<0.01	72.1	83.4	84.7	<0.01
Hyperglycemia	69.9	73.8	74.0	0.25	86.4	80.2	91.4	0.12	66.9	72.7	70.8	0.16
Low HDL-Cholesterol	63.0	64.6	68.5	0.17	40.7	45.7	42.0	0.80	67.1	68.1	73.3	0.09
Hypertriglyceridemia	40.3	46.2	47.7	0.04	54.3	58.0	64.2	0.43	37.7	44.0	44.6	0.07
Hypertension	29.3	32.5	34.4	0.20	38.3	35.8	39.5	0.88	27.6	31.9	33.5	0.15
Full MetS	56.1	63.3	67.6	<0.01	50.6	60.5	71.6	0.02	57.1	64.4	65.8	0.003

Note: Data presented as frequency (%) for the components of MetS and full MetS. T1, T2 and T3 are the three tertiles of T-score (spine) whose respective values as median (Q1, Q3) are −2.70 (−3.1, −2.4), −1.65 (−1.9, −1.3) and −0.30 (−0.7, 0.4) for all participants; −2.20 (−2.7, −1.7), 0.80 (−1.2, −0.5) and 0.55 (0.1, 1.1) for males; −2.80 (−3.2, −2.5), −1.70 (−2.0, −1.5) and −0.40 (−0.8, 0.2) for females. Chi-squared test was used to check the differences of frequencies in different tertiles of T-score. $p < 0.05$ was considered significant. HDL, high density lipoprotein.

Figure 1 shows the average T-score (spine) in individuals with one or more MetS components in males and females. A statistically significant trend was observed in both sexes with average T-score values increasing with increasing MetS components and this remained so even after multiple adjustments.

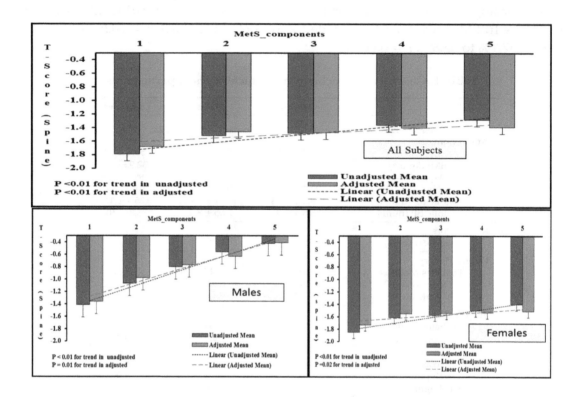

Figure 1. Increasing T-score (spine) values with increasing MetS components according to sex. Note: The figure shows the average T-score (spine) in participants with 1 or more MetS components. The data was generated by univariate analysis by taking T-score (spine) values as dependent variables and "number of components" as factors. The values were adjusted for age, BMI and other risk factors associated with bone loss. $p < 0.05$ was considered as significant.

3.3. Association of T-score with Different Components of MetS and Full MetS.

Table 3 shows the results of a multinomial regression analysis done using T-score (spine) tertiles as dependent variables (with lowest tertile as reference) and different components of MetS as factors. The results are shown as odds ratio (95% confidence interval) and respective p-values representing odds of having different components of metabolic syndrome with different tertiles of T-score. The odds of having full MetS increased significantly from lowest tertile to the highest tertile of T-score in all participants (OR (95% CI) of tertile 2 and 3 at 1.55 (1.2 to 2.0) and 1.57 (1.2 to 2.0), p (trend) < 0.01 as well as in both males and females (1.49 (0.8 to 2.8) and 2.46 (1.3 to 4.7), p (trend) = 0.02 in males and 1.35 (1.0 to 1.7) and 1.45 (1.1 to 1.9), $p < 0.01$ in females) and the odds ratio remained statistically significant even after multiple adjustments with age, BMI and other risk factors associated with bone loss. Among the components of MetS, the odds of hyperglycemia and hypertriglyceridemia increased significantly with T-score tertiles when unadjusted only in all participants, however, the association lost significance after adjusting with confounders. This association was not significant when the data was divided according to sexes. Only the odds of central obesity as a component of MetS increased significantly with T-score tertiles in univariate as well as adjusted models, and this trend was seen when investigated in all participants as well as when the data were divided into different sexes.

Table 3. Odds ratio of full metabolic syndrome and its components at different tertile of T-score (spine) according to sex.

MODEL	ALL TERTILE 1	ALL TERTILE 2	ALL TERTILE 3	ALL p	MALES TERTILE 1	MALES TERTILE 2	MALES TERTILE 3	MALES p	FEMALES TERTILE 1	FEMALES TERTILE 2	FEMALES TERTILE 3	FEMALES p
CENTRAL OBESITY												
a	1	1.96 (1.5-2.6)	2.37 (1.8-3.2)	<0.01	1	2.47 (1.3-4.6)	4.07 (2.1-7.9)	<0.01	1.0	1.94 (1.4-2.7)	2.14 (1.5-2.9)	<0.01
b	1	1.95 (1.5-2.6)	2.44 (1.8-2.3)	<0.01	1	2.58 (1.4-4.9)	4.23 (2.2-8.3)	<0.01	1.0	1.95 (1.4-2.7)	2.21 (1.6-3.1)	<0.01
c	1	1.98 (1.4-2.6)	2.24 (1.6-3.1)	<0.01	1	1.94 (0.8-4.6)	3.06 (1.2-7.4)	0.04	1.0	2.01 (1.4-2.8)	2.27 (1.6-3.3)	<0.01
d	1	1.88 (1.4-2.5)	2.21 (1.6-3.0)	<0.01	1	1.97 (0.8-4.7)	2.95 (1.2-7.1)	0.04	1.0	1.82 (1.3-2.5)	1.98 (1.4-2.8)	<0.01
e	1	1.90 (1.4-2.5)	2.20 (1.6-3.0)	<0.01	1	2.00 (0.8-4.8)	3.07 (1.2-7.5)	0.04	1.0	1.83 (1.3-2.6)	1.97 (1.4-2.8)	<0.01
HYPERGLYCEMIA												
a	1	1.21 (0.9-1.6)	1.23 (0.9-1.6)	0.25	1	0.64 (0.3-1.5)	1.66 (0.6-4.5)	0.12	1.0	1.32 (1.0-1.8)	1.20 (0.9-1.6)	0.16
b	1	1.32 (1.0-1.7)	1.54 (1.2-2.1)	0.01	1	0.82 (0.3-1.9)	2.25 (0.8-6.4)	0.10	1.0	1.40 (1.0-1.9)	1.47 (1.1-2.0)	0.02
c	1	1.28 (1.0-1.8)	1.34 (1.2-2.2)	0.04	1	0.71 (0.3-1.8)	1.71 (0.6-5.1)	0.21	1.0	1.32 (1.0-1.8)	1.44 (1.1-2.0)	0.05
d	1	1.18 (0.9-1.6)	1.29 (0.9-1.7)	0.23	1	0.66 (0.3-1.7)	1.59 (0.5-4.8)	0.24	1.0	1.25 (0.9-1.7)	1.26 (0.9-1.7)	0.29
e	1	1.17 (0.9-1.6)	1.15 (0.8-1.6)	0.57	1	0.62 (0.2-1.7)	1.58 (0.5-5.1)	0.26	1.0	1.25 (0.9-1.7)	1.21 (0.8-1.6)	0.41
LOW HDL-CHOLESTEROL												
a	1	1.07 (0.8-1.4)	1.28 (1.0-1.6)	0.16	1	1.22 (0.6-2.3)	1.05 (0.6-1.9)	0.80	1.0	1.05 (0.8-1.4)	1.35 (1.0-1.8)	0.09
b	1	1.08 (0.8-1.4)	1.32 (1.0-1.7)	0.11	1	1.43 (0.8-2.7)	1.20 (0.6-2.3)	0.55	1.0	1.05 (0.8-1.4)	1.38 (1.0-1.9)	0.08
c	1	1.05 (0.9-1.6)	1.30 (1.0-1.9)	0.32	1	1.19 (0.6-2.3)	1.01 (0.5-1.9)	0.84	1.0	1.02 (0.8-1.4)	1.29 (0.9-1.8)	0.21
d	1	0.96 (0.7-1.2)	1.13 (0.9-1.5)	0.46	1	1.20 (0.6-2.4)	0.90 (0.4-1.8)	0.69	1.0	0.94 (0.7-1.3)	1.30 (0.9-1.7)	0.21
e	1	0.96 (0.7-1.3)	1.15 (0.9-1.5)	0.39	1	1.17 (0.6-2.4)	0.82 (0.4-1.7)	0.59	1.0	0.94 (0.7-1.3)	1.24 (0.9-1.7)	0.18
HYPERTRIGLYCERIDEMIA												
a	1	1.27 (1.0-1.6)	1.35 (1.1-1.7)	0.04	1	1.16 (0.6-2.2)	1.51 (0.8-2.8)	0.43	1.0	1.30 (1.0-1.7)	1.34 (1.0-1.7)	0.06
b	1	1.29 (1.0-1.7)	1.42 (1.1-1.8)	0.02	1	1.25 (0.7-2.4)	1.62 (0.8-3.1)	0.34	1.0	1.30 (1.0-1.7)	1.34 (1.0-1.8)	0.07
c	1	1.25 (1.0-1.7)	1.29 (1.2-1.9)	0.04	1	1.18 (0.6-2.3)	1.47 (0.8-2.9)	0.51	1.0	1.20 (0.9-1.6)	1.24 (0.9-1.7)	0.29
d	1	1.18 (0.9-1.5)	1.22 (0.9-1.6)	0.30	1	1.24 (0.6-2.4)	1.38 (0.7-2.7)	0.64	1.0	1.16 (0.9-1.5)	1.13 (0.8-1.5)	0.56
e	1	1.17 (0.9-1.7)	1.15 (0.9-1.5)	0.46	1	1.16 (0.6-2.3)	1.47 (0.7-2.9)	0.56	1.0	1.16 (0.9-1.5)	1.07 (0.8-1.5)	0.61
HYPERTENSION												
a	1	1.16 (0.9-1.5)	1.27 (1.0-1.6)	0.20	1	0.90 (0.5-1.7)	1.05 (0.6-1.9)	0.88	1.0	1.23 (0.9-1.6)	1.32 (1.0-1.8)	0.15
b	1	1.12 (0.9-1.6)	1.45 (0.9-1.9)	0.06	1	1.07 (0.5-2.1)	1.25 (0.6-2.4)	0.80	1.0	1.27 (0.9-1.7)	1.45 (1.1-1.9)	0.05
c	1	1.20 (0.9-1.7)	1.32 (1.0-1.9)	0.21	1	0.95 (0.5-1.9)	1.10 (0.6-2.2)	0.91	1.0	1.24 (0.9-1.7)	1.37 (1.0-1.9)	0.13
d	1	1.10 (0.8-1.4)	1.24 (0.9-1.6)	0.33	1	0.93 (0.5-1.8)	1.16 (0.6-2.3)	0.79	1.0	1.11 (0.8-1.5)	1.24 (0.9-1.7)	0.40
e	1	1.10 (0.8-1.4)	1.20 (0.9-1.6)	0.50	1	0.90 (0.4-1.8)	1.16 (0.6-2.4)	0.77	1.0	1.11 (0.8-1.5)	1.19 (0.9-1.6)	0.56
FULL METS												
a	1	1.55 (1.2-2.0)	1.57 (1.2-2.0)	<0.01	1	1.49 (0.8-2.8)	2.46 (1.3-4.7)	0.02	1.0	1.35 (1.0-1.7)	1.45 (1.1-1.9)	<0.01
b	1	1.61 (1.2-2.1)	1.74 (1.3-2.3)	<0.01	1	1.82 (0.9-3.5)	3.05 (1.5-6.0)	<0.01	1.0	1.53 (1.2-2.0)	1.59 (1.2-2.1)	<0.01
c	1	1.54 (1.1-2.0)	1.62 (1.2-2.2)	<0.01	1	1.31 (0.6-2.7)	2.10 (1.1-4.4)	0.03	1.0	1.48 (1.1-2.0)	1.48 (1.1-2.0)	<0.01
e	1	1.59 (1.2-2.1)	1.63 (1.2-2.2)	<0.01	1	1.29 (0.6-2.5)	2.12 (1.1-4.6)	0.03	1.0	1.46 (1.1-2.0)	1.47 (1.1-2.0)	<0.01

Note: Data presented as odds ratio (95% confidence interval) (OR (95% CI)) and respective p-values representing odds of having different components of metabolic syndrome at higher tertiles of T-score (spine) compared to the lowest tertile. MetS is full metabolic syndrome; Ref is reference; Ter1, 2 and 3 are different tertiles of T-score. The data was generated by multinomial regression taking T-score tertiles as dependent variables and MetS and its components (present versus absent) as factors. Model "a" is univariate. All other models are additionally adjusted for age (model "b"), BMI (model "c"), all other MetS components (model "d") and risk factors associated with bone loss like family history of diabetes, osteoporosis, arthritis, whether or not suffering from T2DM, thyroid disease, history of broken bones, etc. (model "e"). For full MetS, model "d" is excluded as it is a combination of these five components. $p < 0.05$ is considered significant.

Figure 2 shows the odds ratio and its associated 95% confidence interval of different components of MetS in higher tertiles of T-score (spine) compared with the lowest tertile.

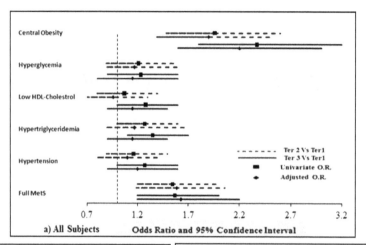

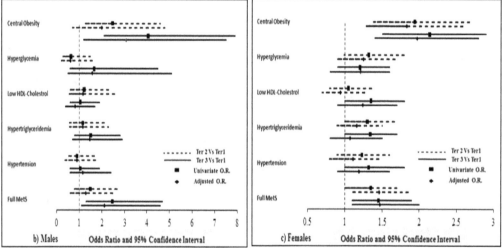

Figure 2. Odds of having full MetS and its components in individuals with higher tertiles of T-score (spine) compared with lowest tertile. Note: The figure shows the odds ratio (OR) and 95% confidence interval representing odds of having different components of metabolic syndrome at higher tertiles of T-score (spine) compared to the lowest tertile. The data was generated by multinomial regression taking T-score tertiles as dependent variables and MetS and its components (present versus absent) as factors. Unadjusted OR; and OR adjusted for age, BMI and risk factors associated with bone loss like family history of diabetes, osteoporosis, arthritis, whether or not suffering from T2DM, thyroid disease, history of broken bones, etc., are represented here.

4. Discussion

The current population-based study aimed to investigate the relationship between MetS and its components with the BMD of the spine. The main novelty of the study is that it is the first large-scale investigation on the association of MetS and BMD in a homogenous Arab ethnic group. This is clinically relevant since it is well established that bone health and risk for certain chronic conditions are influenced by genetics and environment. Several inconsistencies in associations have been found in other studies and one of the main reasons is the differences in population. The study fills this gap as it has never been investigated in this region; a well-structured logistic regression model with multiple adjustments for risk factors associated with bone loss differentiates this study from others on a similar topic. In this study, the authors found a significant positive association of full MetS with BMD spine and this association was independent of sex. The odds ratio of having full MetS, as revealed by logistic regression analysis, increased significantly from the lowest T-score tertile to the highest one and the odds remained significant even after adjustment with multiple confounders and the trend revealed similar association across both sexes. This significant positive association of MetS with BMD seemed to be driven by central obesity as all other components of MetS showed little or no association with increasing tertiles of T-score.

Many recent studies in varied populations were conducted to investigate the associations between MetS, BMD, osteoporosis and fractures. In these studies, the difference in MetS selection criteria, difference in the bone site used to calculate BMD like femoral neck, lumbar spine etc., or the difference in osteoporotic fractures and non-vertebral fractures, played a role in these associations, yet the overall picture of the relationship remains blurred. In one of the earliest studies by Muhlen et al. [17], significantly lower BMD at total hip was associated with MetS in age-adjusted models. Also, in a report by Hwang et al. [18], vertebral BMD was found to be significantly lower in women with MetS compared to non-MetS. Similarly, Jeon et al. [19] suggested higher BMD at the lumbar spine and femoral neck in post-menopausal women with MetS. The results from these studies are in conflict with the present study where a significant positive association was seen between MetS and lumbar BMD. The difference might be because of the lower prevalence of MetS in these studies [17–19] (20.9%, 20.7% and 9.0%, respectively) than the present study (62.3%), suggesting that the participants recruited in these studies were healthier than the current study group. Also, the study participants used by Muhlen et al. were much older than our study (mean age of 74.2 and 74.4 years in men and women, respectively, compared to 58.1 and 56.4 years in this study). The results in the current study are in line with some of the earlier reports [20–22] which suggest women with MetS have a significantly higher BMD than those without MetS. A meta-analysis of a total of 11 studies including 13,122 participants [23] revealed a significant overall association between MetS and increased BMD of spine, in concordance with the present study results.

The present study results of the positive association of full MetS with BMD spine seem to be driven by the component of central obesity as only this component predominantly follows the same pattern in its relationship with BMD spine as the full MetS (Table 3). A positive association of central obesity with BMD at all sites was reported first by Edelstein et al. [24] and since then BMI has been reported as a protective factor against bone loss as concluded by a meta-analysis of 12 studies including 60,000 participants [9]. However, as a flipside to this story, some studies advocate that increased obesity is correlated to low bone mass [25,26]. This paradox in the nature of this relationship of obesity with bone health may be explained by the heterogeneous role of obesity. On one hand higher waist circumference used to calculate central obesity as a component of MetS is associated with higher 17 beta-estradiol levels which may protect bone [27], while on the other hand, intra-abdominal fat or visceral fat may lead to increased bone resorption and hence lower BMD because of its association with pro-inflammatory cytokines [28,29]. Heavy weight is indeed one of the consequences since it is well-established that increased mechanical loading conferred by body weight (e.g., increased BMI or being overweight/obese) has a positive effect on bone formation, regardless of other consequences such as increased risk for other chronic health disorders [30].

The association of other components of MetS with BMD, like full MetS, as reported by many studies in the recent past is also inconclusive. In our study, in all participants, hyperglycemia increased significantly with increasing tertiles of T-score in an unadjusted model but lost significance after adjustment with multiple confounders (Table 3). This observation is supported by some of the earlier reports [31,32] which suggest an indirect effect of hyperglycemia through associated hyperinsulinemia on bone formation, as interaction between insulin, insulin like growth factor-1 and parathyroid hormone has been proposed to have an anabolic effect on bone cells [33]. At the same time, however, long-term diabetes has consistently been shown to be detrimental for bone health and associated fractures [10,34]. A direct effect of hyperglycemia and hyperinsulinemia on bone health and associated fractures would be interesting to investigate. Also, hypertriglyceridemia in our study increased, in all participants, with increased tertiles of T-score in an unadjusted model but lost significance after adjustment. Elevated triglycerides have been suggested to contribute to the overall improvement of qualitative properties of bone by forming a layer between collagen fibers and mineral crystals [35]. We did not observe a significant relationship between other components of MetS and T-score spine, but the results of some other studies present a conflicting picture [36,37].

In our study, no sexual disparity was observed as far as the relationship of MetS and T-score spine was concerned. In both sexes, a positive correlation was found in this relationship and the odds of having MetS increased significantly with higher tertiles of T-score spine even after multiple adjustments. This relationship seems to be driven by the central obesity component in both sexes. Similar to our observations, a meta-analysis conducted on participants showed no gender differences [23]. In contrast, some studies suggest gender disparity in the relationship between MetS and BMI-adjusted BMD, showing a less beneficial effect in men than women [15]. It is difficult to explain this disparity in different studies; however, an explanation might be in the age group of the study participants (e.g., the study that suggests gender differences in the relationship between MetS and BMD was conducted in much younger participants than ours (mean age 56.7 years) and it has been shown that BMD overall decreases as age progresses and the rate of decline in the BMD differs according to sex) [38].

The heterogeneity of the complex relationship between MetS and BMD as seen in various studies before may be explained on the basis of various study-level variables like ethnicity, DXA scanner manufacturer and MetS definition [23]. MetS in Asians may be more influenced by visceral adiposity as compared to Caucasians [39] and hence may explain the positive relationship of MetS and BMD seen in Caucasians rather than Asians. The choice of the DXA scanner used may also play a role in the relationship as the absolute values of BMD differ between instruments from different manufacturers [40]. Also, the differences in the definition of the MetS used in various such studies add to the heterogeneous relationship between MetS and BMD. Abdominal obesity is a necessary factor for the International Diabetes Federation (IDF) criteria of MetS whereas NCEP-ATP III criteria categorizes MetS by having any three of the five components. This difference in MetS definition may dictate the observable positive association of MetS defined by NCEP-ATP III as seen in many studies before including ours rather than when MetS was defined by IDF criteria.

Higher waist circumference (central obesity), is associated with higher 17 β-estradiol levels which is known to improve bone density by inhibiting bone resorption and stimulating bone formation [27]. On the other hand, triglycerides affect osteoblast and osteoclast differentiation, with lower levels associated with osteoporotic bone tissue [41]. Lastly, hyperglycemia and hyperinsulinemia have been demonstrated to exert an anabolic effect on bone cells by interacting insulin-growth factor (IGF)-1 receptors which are known to increase BMD by promoting osteoblast differentiation [42]. It is worthy to note that higher BMD alone cannot account for improved fracture risk since patients with T2DM and those who are obese are still at an increased risk for fragility fractures and associated mortality [43,44]. MetS being a constellation of interconnected physiological, biochemical, clinical and metabolic factors has in itself two contrasting factors: one of which is abdominal obesity known to be protective against osteoporosis and may lead to higher BMD levels [45,46] while at the same time intra-abdominal obesity, hyperglycemia and insulin resistance leads to a low-grade inflammatory state that activates bone resorption [28,47]. This might explain this heterogeneous complex relationship, however, more such studies need to be conducted in different populations to fully elucidate the pathophysiology behind this complexity.

There are several strengths of the current study. First, the sizable study sample of 1587 participants gives this study an edge over many other studies with fewer participants. Secondly, the multi-center recruitment of the study participants used in this study provides a proper representation of a population. Thirdly, this is the first study to report the relationship of MetS with BMD spine in a population with high prevalence of MetS as well as osteoporosis. Apart from these, the use of the most recent definition of MetS, well-calibrated DXA scans performed by a certified bone densitometry technologist and a well-structured logistic regression model analysis adjusted by multiple confounders gave reliable results. The authors, however, acknowledge certain limitations. The cross-sectional nature of this study limits its applicability outside cause and effect of the proposed relationship. A longitudinal study in this population would be interesting to investigate. Some of the biochemical markers that may influence BMD like 25(OH) vitamin D, serum estradiol, follicle stimulating hormone, etc. were not measured in this study. Also, the BMD was measured only at lumbar L–L4 site and hence the proposed relationship with MetS may not hold true for other anatomic sites like femoral neck, total hip, etc.

5. Conclusions

The results of the logistic regression analysis with multiple adjustments conducted in this study suggest a sex-irrespective positive association between MetS and lumbar BMD. The results also suggest that the positive relationship between MetS and lumbar BMD is predominantly driven by the central obesity component of MetS as the rest of the components show little or no association with lumbar BMD, irrespective of sex.

Author Contributions: Conceptualization: K.W., N.M.A.-D., M.S.A., N.J.A.; study execution: K.W., S.M.Y., S.S., Y.A.-S.; sample analysis: K.W., M.G.A.A., E.S.; statistical analysis: K.W., S.D.H.; manuscript writing: K.W.; Manuscript review: N.M.A.-D., S.M.Y., M.G.A.A., S.S., S.D.H., M.S.A., E.S., N.J.A., Y.A.-S., J.-Y.R.

Acknowledgments: The authors would like to thank the research coordinators and nurses at the recruitment centers especially KFMC, KKUH and KSH for their support and technical expertise. Also, the authors thank the CBCD biobank staff, especially Hamza Saber who deserves credit for his meticulous efforts in storing/retrieval of the study samples.

References

1. Maiorino, M.; Bellastella, G.; Giugliano, D.; Esposito, K. From inflammation to sexual dysfunctions: A journey through diabetes, obesity, and metabolic syndrome. *J. Endocrinol. Investig.* **2018**, *41*, 1249–12580. [CrossRef] [PubMed]
2. Darroudi, S.; Fereydouni, N.; Tayefi, M.; Ahmadnezhad, M.; Zamani, P.; Tayefi, B.; Kharazmi, J.; Tavalaie, S.; Heidari-Bakavoli, A.; Azarpajouh, M.R. Oxidative stress and inflammation, two features associated with a high percentage body fat, and that may lead to diabetes mellitus and metabolic syndrome. *BioFactors* **2018**, *45*, 35–42. [CrossRef] [PubMed]
3. Al-Nozha, M.; Al-Khadra, A.; Arafah, M.R.; Al-Maatouq, M.A.; Khalil, M.Z.; Khan, N.B.; Al-Mazrou, Y.Y.; Al-Marzouki, K.; Al-Harthi, S.S.; Abdullah, M.; et al. Metabolic syndrome in saudi arabia. *Saudi Med. J.* **2005**, *26*, 1918–1925. [PubMed]
4. Al-Qahtani, D.A.; Imtiaz, M.L. Prevalence of metabolic syndrome in saudi adult soldiers. *Saudi Med. J.* **2005**, *26*, 1360–1366. [PubMed]
5. Prasad, H.; Ryan, D.A.; Celzo, M.F.; Stapleton, D. Metabolic syndrome: Definition and therapeutic implications. *Postgrad. Med.* **2012**, *124*, 21–30. [CrossRef] [PubMed]
6. Kaur, J. A comprehensive review on metabolic syndrome. *Cardiol. Res. Pract.* **2014**, *2014*, 943162. [CrossRef]
7. Huang, P.L. A comprehensive definition for metabolic syndrome. *Dis. Model. Mech.* **2009**, *2*, 231–237. [CrossRef]
8. Wong, S.; Chin, K.-Y.; Suhaimi, F.; Ahmad, F.; Ima-Nirwana, S. The relationship between metabolic syndrome and osteoporosis: A review. *Nutrients* **2016**, *8*, 347. [CrossRef]
9. De Laet, C.; Kanis, J.; Odén, A.; Johanson, H.; Johnell, O.; Delmas, P.; Eisman, J.; Kroger, H.; Fujiwara, S.; Garnero, P. Body mass index as a predictor of fracture risk: A meta-analysis. *Osteoporos. Int.* **2005**, *16*, 1330–1338. [CrossRef]
10. Janghorbani, M.; Van Dam, R.M.; Willett, W.C.; Hu, F.B. Systematic review of type 1 and type 2 diabetes mellitus and risk of fracture. *Am. J. Epidemiol.* **2007**, *166*, 495–505. [CrossRef]
11. Schwartz, A.V.; Vittinghoff, E.; Bauer, D.C.; Hillier, T.A.; Strotmeyer, E.S.; Ensrud, K.E.; Donaldson, M.G.; Cauley, J.A.; Harris, T.B.; Koster, A. Association of bmd and frax score with risk of fracture in older adults with type 2 diabetes. *JAMA* **2011**, *305*, 2184–2192. [CrossRef] [PubMed]

12. Oei, L.; Zillikens, M.C.; Dehghan, A.; Buitendijk, G.H.; Castaño-Betancourt, M.C.; Estrada, K.; Stolk, L.; Oei, E.H.; van Meurs, J.B.; Janssen, J.A. High bone mineral density and fracture risk in type 2 diabetes as skeletal complications of inadequate glucose control: The rotterdam study. *Diabetes Care* **2013**, *36*, 1619–1628. [CrossRef] [PubMed]

13. Sun, K.; Liu, J.; Lu, N.; Sun, H.; Ning, G. Association between metabolic syndrome and bone fractures: A meta-analysis of observational studies. *BMC Endocr. Disord.* **2014**, *14*, 13. [CrossRef] [PubMed]

14. Yamaguchi, T.; Kanazawa, I.; Yamamoto, M.; Kurioka, S.; Yamauchi, M.; Yano, S.; Sugimoto, T. Associations between components of the metabolic syndrome versus bone mineral density and vertebral fractures in patients with type 2 diabetes. *Bone* **2009**, *45*, 174–179. [CrossRef] [PubMed]

15. Kim, H.; Oh, H.J.; Choi, H.; Choi, W.H.; Lim, S.-K.; Kim, J.G. The association between bone mineral density and metabolic syndrome: A Korean population-based study. *J. Bone Miner. Metab.* **2013**, *31*, 571–578. [CrossRef]

16. Al-Daghri, N.M.; Al-Attas, O.S.; Wani, K.; Sabico, S.; Alokail, M.S. Serum uric acid to creatinine ratio and risk of metabolic syndrome in saudi type 2 diabetic patients. *Sci. Rep.* **2017**, *7*, 12104. [CrossRef] [PubMed]

17. Von Muhlen, D.; Safii, S.; Jassal, S.; Svartberg, J.; Barrett-Connor, E. Associations between the metabolic syndrome and bone health in older men and women: The rancho bernardo study. *Osteoporos. Int.* **2007**, *18*, 1337–1344. [CrossRef]

18. Hwang, D.-K.; Choi, H.-J. The relationship between low bone mass and metabolic syndrome in korean women. *Osteoporos. Int.* **2010**, *21*, 425–431. [CrossRef]

19. Jeon, Y.K.; Lee, J.G.; Kim, S.S.; Kim, B.H.; Kim, S.-J.; Kim, Y.K.; Kim, I.J. Association between bone mineral density and metabolic syndrome in pre- and postmenopausal women. *Endocr. J.* **2011**, *58*, 87–93. [CrossRef]

20. Hernández, J.L.; Olmos, J.M.; Pariente, E.; Martínez, J.; Valero, C.; García-Velasco, P.; Nan, D.; Llorca, J.; González-Macías, J. Metabolic syndrome and bone metabolism: The camargo cohort study. *Menopause* **2010**, *17*, 955–961. [CrossRef]

21. El Maghraoui, A.; Rezqi, A.; El Mrahi, S.; Sadni, S.; Ghozlani, I.; Mounach, A. Osteoporosis, vertebral fractures and metabolic syndrome in postmenopausal women. *BMC Endocr. Disord.* **2014**, *14*, 93. [CrossRef] [PubMed]

22. Muka, T.; Trajanoska, K.; Kiefte-de Jong, J.C.; Oei, L.; Uitterlinden, A.G.; Hofman, A.; Dehghan, A.; Zillikens, M.C.; Franco, O.H.; Rivadeneira, F. The association between metabolic syndrome, bone mineral density, hip bone geometry and fracture risk: The Rotterdam study. *PLoS ONE* **2015**, *10*, e0129116. [CrossRef] [PubMed]

23. Xue, P.; Gao, P.; Li, Y. The association between metabolic syndrome and bone mineral density: A meta-analysis. *Endocrine* **2012**, *42*, 546–554. [CrossRef] [PubMed]

24. Edelstein, S.L.; Barrett-Connor, E. Relation between body size and bone mineral density in elderly men and women. *Am. J. Epidemiol.* **1993**, *138*, 160–169. [CrossRef] [PubMed]

25. Jankowska, E.; Rogucka, E.; Mędraś, M. Are general obesity and visceral adiposity in men linked to reduced bone mineral content resulting from normal ageing? A population-based study. *Andrologia* **2001**, *33*, 384–389. [CrossRef] [PubMed]

26. Moon, S.-S.; Lee, Y.-S.; Kim, S.W. Association of nonalcoholic fatty liver disease with low bone mass in postmenopausal women. *Endocrine* **2012**, *42*, 423–429. [CrossRef] [PubMed]

27. Nelson, L.R.; Bulun, S.E. Estrogen production and action. *J. Am. Acad. Dermatol.* **2001**, *45*, S116–S124. [CrossRef]

28. Hofbauer, L.C.; Schoppet, M. Clinical implications of the osteoprotegerin/rankl/rank system for bone and vascular diseases. *JAMA* **2004**, *292*, 490–495. [CrossRef]

29. Campos, R.M.; de Piano, A.; da Silva, P.L.; Carnier, J.; Sanches, P.L.; Corgosinho, F.C.; Masquio, D.C.; Lazaretti-Castro, M.; Oyama, L.M.; Nascimento, C.M. The role of pro/anti-inflammatory adipokines on bone metabolism in nafld obese adolescents: Effects of long-term interdisciplinary therapy. *Endocrine* **2012**, *42*, 146–156. [CrossRef]

30. Cao, J.J. Effects of obesity on bone metabolism. *J. Orthop. Surg. Res.* **2011**, *6*, 30. [CrossRef]

31. Kinjo, M.; Setoguchi, S.; Solomon, D.H. Bone mineral density in adults with the metabolic syndrome: Analysis in a population-based US sample. *J. Clin. Endocrinol. Metab.* **2007**, *92*, 4161–4164. [CrossRef] [PubMed]

32. Holmberg, A.H.; Nilsson, P.; Nilsson, J.-A.; Akesson, K. The association between hyperglycemia and fracture risk in middle age. A prospective, population-based study of 22,444 men and 10,902 women. *J. Clin. Endocrinol. Metab.* **2008**, *93*, 815–822. [CrossRef] [PubMed]

33. Thrailkill, K.M.; Lumpkin, C.K., Jr.; Bunn, R.C.; Kemp, S.F.; Fowlkes, J.L. Is insulin an anabolic agent in bone? Dissecting the diabetic bone for clues. *Am. J. Physiol. -Endocrinol. Metab.* **2005**, *289*, E735–E745. [CrossRef] [PubMed]

34. Ivers, R.Q.; Cumming, R.G.; Mitchell, P.; Peduto, A.J. Diabetes and risk of fracture: The blue mountains eye study. *Diabetes Care* **2001**, *24*, 1198–1203. [CrossRef] [PubMed]

35. Xu, S.; Jianqing, J.Y. Beneath the minerals, a layer of round lipid particles was identified to mediate collagen calcification in compact bone formation. *Biophys. J.* **2006**, *91*, 4221–4229. [CrossRef]

36. Hanley, D.; Brown, J.; Tenenhouse, A.; Olszynski, W.; Ioannidis, G.; Berger, C.; Prior, J.; Pickard, L.; Murray, T.; Anastassiades, T. Associations among disease conditions, bone mineral density, and prevalent vertebral deformities in men and women 50 years of age and older: Cross-sectional results from the canadian multicentre osteoporosis study. *J. Bone Miner. Res.* **2003**, *18*, 784–790. [CrossRef] [PubMed]

37. Mussolino, M.E.; Gillum, R. Bone mineral density and hypertension prevalence in postmenopausal women: Results from the third national health and nutrition examination survey. *Ann. Epidemiol.* **2006**, *16*, 395–399. [CrossRef]

38. Krall, E.A.; Dawson-Hughes, B.; Hirst, K.; Gallagher, J.; Sherman, S.S.; Dalsky, G. Bone mineral density and biochemical markers of bone turnover in healthy elderly men and women. *J. Gerontol. A Biol. Sci. Med. Sci.* **1997**, *52*, M61–M67. [CrossRef]

39. Abate, N.; Chandalia, M. The impact of ethnicity on type 2 diabetes. *J. Diabetes Complicat.* **2003**, *17*, 39–58. [CrossRef]

40. Pocock, N.A.; Noakes, K.A.; Griffiths, M.; Bhalerao, N.; Sambrook, P.N.; Eisman, J.A.; Freund, J. A comparison of longitudinal measurements in the spine and proximal femur using lunar and hologic instruments. *J. Bone Miner. Res.* **1997**, *12*, 2113–2118. [CrossRef]

41. Dragojevič, J.; Zupan, J.; Haring, G.; Herman, S.; Komadina, R.; Marc, J. Triglyceride metabolism in bone tissue is associated with osteoblast and osteoclast differentiation: a gene expression study. *J. Bone Miner. Metab.* **2013**, *31*, 512–519. [CrossRef] [PubMed]

42. Sundararaghavan, V.; Mazur, M.M.; Evans, B.; Liu, J.; Ebraheim, N.A. Diabetes and bone health: Latest evidence and clinical implications. *Ther. Adv. Musculoskelet. Dis.* **2017**, *9*, 67–74. [CrossRef] [PubMed]

43. Komorita, Y.; Iwase, M.; Idewaki, Y.; Fujii, H.; Ohkuma, T.; Ide, H.; Jodai, K.T.; Yoshinari, M.; Murao, K.A.; Oku, Y. Impact of hip fracture on all-cause mortality in Japanese patients with type 2 diabetes mellitus: The Fukuoka Diabetes Registry. *J. Diabetes Investig.* **2019**. [CrossRef] [PubMed]

44. Tencerova, M.; Frost, M.; Figeac, F.; Nielsen, T.K.; Ali, D.; Lauterlein, J.-J.L.; Andersen, T.L.; Haakonsson, A.K.; Rauch, A.; Madsen, J.S. Obesity-Associated Hypermetabolism and Accelerated Senescence of Bone Marrow Stromal Stem Cells Suggest a Potential Mechanism for Bone Fragility. *Cell Rep.* **2019**, *27*, 2050–2062. [CrossRef] [PubMed]

45. Guh, D.P.; Zhang, W.; Bansback, N.; Amarsi, Z.; Birmingham, C.L.; Anis, A.H. The incidence of co-morbidities related to obesity and overweight: A systematic review and meta-analysis. *BMC Public Health* **2009**, *9*, 88. [CrossRef] [PubMed]

46. Salamat, M.R.; Salamat, A.H.; Janghorbani, M. Association between obesity and bone mineral density by gender and menopausal status. *Endocrinol. Metab.* **2016**, *31*, 547–558. [CrossRef] [PubMed]

47. Smith, B.; Lerner, M.; Bu, S.; Lucas, E.; Hanas, J.; Lightfoot, S.; Postier, R.; Bronze, M.; Brackett, D. Systemic bone loss and induction of coronary vessel disease in a rat model of chronic inflammation. *Bone* **2006**, *38*, 378–386. [CrossRef] [PubMed]

11

Healthy Lifestyle and Incidence of Metabolic Syndrome in the SUN Cohort

Maria Garralda-Del-Villar [1], Silvia Carlos-Chillerón [2,3], Jesus Diaz-Gutierrez [2], Miguel Ruiz-Canela [2,3,4], Alfredo Gea [2,3], Miguel Angel Martínez-González [2,3,4,5], Maira Bes-Rastrollo [2,3,4], Liz Ruiz-Estigarribia [2], Stefanos N. Kales [6] and Alejandro Fernández-Montero [1,3,6,*]

[1]   Department of Occupational Medicine, University of Navarra, 31008 Pamplona, Navarra, Spain; mgarralda.7@alumni.unav.es
[2]   Department of Preventive Medicine and Public Health, University of Navarra, 31008 Pamplona, Navarra, Spain; scarlos@unav.es (S.C.-C.); jdiaz.14@alumni.unav.es (J.D.-G.); mcanela@unav.es (M.R.-C.); ageas@unav.es (A.G.); mamartinez@unav.es (M.A.M.-G.); mbes@unav.es (M.B.-R.); lruiz.29@alumni.unav.es (L.R.-E.)
[3]   IDISNA, Navarra Health Research Institute, 31008 Pamplona, Navarra, Spain
[4]   CIBER Fisiopatología de la Obesidad y Nutrición (CIBER Obn), Instituto de Salud Carlos III, 28029 Madrid, Spain
[5]   Department of Nutrition, Harvard T.H. Chan School of Public Health, Boston, MA 20115, USA
[6]   Department of Environmental Health, Harvard T.H. Chan School of Public Health, Boston, MA 20115, USA; skales@hsph.harvard.edu
*   Correspondence: afmontero@unav.es

Abstract: We assessed the relationship between a healthy lifestyle and the subsequent risk of developing metabolic syndrome. The "Seguimiento Universidad de Navarra" (SUN) Project is a prospective cohort study, focused on nutrition, lifestyle, and chronic diseases. Participants (n = 10,807, mean age 37 years, 67% women) initially free of metabolic syndrome were followed prospectively for a minimum of 6 years. To evaluate healthy lifestyle, nine habits were used to derive a Healthy Lifestyle Score (HLS): Never smoking, moderate to high physical activity (>20 MET-h/week), Mediterranean diet ($\geq$4/8 adherence points), moderate alcohol consumption (women, 0.1–5.0 g/day; men, 0.1–10.0 g/day), low television exposure (<2 h/day), no binge drinking ($\leq$5 alcoholic drinks at any time), taking a short afternoon nap (<30 min/day), meeting up with friends >1 h/day, and working at least 40 h/week. Metabolic syndrome was defined according to the harmonizing definition. The association between the baseline HLS and metabolic syndrome at follow-up was assessed with multivariable-adjusted logistic regressions. During follow-up, we observed 458 (4.24%) new cases of metabolic syndrome. Participants in the highest category of HLS adherence (7–9 points) enjoyed a significantly reduced risk of developing metabolic syndrome compared to those in the lowest category (0–3 points) (adjusted odds ratio (OR) = 0.66, 95% confidence interval (CI) = 0.47–0.93). Higher adherence to the Healthy Lifestyle Score was associated with a lower risk of developing metabolic syndrome. The HLS may be a simple metabolic health promotion tool.

Keywords: healthy lifestyle score; metabolic syndrome; SUN cohort

---

1. Introduction

Metabolic syndrome (MetSyn) is characterized by the clustering of several metabolic abnormalities frequently observed in clinical practice: Abdominal obesity, dyslipidemia, hyperinsulinemia, impaired fasting glucose, and high blood pressure, according to the International Diabetes Federation, the American Heart Association, and the National Heart, Lung, and Blood Institute harmonizing definition [1]. In a prospective cohort study done on middle-aged healthy men, MetSyn was associated with cardiovascular disease and mortality, and a published meta-analysis of longitudinal studies revealed an association between MetSyn and a higher risk of developing type 2 diabetes mellitus, cardiovascular disease, atherosclerosis, and higher all-cause mortality [2,3]. Due to the existence of different definitions for diagnosing this syndrome, prevalence estimates vary. However, it is accepted that the prevalence of MetSyn generally increases as body mass index and age increase [4]. In developed countries, the prevalence of MetSyn is about 25% of the adult population [5–7], and its incidence has been increasing over the last years. In Spain, MetSyn prevalence reached 10% in 2005 [8], and it increased to over 30% by 2012 [9]. Genetics cannot explain these differences alone, and environmental influences play an important role.

Several articles have shown the association between different lifestyle habits and the risk of developing MetSyn according to the harmonizing definition. In this context, eating habits are considered modifiable determinants of MetSyn. Prospective studies (that included participants who were young–middle-aged adults and that considered the harmonizing definition of MetSyn) and a systematic review (that evaluated studies with adults >18 years and that considered the ATPIII definition) analyzing nut consumption, sweet beverages, or adherence to Mediterranean diet patterns, as well as a meta-analysis on this topic (that worked with trials including adults >29 years and used the ATPIII criteria) have proven this association [10–13]. In a prospective study from the "Seguimiento Universidad de Navarra" (SUN) (that included young–middle-aged adults and used the harmonizing definition of MetSyn), physical activity was significantly associated with a lower risk of developing MetSyn [14], whereas, according to a meta-analysis (that analyzed studies whose participants were young–middle-aged adults and that used the MetSyn criteria proposed by the WHO, ATPIII, modified ATPIII, and ACE/AACE) and a longitudinal population-based study (that analyzed 43-year-old adults and used the IDF definition), active smoking and time spent viewing TV were associated with higher risks of MetSyn [15,16]. Several studies evaluating middle-aged adults and using the AHA definition, as well as studies in people who were overweight or obese, have evaluated the effect of the combination of classical healthy life factors on MetSyn (smoking, drinking, dietary habits, and physical activity) with more complex nutritional indexes and have reported them to be significantly associated with MetSyn [17,18]. These previous articles worked with middle-aged adults.

In conclusion, classic healthy lifestyle habits have proven to reduce the risk of developing MetSyn.

In a recent longitudinal study conducted in 2017 in the SUN cohort [19] (in young–middle-aged adults), a new Healthy Lifestyle Score (HLS) was associated with a significant reduction in cardiovascular disease (CVD). This HLS basically included the traditional cardiovascular healthy lifestyle factors (i.e., tobacco, alcohol, diet, and physical activity), and it also took into account other modern life habits including time spent watching television, binge drinking, napping, social life with friends, and number of hours spent working.

Therefore, since it is well known that the MetSyn is a risk factor for CVD, an important question from a public health perspective is whether a healthy lifestyle would also reduce the risk of MetSyn. Our hypothesis was that a higher adherence to the HLS would be associated with a lower risk of MetSyn.

The aim of this study was to prospectively analyze the effectiveness of this new and easy-to-apply HLS in the reduction of MetSyn risk.

2. Materials and Methods

2.1. Study Design

The "Seguimiento Universidad de Navarra" (University of Navarra Follow-Up) Project is a dynamic prospective cohort study that has been conducted in Spain since December 1999 with permanently open recruitment of university graduates. It was designed based on the model of other large cohort studies conducted at the Harvard School of Public Health (the Nurses' Health Study and the Health Professionals Follow-Up Study). Additional details on its objectives, design, and methods have been previously published [20].

Information is mainly gathered through self-reported questionnaires. Participants' information is collected biennially through mailed or electronically mailed questionnaires. Upon completion of the first questionnaire (Q_0), including a total of 554 items used as baseline information, participants receive, every other year, different follow-up questionnaires. These contain important questions to evaluate changes in lifestyle and health-related behaviors, anthropometric measures, incident diseases, and medical conditions. Participants of all ages may be included in the SUN cohort, but they must have had university studies. This inclusion criteria allows for a better control of confounding by education-related variables and by making the interpretation of results easier and therefore adding internal validity to the high-quality information derived from the questionnaires.

2.2. Participants

In our study, a subsample of the SUN cohort was selected. In order to achieve a minimum follow-up of 6 years, only participants who had at least completed the 6-year follow-up questionnaire (Q_6) were included. There were 20,622 participants eligible to be included (SUN participants who responded to the baseline questionnaire (Q_0) before March 2010). We excluded 5080 participants who had either prevalent MetSyn or any MetSyn component at baseline. We also excluded 1399 participants who had extremely low or high total energy intake [21], as well as 1411 participants lost to follow-up (retention rate = 92.7%) and 1985 subjects who did not provide all of the relevant information to diagnose metabolic syndrome at the 6-year follow-up (Figure 1). Therefore, there were 10,807 participants available for analysis.

Informed consent was obtained from all individual participants included in the study by the voluntary completion of the baseline questionnaire once participants understood the specific information needed, the methods used to deliver their data, and the future feedback from the research team. We asked their permission before any follow-up on their medical history. We informed the potential candidates of their right to refuse to participate in the SUN study or to withdraw their consent to participate at any time without reprisal, according to the principles of the Declaration of Helsinki. The Institutional Review Board of the University of Navarra approved these methods.

2.3. Exposure Assessment: Healthy Lifestyle Score Variables

We gathered information from the baseline questionnaires, which collected data on sociodemographic, clinical, anthropometric variables, and lifestyle aspects. Various studies have validated data from the self-reported questionnaires in the SUN cohort: Both anthropometric [22] and physical activity [23] data were analyzed in cohort subgroups. We used the validated 136-question semiquantitative food frequency questionnaire (FFQ) [24] for the evaluation of Mediterranean diet adherence, which was estimated with the Trichopoulou score (0–8 points) [25], (alcohol was excluded). So as to collect information on alcohol consumption, data was obtained through this questionnaire and other additional items related to alcohol consumption in the baseline questionnaire.

In order to assess adherence to a healthy lifestyle, 9 habits of the Healthy Lifestyle Score [19] were used (Table 1), excluding body mass index (BMI), as it is strongly related to MetSyn. The information for this score was gathered from the baseline questionnaire. Each participant received one point for each of the following 9 habits: Never smoking, moderate to high physical activity (>20 MET-h/week), Mediterranean diet ($\geq$4 adherence points), moderate alcohol consumption (women, 0.1–5.0 g/day; men, 0.1–10.0 g/day; abstainers excluded), low television exposure (<2 h/day), no binge drinking ($\leq$5 alcoholic drinks at any time), taking a short afternoon nap (<30 min/day), meeting up with friends >1 h/day, and working at least 40 h/week. This HLS could range from 0 (worst lifestyle) and 9 points (best lifestyle).

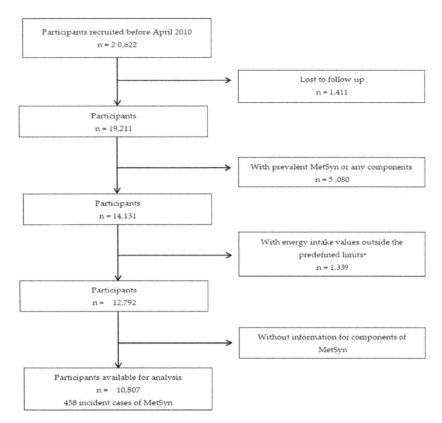

Figure 1. Flow chart depicting the selection process among participants of the Seguimiento Universidad de Navarra (SUN) cohort, 1999–2017; *n*: Number of participants; MetSyn: Metabolic Syndrome. [a] Total energy intake outside predefined limits (<800 or >4000 kcal/day for men, and <500 or >3500 kcal/day for women) [21].

2.4. Outcome Assessment: Metabolic Syndrome and Assessment of Other Variables

The study outcome was incidence of MetSyn. We followed the harmonized definition of MetSyn according to the International Diabetes Federation; the National Heart, Lung, and Blood Institute; the American Heart Association; the World Heart Federation; the International Atherosclerosis Society; and the International Association for the Study of Obesity. According to this definition, metabolic syndrome consists of at least three abnormal findings out of the following 5 criteria [1]: (i) Central adiposity ($\geq$94 cm for men and $\geq$80 cm for women, cut-off points for European populations); (ii) elevated triglycerides (TAG) ($\geq$150 mg/dL or presence of pharmacological treatment for hypertriglyceridemia); (iii) reduced high-density lipoprotein cholesterol (HDL-cholesterol) (<40 mg/dL for men and <50 mg/dL for women or presence of pharmacological treatment for reduced HDL-cholesterol); (iv) elevated blood pressure (systolic $\geq$130 mmHg or diastolic $\geq$85 mmHg or presence of pharmacological treatment for hypertension in patients with a history of this disease); and (v) fasting glucose metabolism ($\geq$100 mg/dL or pharmacological treatment for hyperglycemia).

To obtain the clinical criteria needed for the diagnosis of MetSyn, we used self-reported information provided by participants during the follow-up questionnaires. In the 6-year and 8-year follow-up questionnaires (Q_6 and Q_8), self-reported data about these specific MetSyn criteria were collected. All participants were sent a measuring tape with the Q_6 and Q_8 follow-up questionnaires, together with an explanation on how to measure their waist circumference by using the horizontal plane, midway between the inferior margin of the ribs and the superior border of the iliac crest [26]. Accuracy and validation of all self-reported data on MetSyn components had been previously analyzed in a specific subsample study from the SUN Project of 287 participants [27]. All the analytical parameters used in the validation of self-reported metabolic syndrome components were obtained from the Clinical Analyses Service of Clínica Universidad de Navarra (CUN). The analyses of glucose,

HDL-cholesterol, total cholesterol, and triglycerides were measured in blood serum with the analyzer equipment Roche/Hitachi Modular Analytics, and through spectrophotometry by the enzymatic colorimetric method with glucose oxidase and p-aminophenazone (GOD-PAP). High intraclass correlations were found for waist circumference ($r = 0.86$, 95% confidence interval (CI): 0.80–0.90) and triglycerides ($r = 0.71$, 95% CI: 0.61–0.79), whereas moderate intraclass correlations were found (between 0.46 and 0.63) for the other factors. An additional study, which compared the validity of self-reported diagnosed MetSyn and MetSyn diagnosed by the medical records of the participants, was conducted in another subsample of the SUN Project [28]. Using ATP III criteria, 91.2% of MetSyn and 92.2% (95% CI: 85.7–96.4) of non-MetSyn cases were confirmed.

An incident case of MetSyn was defined when a participant, free of this condition or any of its components at baseline, met three or more of the criteria after at least 6 years of follow-up.

Table 1. Healthy Lifestyle Score (HLS) [a].

	Score
Not smoking	
Never a smoker	1
Smoker (current and former)	0
Physical activity (MET-h/week)	
Physically active (>20 MET-h/week)	1
Not physically active (≤20 MET-h/week)	0
Mediterranean diet pattern (Trichopoulou score excluding alcohol) [b]	
High adherence (≥4)	1
Low adherence (<4)	0
Moderate alcohol consumption	
Moderate consumption (women, 0.1–5.0 g/day; men, 0.1–10.0 g/day)	1
Abstention or high consumption (women >5 g/day; men >10 g/day)	0
Low time spent watching television	
Low television watching (<2 h/day)	1
High television watching (≥2 h/day)	0
Avoidance of binge drinking	
No binge drinking (≤5 alcoholic drinks at any time)	1
Binge drinking (>5 alcoholic drinks at any time)	0
Having a short afternoon nap	
Short afternoon nap (0.1–0.5 h/day)	1
Not having an afternoon nap or having a long nap (>0.5 h/day)	0
Time with friends	
Spending time with friends (>1 h/day)	1
Not spending time with friends (≤1 h/day)	0
Time working	
Full-time work (≥40 h/week)	1
Less than full-time work (<40 h/week)	0

[a] Body mass index was excluded, as it is a component of metabolic syndrome. [b] Score from 0 to 8, because alcohol consumption was excluded.

2.5. Ascertainment of Covariates

The baseline questionnaire also collected information of potential confounding factors between HLS and MetSyn such as sociodemographic characteristics (sex, age, and education level), sleep, medical history (prevalence of cancer, cardiovascular disease, and depression), dietary factors (following a special diet and total energy intake (Kcals/day)), and anthropometric data (BMI). Our approach was to use the consideration of a priori causal knowledge to suggest which were the most relevant variables to be adjusted for. Causal diagrams were used to encode qualitative a priori subject matter knowledge. We did not use merely statistical criteria, because this statistics-only approach has been discouraged [29–31]. For instance, in reference to the prevalence of cancer, it may lead to weight loss and therefore be associated with MetSyn. Besides, it can be related to a change in diet and lifestyle, and these can influence MetSyn.

2.6. Statistical Analyses

According to their baseline HLS, participants were classified into 5 groups to ensure an appropriate sample distribution with sufficient participants and incident cases in each category. Thus, we merged extreme categories, and the distribution of these five categories was 0–3, 4, 5, 6, and 7–9 points. Logistic regression models were fit to assess the risk of metabolic syndrome (MetSyn) after a 6-year follow-up according to HLS categories. Odds ratios (ORs) and their 95% confidence intervals (95% CIs) were calculated considering the lowest category (0–3) as the reference. Linear trend tests were calculated by assigning the median score of each category to all participants in that category and treating this variable as a continuous variable.

For all the analyses, we fitted a crude model, an age- and sex-adjusted model, and a multivariable adjusted model using the following covariates as confounding factors: Age, sex, depression (yes/no), education level (technical/nongraduated, graduated, postgraduate, master's, doctorate), cardiovascular disease (yes/no), prevalent cancer (yes/no), following any special diet (yes/no), body mass index (kg/m^2), energy intake (kcal/day), hours of sleep (h/day), and year of questionnaire completion.

Additional multivariable adjusted analyses were conducted to test the association between the HLS categories and each of the individual criteria for MetSyn.

To assess the individual contribution of each specific factor of the HLS score to the risk of MetSyn, logistic regression models were fitted for each of the nine indicators of healthy life habits, adjusting for the effect of the rest of the elements that constituted the index. The reference category was the absence of the habit of healthy life (score 0 on the specific element).

We used the imputation approach because we had some missing information in important variables such as time spent watching TV, having a short afternoon nap, and time spent with friends. This statistical technique tries to overcome the problem that single imputed values are not actually observed but predicted values, and attributes the most probable value [32]. To carry out the imputation approach, we took into account potential confounding factors, each of the other components of Healthy Lifestyle Score, and each one of the components of MetSyn.

Sensitivity analyses were performed to ensure the robustness of the results in different scenarios. We repeated the analyses stratifying by age ($\geq$45) and sex and without imputation of the lost variables.

All p-values presented are two-tailed, and $p < 0.05$ was considered to be statistically significant. Analyses were performed using STATA/SE version 12.0.

3. Results

The main characteristics of participants according to the HLS categories are shown in Table 2. Compared to subjects who had lower HLSes (0–3 points), those who had the highest score (7–9 points) were less likely to be women, consumed less alcohol per day, had less prevalent depression, were more likely to follow a special diet, and had a slightly higher total energy intake per day. There were no differences in age, baseline BMI, and the prevalence of CVD and cancer.

Of the participants, 458 (4.24%) (272 men, 186 women) initially free of metabolic syndrome (MetSyn) were newly diagnosed as incident cases during the 6-year follow-up. Those who had high HLSes (7 to 9 points) had a significant 34% lower risk of developing MetSyn than those who had lower HLSes (0 to 3), after adjusting for other factors related to MetSyn (Table 3).

Table 4 shows the multivariable-adjusted ORs for each component of MetSyn across HLS categories after the 6-year follow-up. With the exception of HDL-cholesterol, all point estimates of ORs for the upper versus lower category of the HLS suggested inverse associations. However, only the associations with waist circumference and elevated blood pressure showed statistically significant associations (p for trend < 0.05).

Table 2. Baseline characteristics of participants according to the number of Healthy Lifestyle Factors (HLFs) (the SUN cohort).

Number of Healthy Lifestyle Factors	0–3	4	5	6	7–9	p-Value
Participants, n	1468	1993	2599	2525	2222	
Sex, women (%)	69.8	68.0	68.3	66.3	63.7	<0.001
Age, years	35.8 ± 10.6	36.5 ± 11	35.9 ± 10.7	35.9 ± 10.8	34.2 ± 10	<0.001
Body mass index in men	24.9 ± 2.5	24.6 ± 2.3	24.6 ± 2.3	24.6 ± 2.2	24.3 ± 2.3	<0.001
Body mass index in women	22.0 ± 2.5	21.9 ± 2.5	21.9 ± 2.5	21.6 ± 2.4	21.6 ± 2.4	<0.001
Smoking, packs per year	8.8 ± 10.2	7.1 ± 9.4	5.4 ± 8.1	4.21 ± 7.8	1.9 ± 5.8	<0.001
Physical activity, MET-h/week	16.1 ± 15.2	21.4 ± 19.3	25.1 ± 21.8	30.3 ± 25	36.7 ± 26	<0.001
Mediterranean diet pattern [a]	3.04 ± 1.54	3.56 ± 1.7	3.89 ± 1.73	4.24 ± 1.69	4.71 ± 1.49	<0.001
Alcohol consumption, g/day	8.0 ± 11.1	6.9 ± 9.4	6.2 ± 8.7	5.1 ± 7.1	3.9 ± 5.1	<0.001
Watching television, h/day	2.27 ± 1.51	1.81 ± 1.4	1.58 ± 1.31	1.33 ± 1.11	1.09 ± 0.83	<0.001
No binge drinking (%) [b]	44.3	60.7	71	77.2	86.6	<0.001
Afternoon nap, min/day	0.3 ± 0.45	0.27 ± 0.39	0.25 ± 0.34	0.22 ± 0.29	0.22 ± 0.22	<0.001
Meeting up with friends, h/day	1.11 ± 1	1.24 ± 1.05	1.34 ± 1.09	1.39 ± 1	1.54 ± 1.03	<0.001
Working ≥40 h/week (%)	25.4	37.7	49.2	60.6	76.3	<0.001
Sleeping, h/day	7.5 ± 1.1	7.4 ± 1	7.4 ± 1	7.4 ± 0.9	7.4 ± 0.9	0.011
Depression disease (%)	12.7	11.2	10.7	9.2	9.3	0.001
Prevalent cardiovascular disease (%) [c]	1.43	2.06	1.89	1.43	1.53	0.512
Prevalent cancer (%)	3.07	3.21	2.89	3.05	2.43	0.826
Education level						<0.001
No college (%)	8.86	9.13	8.96	10.18	10.26	
College (%)	26.6	22.9	25.2	23.1	21.1	
Postgraduate (%)	51.2	51.9	49.5	47.9	49.1	
Master's (%)	5.93	7.02	7.7	8.08	8.51	
Doctorate (%)	7.43	9.03	8.66	10.73	10.98	
On any special diet (%)	4.36	6.77	5.73	6.81	7.25	0.003
Caloric consumption	2282 ± 607	2302 ± 594	2359 ± 603	2392 ± 606	2428 ± 593	<0.001

[a] Trichopoulou score (from 0 to 8, with alcohol consumption excluded). [b] Less than 5 alcoholic drinks at any time. [c] Atrial fibrillation, paroxysmal tachycardia, coronFary artery bypass surgery or another revascularization procedure, heart failure, aortic aneurysm, pulmonary embolism, or peripheral venous thrombosis.

Table 3. Incidence of metabolic syndrome at 6-year follow-up, according to the number of Healthy Lifestyle Score factors (the SUN cohort). OR: Odds ratio; CI: Confidence interval.

	Number of Healthy Lifestyle Factors					
	0–3	4	5	6	7–9	p for Trend
Participants, n	1468	1993	2599	2525	2222	
Incident cases	80	92	109	103	74	
Crude OR (95% CI)	1 (ref.)	0.86 (0.64–1.17)	0.73 (0.54–0.98)	0.75 (0.56–1.01)	0.57 (0.42–0.80)	0.002
OR adjusted for age and sex (95% CI)	1 (ref.)	0.77 (0.56–1.05)	0.68 (0.50–0.93)	0.69 (0.51–0.94)	0.60 (0.43–0.83)	0.003
Multivariable adjusted OR [a]	1 (ref.)	0.82 (0.59–1.13)	0.72 (0.52–0.98)	0.76 (0.77–1.05)	0.66 (0.47–0.93)	0.027

ref: reference category. [a] Adjusted for age, sex, depression, education level, cardiovascular disease, prevalent cancer, following any special diet, body mass index, energy intake, hours of sleep, year of questionnaire completion.

Figure 2 shows the multivariable-adjusted ORs across the 9 habits of the HLS and the risk of MetSyn. Only low television exposure (<2 h/day) and a short afternoon nap (<30 min/day) were significantly related to the incidence of MetSyn.

In the stratified analysis, we found a significant inverse association between HLS and MetSyn in men and in those older than 55 years, but we did not find any significant interaction (Figure 3).

When we performed the analyses without imputation, the results did not change in magnitude, but they were no longer significant (OR = 0.67, 95% CI = 0.44–1.02).

Table 4. Odds ratios and 95% confidence intervals for each component of metabolic syndrome at the 6-year follow-up, according to the number of HLFs (the SUN Cohort).

	Number of Healthy Lifestyle Factors					
	0–3	4	5	6	7–9	p for Trend
Waist Circumference (>94 cm men, 80 cm women) [a]	1 (ref.)	0.88 (0.75–1.02)	0.74 (0.64–0.86)	0.74 (0.64–0.86)	0.68 (0.58–0.79)	<0.001
Elevated triglycerides (>150 mg/dL) [a]	1 (ref.)	0.84 (0.64–1.12)	0.80 (0.62–1.07)	0.72 (0.54–0.95)	0.87 (0.66–1.16)	0.213
Reduced HDL-cholesterol (<40 mg/dL) [a]	1 (ref.)	1.00 (0.73–1.38)	1.27 (0.95–1.70)	1.10 (0.81–1.49)	1.10 (0.80–1.51)	0.483
Elevated blood pressure (systolic >130 or diastolic >85 mmHg) [a]	1 (ref.)	1.02 (0.85–1.24)	0.93 (0.78–1.12)	0.89 (0.74–1.07)	0.86 (0.71–1.05)	0.033
Elevated glucose (>100 mg/dL) [a]	1 (ref.)	0.82 (0.64–1.05)	0.86 (0.68–1.09)	0.93 (0.74–1.17)	0.73 (0.57–0.94)	0.127

ref: reference category. [a] Adjusted for age, sex, depression, education level, cardiovascular disease, prevalent cancer, following any special diet, body mass index, energy intake, hours of sleep, year of questionnaire completion. HDL-cholesterol: High-density lipoprotein cholesterol.

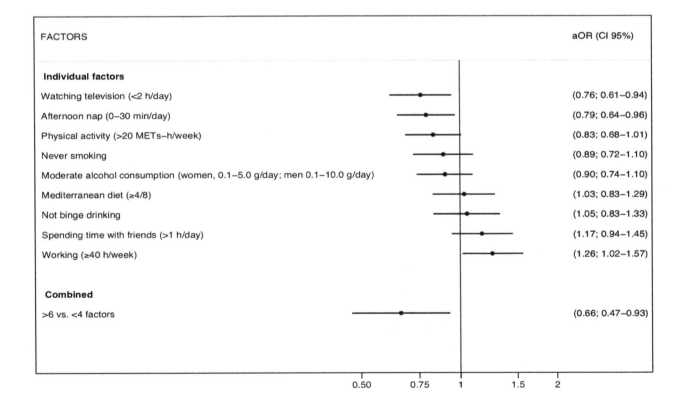

Figure 2. Risk of metabolic syndrome for each factor of the Healthy Lifestyle Score (the SUN cohort); aOR: Adjusted odds ratio; CI: Confidence interval.

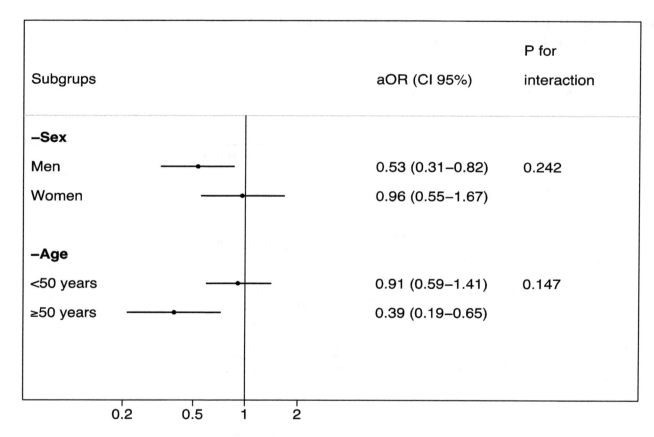

Subgrups		aOR (CI 95%)	P for interaction

–Sex
Men | 0.53 (0.31–0.82) | 0.242
Women | 0.96 (0.55–1.67)

–Age
<50 years | 0.91 (0.59–1.41) | 0.147
≥50 years | 0.39 (0.19–0.65)

0.2   0.5   1   2

Figure 3. Risk of metabolic syndrome in the highest category compared to the lowest category of the Healthy Lifestyle Score. Stratified analyses (the SUN cohort); aOR: Adjusted odds ratio; CI: Confidence interval.

4. Discussion

This prospective study of initially healthy young–middle-aged Mediterranean university graduates showed that a high adherence to a Healthy Lifestyle Score (7 to 9 points) was associated with a lower risk of incident MetSyn after 6 years of follow-up compared to participants with the lowest number of healthy lifestyle factors (0 to 3). Regarding the components of MetSyn, the highest inverse association of this HLS was observed for a high waist circumference and blood pressure. Although we observed a strong and consistent association, only two healthy lifestyle factors, reduced time watching TV and napping less than 30 min, were significantly associated with a risk reduction of MetSyn. This finding suggests that the synergistic effect of the combination of several lifestyle factors is probably more important than the individual effect of each one of them when considered individually.

The HLS has already been shown to present a strong inverse association with cardiovascular disease in this same cohort [19]. Our study is of interest given that MetSyn is not only a risk factor for cardiovascular diseases, but also for type 2 diabetes, atherosclerosis, and all-cause mortality [17,18], among others.

Our findings were consistent with several previous studies supporting the beneficial impact of combinations of healthy lifestyle behaviors on the primary prevention of MetSyn. These studies demonstrated that the risk of MetSyn decreased as the number of lifestyle factors increased, suggesting that a constellation of factors rather than a single factor is more associated with decreased risks of MetSyn [17,18,33,34].

Our findings were also consistent with previous studies demonstrating an association between lifestyle scores and health-related outcomes, such as mortality [35] and cardiovascular diseases [19]. A recent prospective cohort study conducted in the United States showed that five healthy lifestyle-related factors—physical activity (>30 min/day of moderate or vigorous activities), a healthy diet, moderate alcohol consumption, never smoking, and a normal BMI (18.5 to 24.9 kg/m²)—are associated with lower risk of all-cause mortality (hazard ratio (HR) 0.26 (95% CI, 0.22–0.31)), cancer mortality (HR 0.35 (95% CI, 0.27–0.45)), and CVD mortality (HR 0.18 (95% CI, 0.12–0.26)) compared to participants with zero low-risk factors [36]. Similar findings of reduced mortality were demonstrated in another prospective cohort study of Spanish older adults, investigating the combined impact between three traditional (diet, physical activity, and smoking) and three nontraditional health behaviors (social interaction, sedentary time, and sleep duration) on mortality [37].

Our HLS combined indicators of lifestyle habits (never smoking, physical activity, Mediterranean diet, and moderate alcohol consumption) with other factors not typically included in risk scores (television exposure <2 h/day, no binge drinking, taking a short afternoon nap (<30 min), meeting up with friends for more than 1 h/day, and working at least 40 h/week).

According to the literature, and consistent with our results, smoking is associated with a higher risk of developing MetSyn [15,38,39]. Physical activity is also associated with a reduction in the risk of MetSyn [14,40–42]: However, we did not find a significant association between physical activity and MetSyn, only a trend.

Many studies have shown, in agreement with our results, the association between the Mediterranean dietary pattern and the risk of MetSyn [43–46]. However, this finding did not reach statistical significance. A potential explanation for these results may rely on the fact that our population was composed of healthy young–middle-aged Mediterranean university graduates, as shown in Table 2. In addition, the Mediterranean diet score proposed by Trichopoulou et al. [25,47] included alcohol intake: Nevertheless, in our study this was considered a separate lifestyle element because the literature suggests that excessive consumption is related to an increased risk of MetSyn [48,49]. Inconsistent with the literature, our results showed that avoidance of "binge drinking" was not associated with a lower risk of MetSyn. However, this could be explained by the fact that we defined avoidance of binge drinking as never having had more than five alcoholic drinks in a single occasion. Therefore, since the prevalence of binge drinking in Spain has been found to be moderately high [50,51], people with healthy lifestyle habits were included in the unhealthy allocation, potentially leading to a non-differential misclassification bias.

Consistent with our results, some studies have reported the relation between TV viewing and MetSyn [52], as TV viewing may displace physical activity. A meta-analysis [53] demonstrated a J-curve relation between nap time and the risk of MetSyn. This study proved that longer than 40 min/day napping was associated with an increased risk of MetSyn.

Social relationships have been suggested as a protective factor, as they are positively related to minutes of physical activity per week and days of physical activity per week. However, they have been positively associated with number of servings of wine per week and increased high-density lipoprotein cholesterol [54], which may explain why our results showed no protection related to social relationships (variable: Spending time with friends) and MetSyn.

Finally, even if O'Reilly and Rosato found that professionals or managers who worked more than 40 h/week had a lower risk of death [55], which may be explained by maintaining a healthy lifestyle [56], other articles have not found a significant association [57]. In our study, working ≥40 h/week was associated with a higher risk of metabolic syndrome (OR 1.26; 95% CI 1.02–1.57): However, the results should be examined carefully, since our population consisted of university graduates whose work may be related to sedentary, seated jobs.

As expected, and consistent with the literature, adherence to various lifestyle habits showed a greater synergistic effect than a single habit in particular. Therefore, if individuals are concerned about their health, the total number of healthy habits should be increased [58].

It is important when interpreting our results to emphasize that the variables that made up this HLS were categorized in a dichotomous way. Most studies divide these variables into more categories to find greater differences between the extremes. This may be the reason why the differences found between healthy lifestyle factors analyzed individually (regarding the risk of MetSyn (Figure 2)) were more modest than in other investigations [38,44].

Therefore, healthy lifestyle scores can potentially be used as health promotion tools, which help people make health-conscious decisions regarding their behaviors. Future research should be conducted in different scenarios to better analyze the potential effects of HLSes on healthy behaviors and health outcomes.

The present study had several limitations. We observed an incidence of 4.24% of MetSyn. This incidence was lower than that described in the general population [8], but expected in a cohort of young adults with low baseline body mass index, a high educational level and, especially, after selecting only participants without any criteria for MetSyn at the baseline. As is the case in most cohort studies, the sample was not representative of the total population, and generalizing the results should be interpreted carefully. Another potential limitation was the self-reported data collection. Nevertheless, previously published validation studies were carried out in the SUN study, which evaluated the validity of our methods and the quality of the self-reported data by our highly trained volunteers. In any case, this would be expected to be nondifferential and would make the bias more likely to tend to null. Moreover, our analyses assumed that baseline habits remained stable throughout the 6-year follow-up, yet there might have been some changes, which would probably have led to underestimating the protective effects of the HLS. On top of this, as participants were young–middle-aged graduates and had few risk factors, there were few incidence cases. This could be associated with a lower statistical power. However, despite missing values of lifestyle behaviors being imputed, the magnitude of the results hardly changed.

The strengths of the present study included its dynamic participation, prospective design, long follow-up period, and high retention rate. As it is an open cohort, the number of participants is large and constantly increasing, which leads to more powerful results. Finally, validation studies were available for some variables, the outcomes were confirmed using medical records, and the findings were adjusted for a large number of covariables, therefore reducing the existence of potential confounding bias, although we cannot rule out the existence of residual confounding.

5. Conclusions

In summary, in this prospective cohort study of healthy young–middle-aged Mediterranean university graduates, a significant association was found between higher Healthy Lifestyle Scores and a reduction in the risk of incident metabolic syndrome. These results suggest the importance of promoting a comprehensive HLS to maintain metabolic health and allow for rapid evaluation in clinical practice. Further longitudinal and intervention studies in the general population should be conducted to confirm this relationship and to enable extrapolation.

Author Contributions: Each participated sufficiently in the conception and design of the work, in the analysis of the data, writing, and editing of the manuscript. M.G.-D.-V. contributed to data research, extracted data, performed data analysis, and drafted the manuscript. S.C.-C., S.N.K., and J.D.-G. reviewed the data analysis and contributed to the discussion and revision of the manuscript and intellectual revision of the manuscript. A.G., L.R.-E., M.B.-R., M.A.M.-G., and M.R.-C. reviewed the data analysis and contributed to the discussion and revision of the manuscript. A.F.-M. contributed to the design, the generation of the database, the data analysis, and the intellectual revision of the manuscript. This article's contents have not been previously presented elsewhere.

Acknowledgments: We thank the collaboration of other members of the SUN Group: Alvarez-Alvarez, I.; Alonso, A.; Balaguer, A.; Barrio López, M.T.; Basterra-Gortari, F.J.; Benito Corchón, S.; Beunza, J.J.; Carmona, L.; Cervantes, S.; de Irala Estévez, J.; de la Fuente-Arrillaga, C.; de la Rosa, P.A.; Delgado Rodríguez, M.; Donat Vargas, C.L.; Galbete Ciáurriz, C.; García López, M.; Gómez-Donoso, C.; Goñi Ochandorena, E.; Guillén Grima, F.; Hernández, A.; Lahortiga, F.; Llorca, J.; López del Burgo, C.; Marí Sanchís, A.; Martí del Moral, A.; Martín-Calvo, N.; Martínez, J.A.; Núñez-Córdoba, J.M.; Pérez de Ciriza, P.; Pimenta, A.M.; Razquin C, Rico-Campà, A., Romanos, A.; Ruiz Zambrana, A.; Sánchez Adán, D.; Sánchez-Villegas, A.; Sayón-Orea, C.; Toledo, E.; Vázquez Ruiz, Z.; and Zazpe, I. All of them contributed to the building of this cohort and to the validation of the questionnaires used in this study.

References

1. Alberti, K.G.M.M.; Eckel, R.H.; Grundy, S.M.; Zimmet, P.Z.; Cleeman, J.I.; Donato, K.A.; Fruchart, J.-C.; James, W.P.T.; Loria, C.M.; Smith, S.C. Harmonizing the Metabolic Syndrome. *Circulation* **2009**, *120*, 1640–1645. [CrossRef] [PubMed]

2. Lakka, H. The Metabolic Syndrome and Total and Cardiovascular Disease Mortality in Middle-aged Men. *JAMA* **2002**, *288*, 2709. [CrossRef] [PubMed]

3. Gami, A.S.; Witt, B.J.; Howard, D.E.; Erwin, P.J.; Gami, L.A.; Somers, V.K.; Montori, V.M. Metabolic Syndrome and Risk of Incident Cardiovascular Events and Death. *J. Am. Coll. Cardiol.* **2007**, *49*, 403–414. [CrossRef] [PubMed]

4. Ervin, R.B. Prevalence of metabolic syndrome among adults 20 years of age and over, by sex, age, race and ethnicity, and body mass index: United States, 2003–2006. *Natl. Health Stat. Rep.* **2009**, 1–7.

5. Ford, E.S.; Giles, W.H.; Dietz, W.H. Prevalence of the Metabolic Syndrome Among US Adults. *JAMA* **2002**, *287*, 356. [CrossRef] [PubMed]

6. Lim, S.; Shin, H.; Song, J.H.; Kwak, S.H.; Kang, S.M.; Won Yoon, J.; Choi, S.H.; Cho, S.I.; Park, K.S.; Lee, H.K.; et al. Increasing Prevalence of Metabolic Syndrome in Korea: The Korean National Health and Nutrition Examination Survey for 1998–2007. *Diabetes Care* **2011**, *34*, 1323–1328. [CrossRef] [PubMed]

7. Delavari, A.; Forouzanfar, M.H.; Alikhani, S.; Sharifian, A.; Kelishadi, R. First Nationwide Study of the Prevalence of the Metabolic Syndrome and Optimal Cutoff Points of Waist Circumference in the Middle East: The National Survey of Risk Factors for Noncommunicable Diseases of Iran. *Diabetes Care* **2009**, *32*, 1092–1097. [CrossRef] [PubMed]

8. Laclaustra, M.; Ordoñez, B.; Leon, M.; Andres, E.M.; Cordero, A.; Pascual-Calleja, I.; Grima, A.; Luengo, E.; Alegria, E.; Pocovi, M.; et al. Metabolic syndrome and coronary heart disease among Spanish male workers: A case-control study of MESYAS. *Nutr. Metab. Cardiovasc. Dis.* **2012**, *22*, 510–516. [CrossRef]

9. Fernández-Bergés, D.; Cabrera de León, A.; Sanz, H.; Elosua, R.; Guembe, M.J.; Alzamora, M.; Vega-Alonso, T.; Félix-Redondo, F.J.; Ortiz-Marrón, H.; Rigo, F.; et al. Metabolic Syndrome in Spain: Prevalence and Coronary Risk Associated With Harmonized Definition and WHO Proposal. DARIOS Study. *Rev. Esp. Cardiol.* **2012**, *65*, 241–248. [CrossRef]

10. Yamaoka, K.; Tango, T. Effects of lifestyle modification on metabolic syndrome: A systematic review and meta-analysis. *BMC Med.* **2012**, *10*, 138. [CrossRef]

11. Fernández-Montero, A.; Bes-Rastrollo, M.; Beunza, J.J.; Barrio-Lopez, M.T.; De La Fuente-Arrillaga, C.; Moreno-Galarraga, L.; Martínez-González, M.A. Nut consumption and incidence of metabolic syndrome after 6-year follow-up: The SUN (Seguimiento Universidad de Navarra, University of Navarra Follow-up) cohort. *Public Health Nutr.* **2013**, *16*, 2064–2072. [CrossRef] [PubMed]

12. Barrio-Lopez, M.T.; Martinez-Gonzalez, M.A.; Fernandez-Montero, A.; Beunza, J.J.; Zazpe, I.; Bes-Rastrollo, M. Prospective study of changes in sugar-sweetened beverage consumption and the incidence of the metabolic syndrome and its components: The SUN cohort. *Br. J. Nutr.* **2013**, *110*, 1722–1731. [CrossRef] [PubMed]

13. Esposito, K.; Kastorini, C.-M.; Panagiotakos, D.B.; Giugliano, D. Mediterranean diet and metabolic syndrome: An updated systematic review. *Rev. Endocr. Metab. Disord.* **2013**, *14*, 255–263. [CrossRef] [PubMed]

14. Hidalgo-Santamaria, M.; Fernandez-Montero, A.; Martinez-Gonzalez, M.A.; Moreno-Galarraga, L.; Sanchez-Villegas, A.; Barrio-Lopez, M.T.; Bes-Rastrollo, M. Exercise Intensity and Incidence of Metabolic Syndrome: The SUN Project. *Am. J. Prev. Med.* **2017**, *52*, e95–e101. [CrossRef] [PubMed]

15. Sun, K.; Liu, J.; Ning, G. Active Smoking and Risk of Metabolic Syndrome: A Meta-Analysis of Prospective Studies. *PLoS ONE* **2012**, *7*, e47791. [CrossRef] [PubMed]

16. Wennberg, P.; Gustafsson, P.E.; Howard, B.; Wennberg, M.; Hammarström, A. Television viewing over the life course and the metabolic syndrome in mid-adulthood: A longitudinal population-based study. *J. Epidemiol. Community Health* **2014**, *68*, 928–933. [CrossRef] [PubMed]

17. Chang, S.-H.; Chen, M.-C.; Chien, N.-H.; Wu, L.-Y. CE: Original Research: Examining the Links between Lifestyle Factors and Metabolic Syndrome. *Am. J. Nurs.* **2016**, *116*, 26–36. [CrossRef] [PubMed]

18. Sotos-Prieto, M.; Bhupathiraju, S.N.; Falcón, L.M.; Gao, X.; Tucker, K.L.; Mattei, J. A Healthy Lifestyle Score Is Associated with Cardiometabolic and Neuroendocrine Risk Factors among Puerto Rican Adults. *J. Nutr.* **2015**, *145*, 1531–1540. [CrossRef]

19. Díaz-Gutiérrez, J.; Ruiz-Canela, M.; Gea, A.; Fernández-Montero, A.; Martínez-González, M.Á. Association between a Healthy Lifestyle Score and the Risk of Cardiovascular Disease in the SUN Cohort. *Rev. Esp. Cardiol.* **2018**, *71*, 1001–1009. [CrossRef]

20. Carlos, S.; De La Fuente-Arrillaga, C.; Bes-Rastrollo, M.; Razquin, C.; Rico-Campà, A.; Martínez-González, M.A.; Ruiz-Canela, M. Mediterranean Diet and Health Outcomes in the SUN Cohort. *Nutrients* **2018**, *10*, 439. [CrossRef]

21. Willett, W. *Nutritional Epidemiology (pp. 74–100)*, 3rd ed.; Oxford University Press: New York, NY, USA, 2013.

22. Bes-Rastrollo, M.; Pérez-Valdivieso, J.R.; Sánchez-Villegas, A.; Alonso, A.; Martínez-González, M.Á. Validación del peso e índice de masa corporal auto-declarados de los participantes de una cohorte de graduados universitarios. *Rev. Esp. Obes.* **2005**, *3*, 352–358.

23. Martínez-González, M.A.; López-Fontana, C.; Varo, J.J.; Sánchez-Villegas, A.; Martinez, J.A. Validation of the Spanish version of the physical activity questionnaire used in the Nurses' Health Study and the Health Professionals' Follow-up Study. *Public Health Nutr.* **2005**, *8*, 920–927. [CrossRef] [PubMed]

24. De la Fuente-Arrillaga, C.; Vázquez Ruiz, Z.; Bes-Rastrollo, M.; Sampson, L.; Martinez-González, M.A. Reproducibility of an FFQ validated in Spain. *Public Health Nutr.* **2010**, *13*, 1364–1372. [CrossRef] [PubMed]

25. Trichopoulou, A.; Costacou, T.; Bamia, C.; Trichopoulos, D. Adherence to a Mediterranean Diet and Survival in a Greek Population. *N. Engl. J. Med.* **2003**, *348*, 2599–2608. [CrossRef] [PubMed]

26. Klein, S.; Allison, D.B.; Heymsfield, S.B.; Kelley, D.E.; Leibel, R.L.; Nonas, C.; Kahn, R. Waist Circumference and Cardiometabolic Risk: A Consensus Statement from Shaping America's Health: Association for Weight Management and Obesity Prevention; NAASO, The Obesity Society; the American Society for Nutrition; and the American Diabetes Associat. *Diabetes Care* **2007**, *30*, 1647–1652. [CrossRef] [PubMed]

27. Fernández-Montero, A.; Beunza, J.J.; Bes-Rastrollo, M.; Barrio, M.T.; de la Fuente-Arrillaga, C.; Moreno-Galarraga, L.; Martínez-González, M.A. Validity of self-reported metabolic syndrome components in a cohort study. *Gac. Sanit.* **2011**, *25*, 303–307. [CrossRef] [PubMed]

28. Barrio-Lopez, M.T.; Bes-Rastrollo, M.; Beunza, J.J.; Fernandez-Montero, A.; Garcia-Lopez, M.; Martinez-Gonzalez, M.A. Validation of metabolic syndrome using medical records in the SUN cohort. *BMC Public Health* **2011**, *11*, 867. [CrossRef]

29. Williamson, E.J.; Aitken, Z.; Lawrie, J.; Dharmage, S.C.; Burgess, J.A.; Forbes, A.B. Introduction to causal diagrams for confounder selection. *Respirology* **2014**, *19*, 303–311. [CrossRef]

30. Flanders, W.D.; Eldridge, R.C. Summary of relationships between exchangeability, biasing paths and bias. *Eur. J. Epidemiol.* **2015**, *30*, 1089–1099. [CrossRef]

31. Hernan, M.A. Causal Knowledge as a Prerequisite for Confounding Evaluation: An Application to Birth Defects Epidemiology. *Am. J. Epidemiol.* **2002**, *155*, 176–184. [CrossRef]

32. Groenwold, R.H.H.; Donders, A.R.T.; Roes, K.C.B.; Harrell, F.E.; Moons, K.G.M. Dealing with Missing Outcome Data in Randomized Trials and Observational Studies. *Am. J. Epidemiol.* **2012**, *175*, 210–217. [CrossRef] [PubMed]

33. Lee, J.A.; Cha, Y.H.; Kim, S.H.; Park, H.S. Impact of combined lifestyle factors on metabolic syndrome in Korean men. *J. Public Health* **2016**, *39*, 82–89. [CrossRef] [PubMed]

34. Mitchell, B.L.; Smith, A.E.; Rowlands, A.V.; Parfitt, G.; Dollman, J. Associations of physical activity and sedentary behaviour with metabolic syndrome in rural Australian adults. *J. Sci. Med. Sport* **2018**, *21*, 1232–1237. [CrossRef] [PubMed]

35. Khaw, K.-T.; Wareham, N.; Bingham, S.; Welch, A.; Luben, R.; Day, N. Combined Impact of Health Behaviours and Mortality in Men and Women: The EPIC-Norfolk Prospective Population Study. *PLoS Med.* **2008**, *5*, e12. [CrossRef]

36. Li, Y.; Pan, A.; Wang, D.D.; Liu, X.; Dhana, K.; Franco, O.H.; Kaptoge, S.; Di Angelantonio, E.; Stampfer, M.; Willett, W.C.; et al. Impact of Healthy Lifestyle Factors on Life Expectancies in the US Population. *Circulation* **2018**, *138*, 345–355. [CrossRef] [PubMed]

37. Martínez-Gómez, D.; Guallar-Castillón, P.; León-Muñoz, L.M.; López-García, E.; Rodríguez-Artalejo, F. Combined impact of traditional and non-traditional health behaviors on mortality: A national prospective cohort study in Spanish older adults. *BMC Med.* **2013**, *11*, 47. [CrossRef] [PubMed]

38. Kim, B.J.; Kim, B.S.; Sung, K.C.; Kang, J.H.; Lee, M.H.; Park, J.R. Association of Smoking Status, Weight Change, and Incident Metabolic Syndrome in Men: A 3-Year Follow-Up Study. *Diabetes Care* **2009**, *32*, 1314–1316. [CrossRef]

39. Nakanishi, N.; Takatorige, T.; Suzuki, K. Cigarette smoking and the risk of the metabolic syndrome in middle-aged Japanese male office workers. *Ind. Health* **2005**, *43*, 295–301. [CrossRef]

40. Pattyn, N.; Cornelissen, V.A.; Eshghi, S.R.T.; Vanhees, L. The Effect of Exercise on the Cardiovascular Risk Factors Constituting the Metabolic Syndrome. *Sports Med.* **2013**, *43*, 121–133. [CrossRef]

41. Strasser, B. Physical activity in obesity and metabolic syndrome. *Ann. N. Y. Acad. Sci.* **2013**, *1281*, 141–159. [CrossRef]

42. Zhang, D.; Liu, X.; Liu, Y.; Sun, X.; Wang, B.; Ren, Y.; Zhao, Y.; Zhou, J.; Han, C.; Yin, L.; et al. Leisure-time physical activity and incident metabolic syndrome: A systematic review and dose-response meta-analysis of cohort studies. *Metabolism* **2017**, *75*, 36–44. [CrossRef] [PubMed]

43. Ahluwalia, N.; Andreeva, V.A.; Kesse-Guyot, E.; Hercberg, S. Dietary patterns, inflammation and the metabolic syndrome. *Diabetes Metab.* **2013**, *39*, 99–110. [CrossRef] [PubMed]

44. Kastorini, C.M.; Milionis, H.J.; Esposito, K.; Giugliano, D.; Goudevenos, J.A.; Panagiotakos, D.B. The effect of mediterranean diet on metabolic syndrome and its components: A meta-analysis of 50 studies and 534,906 individuals. *J. Am. Coll. Cardiol.* **2011**, *57*, 1299–1313. [CrossRef] [PubMed]

45. Kesse-Guyot, E.; Ahluwalia, N.; Lassale, C.; Hercberg, S.; Fezeu, L.; Lairon, D. Adherence to Mediterranean diet reduces the risk of metabolic syndrome: A 6-year prospective study. *Nutr. Metab. Cardiovasc. Dis.* **2013**, *23*, 677–683. [CrossRef] [PubMed]

46. Grosso, G.; Mistretta, A.; Marventano, S.; Purrello, A.; Vitaglione, P.; Calabrese, G.; Drago, F.; Galvano, F. Beneficial Effects of the Mediterranean Diet on Metabolic Syndrome. *Curr. Pharm. Des.* **2014**, *20*, 5039–5044. [CrossRef] [PubMed]

47. Martínez-González, M.A.; Hershey, M.S.; Zazpe, I.; Trichopoulou, A. Transferability of the Mediterranean Diet to Non-Mediterranean Countries. What Is and What Is Not the Mediterranean Diet. *Nutrients* **2018**, *9*, 1226. [CrossRef]

48. Sun, K.; Ren, M.; Liu, D.; Wang, C.; Yang, C.; Yan, L. Alcohol consumption and risk of metabolic syndrome: A meta-analysis of prospective studies. *Clin. Nutr.* **2014**, *33*, 596–602. [CrossRef]

49. Im, H.-J.; Park, S.-M.; Choi, J.-H.; Choi, E.-J. Binge Drinking and Its Relation to Metabolic Syndrome in Korean Adult Men. *Korean J. Fam. Med.* **2014**, *35*, 173. [CrossRef]

50. Valencia-Martín, J.L.; Galán, I.; Rodríguez-Artalejo, F. Binge Drinking in Madrid, Spain. *Alcohol. Clin. Exp. Res.* **2007**, *31*, 1723–1730. [CrossRef]

51. Soler-Vila, H.; Galán, I.; Valencia-Martín, J.L.; León-Muñoz, L.M.; Guallar-Castillón, P.; Rodríguez-Artalejo, F. Binge Drinking in Spain, 2008–2010. *Alcohol. Clin. Exp. Res.* **2014**, *38*, 810–819. [CrossRef]

52. Tremblay, M.S.; LeBlanc, A.G.; Kho, M.E.; Saunders, T.J.; Larouche, R.; Colley, R.C.; Goldfield, G.; Gorber, S.C. Systematic review of sedentary behaviour and health indicators in school-aged children and youth. *Int. J. Behav. Nutr. Phys. Act.* **2011**, *8*, 98. [CrossRef] [PubMed]

53. Yamada, T.; Shojima, N.; Yamauchi, T.; Kadowaki, T. J-curve relation between daytime nap duration and type 2 diabetes or metabolic syndrome: A dose-response meta-analysis. *Sci. Rep.* **2016**, *6*, 38075. [CrossRef] [PubMed]

54. Fischer Aggarwal, B.A.; Liao, M.; Mosca, L. Physical Activity as a Potential Mechanism through Which Social Support May Reduce Cardiovascular Disease Risk. *J. Cardiovasc. Nurs.* **2008**, *23*, 90–96. [CrossRef] [PubMed]

55. O'Reilly, D.; Rosato, M. Worked to death? A census-based longitudinal study of the relationship between the numbers of hours spent working and mortality risk. *Int. J. Epidemiol.* **2013**, *42*, 1820–1830. [CrossRef] [PubMed]

56. Kivimaki, M.; Nyberg, S.T.; Fransson, E.I.; Heikkila, K.; Alfredsson, L.; Casini, A.; Clays, E.; De Bacquer, D.; Dragano, N.; Ferrie, J.E.; et al. Associations of job strain and lifestyle risk factors with risk of coronary artery disease: A meta-analysis of individual participant data. *Can. Med. Assoc. J.* **2013**, *185*, 763–769. [CrossRef] [PubMed]

57. Pimenta, A.M.; Bes-Rastrollo, M.; Sayon-Orea, C.; Gea, A.; Aguinaga-Ontoso, E.; Lopez-Iracheta, R.; Martinez-Gonzalez, M.A. Working hours and incidence of metabolic syndrome and its components in a Mediterranean cohort: The SUN project. *Eur. J. Public Health* **2015**, *25*, 683–688. [CrossRef]

58. Spring, B.; Moller, A.C.; Coons, M.J. Multiple health behaviours: Overview and implications. *J. Public Health* **2012**, *34*, i3–i10. [CrossRef]

12

Metabolomic Salivary Signature of Pediatric Obesity Related Liver Disease and Metabolic Syndrome

Jacopo Troisi [1,2,3,4,*], Federica Belmonte [1], Antonella Bisogno [1], Luca Pierri [1], Angelo Colucci [1,2], Giovanni Scala [4], Pierpaolo Cavallo [5], Claudia Mandato [6], Antonella Di Nuzzi [1], Laura Di Michele [1], Anna Pia Delli Bovi [1], Salvatore Guercio Nuzio [1] and Pietro Vajro [1,7]

[1] Department of Medicine and Surgery and Dentistry, "Scuola Medica Salernitana", Pediatrics Section University of Salerno, 84081 Baronissi (Salerno), Italy; fecu91@gmail.com (F.B.); a.bisogno91@gmail.com (A.B.); luca.pierri@hotmail.com (L.P.); angelocolucci2@gmail.com (A.C.); antonelladinuzzi@gmail.com (A.D.N.); lauradimichele05091993@gmail.com (L.D.M.); delliboviannapia@gmail.com (A.P.D.B.); sguercio.nuzio@gmail.com (S.G.N.); pvajro@unisa.it (P.V.)

[2] Theoreo srl, Via degli Ulivi 3, 84090 Montecorvino Pugliano (SA), Italy

[3] European Biomedical Research Institute of Salerno (EBRIS), Via S. de Renzi, 3, 84125 Salerno, Italy

[4] Hosmotic srl, Via R. Bosco 178, 80069 Vico Equense (NA), Italy; scala@hosmotic.com

[5] Department of Physics, University of Salerno, 84084 Fisciano (Salerno), Italy; pcavallo@unisa.it

[6] Department of Pediatrics, Children's Hospital Santobono-Pausilipon, 80129 Naples, Italy; cla.mandato@gmail.com

[7] European Laboratory of Food Induced Intestinal Disease (ELFID), University of Naples Federico II, 80100 Naples, Italy

* Correspondence: troisi@theoreosrl.com

Abstract: Pediatric obesity-related metabolic syndrome (MetS) and nonalcoholic fatty liver disease (NAFLD) are increasingly frequent conditions with a still-elusive diagnosis and low-efficacy treatment and monitoring options. In this study, we investigated the salivary metabolomic signature, which has been uncharacterized to date. In this pilot-nested case-control study over a transversal design, 41 subjects (23 obese patients and 18 normal weight (NW) healthy controls), characterized based on medical history, clinical, anthropometric, and laboratory data, were recruited. Liver involvement, defined according to ultrasonographic liver brightness, allowed for the allocation of the patients into four groups: obese with hepatic steatosis ([St+], $n = 15$) and without hepatic steatosis ([St−], $n = 8$), and with ($n = 10$) and without ($n = 13$) MetS. A partial least squares discriminant analysis (PLS-DA) model was devised to classify the patients' classes based on their salivary metabolomic signature. Pediatric obesity and its related liver disease and metabolic syndrome appear to have distinct salivary metabolomic signatures. The difference is notable in metabolites involved in energy, amino and organic acid metabolism, as well as in intestinal bacteria metabolism, possibly reflecting diet, fatty acid synthase pathways, and the strict interaction between microbiota and intestinal mucins. This information expands the current understanding of NAFLD pathogenesis, potentially translating into better targeted monitoring and/or treatment strategies in the future.

Keywords: pediatric obesity; nonalcoholic fatty liver disease; metabolic syndrome; saliva; metabolomics; gas-chromatography mass spectrometry

1. Introduction

The incidence of obesity and its related conditions, including metabolic syndrome (MetS) and non-alcoholic fatty liver disease (NAFLD), has dramatically increased worldwide in all age groups including pediatrics [1]. Pediatric obesity definitely is an early risk factor for adult morbidity and mortality [2,3]. Due to the existence of a well-established tracking phenomenon, the early detection and treatment of MetS and fatty liver in childhood represents a valuable tool to prevent further health complications and to minimize the global socioeconomic burden of hepato-metabolic and cardiovascular obesity-associated complications in adulthood [4]. Although the exact definition of MetS is still debated regarding the pediatric population, most researchers agree (a) that it includes hypertension, hyperglycemia, dyslipidemia together with visceral obesity, and (b) that NAFLD has to be considered its hepatic component.

Metabolomics has recently started to pave the way to a better pathomechanistic understanding of these hepatometabolic complications, leading to a more efficient diagnosis and better therapeutic approaches. In this regard, studies have shown that high urinary/blood levels of aromatic (AAA) ± branched chain (BCAA) amino acids are known to be associated with insulin resistance (IR) and the risk of obesity-related MetS [5–8].

Lipid metabolism, tyrosine [9], alanine and the urea cycle [5], acylcarnitine catabolism ± changes in nucleotides, lysolipids, and inflammation markers [10], and several other components [11–13] also appear to be implicated in obesity and its related disorders.

We have recently shown a complex network of urinary molecules prevalently represented by intestinally-derived bacterial products [14] which are correlated with the clinical phenotype and can differentiate between normal weight and obese children, distinguishing between those with and without liver involvement, based also on the characteristics of their gut-liver axis (GLA) function [15].

To identify an even more easily accessible and readily obtained biofluid for possible minimally invasive disease recognition [16], few studies have shown saliva suitability for investigations of individual metabolites of oxidative stress in obesity [17] and obesity-related MetS/NAFLD [4,18]. We showed that salivary testing of uric acid, glucose, insulin and HOMA together with selected anthropometric parameters may help to identify noninvasively obese children with hepatic steatosis and/or having MetS components [4]. However, salivary metabolomics studies in this respect are lacking.

Based on these and a few other urine-and/or plasma-based metabolomic studies of pediatric obesity and MetS [15,19–21], we hypothesized that differences in the metabolite profiling of lean and obese children with and without NAFLD/MetS might also be evident in saliva, which might be ideal to screen noninvasively obese children at a higher risk of hepatometabolic complications. Prospectively, better delineation of individual or clusters of specific metabolites could serve as diagnostic biomarkers to be further investigated in future studies appraising even early stages of these comorbidities.

2. Materials and Methods

2.1. Population and Study Design

Among 46 consecutive subjects (aged 7–15 years) seen at our obesity clinic or planned for only minor surgery, 41 with verified good oral health and not taking medications were enrolled in a nested case-control study over a transversal design. Eighteen had a normal weight (NW; body mass index (BMI) < 85th percentile) and 23 were obese (BMI > 95th percentile). The patients were characterized based on clinical, anthropometric (blood pressure, BMI, waist circumference (WC), and neck circumference (NC)), laboratory (serum alanine aminotransferase (ALT), aspartate aminotransferase (AST), total and high-density lipoprotein (HDL) cholesterol, triglycerides, uric acid (UA), glucose, and insulin) parameters. An ultrasound (US) was used to determine the presence [St+] or absence [St−] of hepatic steatosis [22,23]. Blood tests were performed using a standard laboratory analyzer (Abbott Diagnostics, Santa Clara, CA, USA).

ALT upper normal values referred either to the customary normal range cut-off value of 40 IU/L or more precise SAFETY study cut-off pediatric values of 25.8 and 22.0 IU/L for boys and girls, respectively [24].

Patients with hepatic steatosis and/or transaminases >1.5 times the upper customary normal values were screened for celiac disease, Wilson disease, autoimmune hepatitis, and major and minor hepatotropic viruses [25]. According to the International Diabetes Foundation (IDF), MetS was defined as the presence of at least three of the following parameters: WC >95th percentile; triglycerides >150 mg/dL; blood glucose >100 mg/dL; systolic blood pressure (SBP) >95th percentile; and HDL cholesterol <40 mg/dL [26].

2.2. Saliva Samples

Each subject was asked to refrain from eating, drinking and brush tooting procedures for at least 1 h before saliva collection. Then he/she underwent a morning, whole saliva sampling using a saliva cotton roll commercial collection device (Salivette®; Sarstedt, Nümbrecht, Germany). As recommended by the manufacturer, to stimulate salivation patients, patients were asked to roll and gently chew the cotton swab in their mouth for 60–90 s. Then the swab was spitted in the collection tube of the kit and centrifuged within 1 h at $2000 \times g$ for 2 min. The collected clear, fluid saliva sample was aliquoted without any further processing and frozen at $-80\,^{\circ}$C until samples' analysis, as previously described [4].

2.3. Ethical Approval

The study complied with the terms of the Declaration of Helsinki of 1975 (as revised in 2013) [27] for the investigation of human subjects, with written informed consent from patients and their families. All participants agreed to participate in this study and contribute saliva samples for metabolomic analysis. All samples were collected in accordance with the ethical guidelines mandated by and approved by our institutional Health Research Ethics Board. The study protocol was approved by the Ethics Review Committee of the University Hospital S. Giovanni di Dio e Ruggi d'Aragona of Salerno (Prot. No 18.02.2013/98).

2.4. Untargeted Metabolomics Analysis

2.4.1. Metabolites Extraction and Derivatization

Metabolome extraction, purification and derivatization were carried out using the MetboPrep GC kit (Theoreo srl, Montecorvino Pugliano (SA), Italy) according to the manufacturer's instructions.

2.4.2. GC-MS Analysis

GC-MS analysis was performed on the derivatized extracted metabolome according to Troisi et al. [15] with a few minor changes. Briefly, 2 μL of the sample solution was injected into the GC-MS system (GC-2010 Plus gas chromatograph coupled to a 2010 Plus single quadrupole mass spectrometer; Shimadzu Corp., Kyoto, Japan) equipped with a 30-m, 0.25-mm ID CP-Sil 8 CB fused silica capillary GC column with 1.00-μm film thickness from Agilent (Agilent, J&W Scientific, Folsom, CA, USA), using He as a carrier gas. The initial oven temperature of 100 °C was maintained for 1 min and then raised by 6 °C/min to 320 °C with a further 2.33 min of hold time. The gas flow was set to obtain a constant linear velocity of 39 cm/s, and injections were performed in the splitless mode. The mass spectrometer was operated in electron impact (70 eV) in the full-scan mode in the interval of 35–600 m/z with a scan velocity of 3333 amu/s and a solvent cut-off time of 4.5 min. The complete GC analysis duration was 40 min. Untargeted metabolites were identified by comparing the mass spectrum of each peak with the NIST library collection (NIST, Gaithersburg, MD, USA).

2.4.3. Metabolites Identification

Of the over 240 signals per sample produced by GC-MS analysis, only 222 were investigated further because they were consistently found in at least 85% of samples.

To identify metabolites under the peaks, the Kovats' index [28] difference max tolerance was set at 10, while the minimum matching for the NIST library search was set at 85%. The results were summarized in a comma-separate matrix file and loaded in the appropriate software for statistical manipulation. The chromatographic data for PLS-DA analysis were tabulated with one sample per row and one variable (metabolite) per column. The normalization procedures consisted of data transformation and scaling. Data transformation was made by generalized log transformation and data scaling by autoscaling (mean-centered and divided by standard deviation of each variable) [29]. Relevant metabolites selected using statistical analysis were further confirmed with an analytical standard purchased from Sigma-Aldrich (Milan, Italy) as indicated in the Metabolomic Standard Initiative reports [30].

2.5. Statistical Analysis

2.5.1. Demographical and Clinical Data

Statistical analysis was performed using Statistica software (StatSoft, Tulsa, OK, USA) and Minitab (Minitab Inc., State College, PA, USA). The normal distribution of data was verified using the Shapiro–Wilks test. Because the data were normally distributed, we used one-way ANOVA with Tukey's post-hoc test for intergroup comparisons. A result with $p < 0.05$ was considered statistically significant.

2.5.2. Metabolomics Univariate Data Analysis

Metabolite concentration differences among the classes (NW, OB[St+] and OB[St−]) were evaluated in terms of fold change (FC) and p-value (assessed using Student's t-test because the metabolite amount was previously normalized).

The volcano plot representation was used to encounter both criteria. Metabolites with high FC (>1 or <−1) and lower p-value (<0.05) were selected as the most relevant.

2.5.3. Metabolomic Multivariate Data Analysis

Partial least squares discriminant analysis (PLS-DA) was performed on the internal standard peak area [31] normalized chromatogram using R (Foundation for Statistical Computing, Vienna, Austria). Mean centering and unit variance scaling were applied for all analyses. Class separation was archived by PLS-DA, which is a supervised method that uses multivariate regression techniques to extract, via linear combinations of original variables (X), the information that can predict class membership (Y). PLS regression was performed using the *plsr* function included in the R pls package [32]. Classification and cross-validation were performed using the wrapper function included in the caret package [33]. A permutation test was performed to assess the significance of class discrimination. In each permutation, a PLS-DA model was built between the data (X) and permuted class labels (Y) using the optimal number of components determined by cross validation for the model based on the original class assignment. Two types of test statistics were used to measure class discrimination. The first is based on prediction accuracy during training. The second used separation distance based on the ratio of the between groups sum of the squares and the within group sum of squares (B/W-ratio). If the observed test statistics were part of the distribution based on the permuted class assignments, class discrimination cannot be considered significant from a statistical point of view [34]. Variable importance in projection (VIP) scores were calculated for each component. A VIP score is a weighted sum of squares of the PLS loadings, considering the amount of explained Y-variation in each dimension.

The metabolic pathway was constructed using the MetScape application [35] of the software Cytoscape [36].

3. Results

The demographic and clinical laboratory characteristics of the case and control subjects are reported in Table 1. None of the NW controls had either biochemical or US hepato-metabolic abnormalities.

Table 1. Characteristics of the study population.

Anthropometric and Laboratory Parameters	Controls (n = 18)	Obese with Steatosis (n = 15)	Obese without Steatosis (n = 8)	All Obese (n = 23)
Gender (M/F)	13/5	10/5	4/4	14/9
Age (years)	10.53 ± 2.57	12.48 ± 2.77 *	12.51 ± 2.79 *	12.49 ± 2.71 *
Weight (kg)	37.42 ± 11.26	79.99 ± 28.76 *	71.9 ± 17.31 *	77.18 ± 25.24 *
Height (cm)	140.17 ± 15.17	153.41 ± 19.27 *	157.45 ± 11.97 *	154.52 ± 16.88 *
BMI (kg/cm^2)	18.52 ± 2.92	32.80 ± 6.94 *	28.93 ± 5.58 *	31.45 ± 6.65 *
BMI percentile	23.75 ± 34.25	95.14 ± 0.53 *	95.67 ± 1.03 *	95.40 ± 1.05 *
Waist circumference (cm)	61.14 ± 7.11	93.27 ± 12.68 *	86.00 ± 14.53 *	90.74 ± 13.49 *
WC percentile	65.85 ± 24.58	94.98 ± 0.97 *	94.38 ± 1.77 *	94.78 ± 1.04 *
Cm WC > 95th percentile	0	21.03 ± 10.57 *	14.00 ± 10.99 *	18.59 ± 11.01 *
WtHR	0.43 ± 0.03	0.61 ± 0.05 *	0.55 ± 0.08 *	0.59 ± 0.07 *
Neck circumference (cm)	27.67 ± 2.41	36.05 ± 4.33 *	34.69 ± 4.08 *	35.58 ± 4.20 *
NC percentile	44.12 ± 33.22	95.57 ± 5.35 *	92.61 ± 3.15	94.09 ± 4.26 *
Cm NC > 95th percentile	0	3.71 ± 2.77 *	2.41 ± 2.75 *	3.26 ± 2.77 *
SBP (mmHg)	95.98 ± 11.95	127.47 ± 8.95 *	125.63 ± 20.23 *	126.83 ± 13.49 *
SBP percentile	50.00 ± 0	86.93 ± 19.36 *	83.50 ± 20.96 *	85.74 ± 19.52 *
DBP (mmHg)	55.00 ± 10.77	61.53 ± 10.42 *	60.75 ± 11.70 *	61.26 ± 10.62 *
DBP percentile	50.00 ± 0	56.00 ± 15.83 *	55.00 ± 14.14 *	55.65 ± 14.95 *
ALT (U/L)	17.33 ± 4.31	50.17 ± 28.75 *	34.50 ± 37.74 *	44.72 ± 32.21 *
AST (U/L)	24.72 ± 4.87	46.19 ± 28.58 *	19.75 ± 5.85	37.00 ± 26.39 *
Total cholesterol (mg/dL)	148.78 ± 16.38	158.17 ± 21.91 *	162.00 ± 24.20 *	159.50 ± 22.26 *
HDL (mg/dL)	56.94 ± 14.45	45.07 ± 10.21 *	48.00 ± 5.50 *	46.09 ± 8.83 *
Triglyceride (mg/dL)	Not available	90.59 ± 26.97	138.63 ± 91.90	107.30 ± 60.80
Blood glucose (mg/dL)	83.17 ± 6.61	88.59 ± 10.36 *	90.00 ± 10.34 *	89.08 ± 10.14 *
Salivary glucose (μM)	3338.36 ± 1274.73	3167.86 ± 1192.75	2647.09 ± 1227.77	2986.70 ± 1203.86
Blood insulin (U/L)	10.27 ± 5.22	24.24 ± 10.95 *	19.60 ± 6.63 *	22.62 ± 9.77 *
Salivary insulin (nM)	5.79 ± 2.85	20.89 ± 8.69 *	17.26 ± 6.37 *	19.60 ± 8.00 *
Blood HOMA-IR	2.01 ± 1.16	5.34 ± 2.60 *	4.11 ± 2.16 *	4.91 ± 2.48 *
Salivary HOMA-IR	119.7 ± 73.99	401.81 ± 231.17 *	278.79 ± 162.48 *	358.20 ± 215.35 *
Blood uric acid (mg/dL)	4.04 ± 0.76	5.06 ± 1.23 *	4.42 ± 0.92 *	4.84 ± 1.15 *
Salivary uric acid (μM)	143.46 ± 4.53	157.29 ± 13.04 *	156.45 ± 15.31 *	157.00 ± 13.53 *

Abbreviations = ALT: alanine transaminase; AST: aspartate transaminase; BMI: Body Mass Index; DBP: diastolic blood pressure; HDL: high density lipoproteins; HOMA-IR: Homeostasis Assessment Model—Insulin Resistance WC: waist circumference; NC: neck circumference; SBP: systolic blood pressure; WtHR: Waist to Height Ratio; * p value < 0.05 compared to controls.

More than 50% of obese children (n = 15) had ultrasonographic (US) signs of NAFLD and hypertransaminasemia not due to the most common causes of liver diseases, as well as significantly higher values of systolic blood pressure (127 ± 9 vs. 96 ± 11 mm Hg, p = 0.0003) and glycemia (88.6 ± 10.4 vs. 83.2 ± 6.6 mg/dL, p = 0.002) compared with NW subjects. Twenty-one patients had no component of MetS, 7 had at least one component, 10 had two or three components, and only 3 had more than three components (Table 2).

As shown in Figure 1, the PLS-DA score plots clearly differentiated between obese (OB) and normal weight (NW) children (Figure 1A1) and between OB with and without steatosis and NW controls (Figure 1B1). Twelve and 13 metabolites with a VIP-score > 2 separated NW/OB and NW/OB[St+]/OB[St−], respectively (Figure 1A2,B2). A third PLS-DA model (Figure 1C1) separated children according to MetS via five metabolites that had a VIP-score >2 (Figure 1C2).

As shown in Figure 1 and Table 3, compared with NW subjects, the saliva of obese children had higher levels of palmitic acid, myristic acid, urea, N-acetyl galactosamine, maltose, gluconic acid and isoleucine and lower levels of hydroxy butyric acid and malic acid, which were prevalent in those without steatosis and lauric acid, maltose and methyl maleic acid, which were prevalent in those with steatosis.

Table 2. Metabolic Syndrome components in obese patients with and without hepatic steatosis.

	Number (%) of Obese Patients with Hepatic Steatosis	Number (%) of Obese Patients without Hepatic Steatosis	Total (%)
Sample size	15(65%)	8(35%)	23(100%)
Waist circumference >90th percentile	15(65%)	7(30%)	22(95%)
Glucose blood levels >100 mg/dL	4(17%)	2(9%)	6(26%)
Blood pressure >95th percentile	10(43%)	4(17%)	14(60%)
HDL <40 mg/dL	3(13%)	0(0%)	3(13%)
TG >150 mg/dL	2(9%)	3(13%)	5(22%)
HOMA-IR > 3	13(57%)	5(22%)	18(79%)
Numbers of patients fulfilling MetS Criteria: (WC > 90th percentile and more than two out of four other criteria)	7(30%)	3(13%)	10(43%)

Abbreviations = HDL: high density lipoproteins; HOMA-IR: Homeostasis Assessment Model – Insulin Resistance; MetS: Metabolic Syndrome; TG: Triglycerides; WC: waist circumference

Table 3. Variables important in projection (VIP) metabolites fold changes in patients versus controls' saliva.

VIP	NW (n = 18) [a]	OB[St−] (n = 15)	OB[St+] (n = 8)	p-Value [b]	MetS− (n = 38) [a]	MetS+ (n = 3)	p-Value [c]
Hydroxy butyric acid	0.00697	−0.14	−0.62 *	NS	0.00622	−1.02	NS
Palmitic acid [d]	0.00088	4.46 ***	8.06 **	NS	0.00398	−0.74	NS
Myristic acid	0.00092	3.71 **	7.58 *	NS	0.00375	−0.66	NS
Lauric acid	0.00061	−7.21 **	−3.35	NS	0.00267	0.73	NS
Urea	0.00093	4.15 **	7.65 **	NS	0.00404	−0.71	NS
N-acetyl galactosamine	0.00088	3.72 **	7.60 *	NS	0.00375	−0.66	NS
Malic acid	0.17825	−0.98	−0.98	NS	0.09066	0.96	NS
Methyl maleic acid	0.01375	−0.72	−0.24	NS	0.01164	0.81	NS
Maltose	0.07047	−0.54	−0.25	NS	0.05846	0.24	NS
Xylose	0.00864	−0.62	−0.34	NS	0.00681	0.27	NS
Butanediol	0.00070	−6.16 **	−2.79	NS	0.00272	0.34	NS
Proline	0.00999	−0.56	−0.25	NS	0.00752	−1.02	NS
Tartaric acid	0.06401	0.52	0.40	NS	0.04729	−0.40	NS

* indicates a p-value < 0.05 compared to NW, ** indicates a p-value < 0.01 compared to NW, *** indicates a p-value < 0.001 compared to NW, NS indicates a p-value > 0.05. [a] Normalized chromatographic peak area; [b] p-values of OB[St+]/OB[St−] comparison; [c] p-values of MetS−/MetS+ comparison; [d] Metabolite selected by both PLS-DA models. Abbreviations: MetS−: No metabolic syndrome diagnosis; MetS+: Diagnosis of metabolic syndrome; NW: Normal Weight; OB[St+]: Obese without steatosis; OB[St+]: Obese with Steatosis; PLS-DA: Partial Least Squares Discriminant Analysis; VIP: Variable Important in Projections

The volcano plot representation and histogram of the metabolites selected using volcano plot analysis (FC > 1 or < −1, p < 0.05) of the OB patients compared with NW (Figure S1-A1) and of the OB[St+] patients compared with the OB[St−] patients (Figure S1-A2) is reported in supplementary Figure S1.

The levels of valine, mannose, acetopyruvic acid, palmitic acid, triethylene glycol, gluconic acid, citric acid, scyllo-inositol, deoxyglucose, psicopyranose, myo-inositol and cycloserine were higher in OB patients (Figure 2B1). Conversely, the levels of 1,2,3-butanetriol, 2-oxovaleric acid, 2-palmitoylglycerol, Di-n-octyl phthalate, itaconic acid, methyl galactoside, stearic acid, 2-piperidinone, maltose, 2-deoxy-D-ribose, pentane dioic acid, glycerol, pentitol, glyceric acid, methyl maleic acid, 2-deoxypentofuranose, β-hydroxy pyruvic acid, 2-hydroxy- methylcyclopentanol, and L-serine were higher in NW patients (Figure S1-B1). OB[St+] patients had higher levels of D-glucuronic acid γ-lactone, 2′-deoxyribolactone, 2-hydroxyisocaproic acid, pyroglutamic acid, and propanoic acid. Instead, OB[St−] patients had higher levels of butanoic acid, maltose, thiamine, glucopyranose, 2-hydroxybutyric acid, and mannose (Figure S1-B).

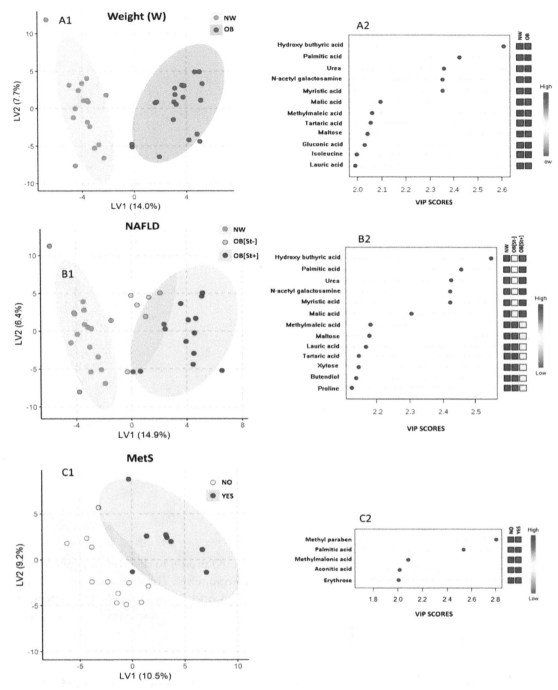

Figure 1. Partial least square discriminant analysis (PLS-DA) models to discriminate children according to Body Mass Index (BMI) (**A1**) and Non Alcoholic Fatty Liver Disease (NAFLD) (**B1**), as unique parameters investigated. The explained variance of each component is shown in parenthesis on the corresponding axis. In panel **A1**, the green ellipse contains normal weight children, while the red one contains the obese children. In panel **B1**, the purple circles represent the obese children with NAFLD (OB[St+]), the pink circles represent obese children without NAFLD (OB[St−]), while green circles represent the normal weight controls (NW). In panel **C1**, the blue circles represent the children with a diagnosis of metabolic syndrome (MetS), while the yellow ones represent the children without MetS diagnosis. The first 12, 13 and 5 variables important in projection (VIP) identified by the corresponding PLS-DA are shown in Panels **A2**, **B2** and **C2** respectively. The number of VIPs was established by setting the VIP-score ≥ 2 as a cut off value. In all cases, the colored boxes on the right indicate the relative amount of the corresponding metabolite in each group under study.

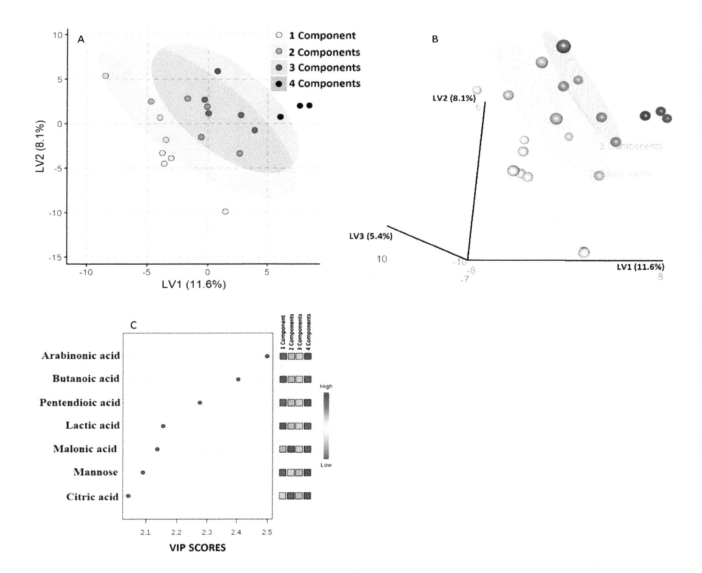

Figure 2. Partial least squares discriminant analysis (PLS-DA) model to discriminate obese children according to the number of Metabolic Syndrome (MetS) components. The explained variance of each component is shown on the corresponding axis. In panels **A** and **B**, the color darkness progression denotes the MetS components increase. The seven metabolites with a variable important in projection score (VIP-score) higher than 2 are shown in Panel **C**.

Figure 2 represents the PLS-DA model regarding the aggregation of saliva samples by the number of MetS components.

A clear-cut class separation was achieved, following the increase in the number of MetS components (Figure 2A,B). The metabolites with a VIP-score > 2 were as follows: arabinoic, butanoic, pentendioic, lactic, malonic and citric acid and mannose (Figure 2C).

Obese patients were also aggregated considering the serum ALT concentration. Figure 3A reports on the PLS-DA model when the serum ALT level higher than 40 mg/mL was considered hypertransaminasemia. Nine metabolites (butentriol, methyl valeric acid, pentanedioic acid, valine, hydroxy butanoic acid, mannose, di-n-octyl-phthalate and stearic and glyceric acid) showed a VIP-score higher than 2 (Figure 3C).

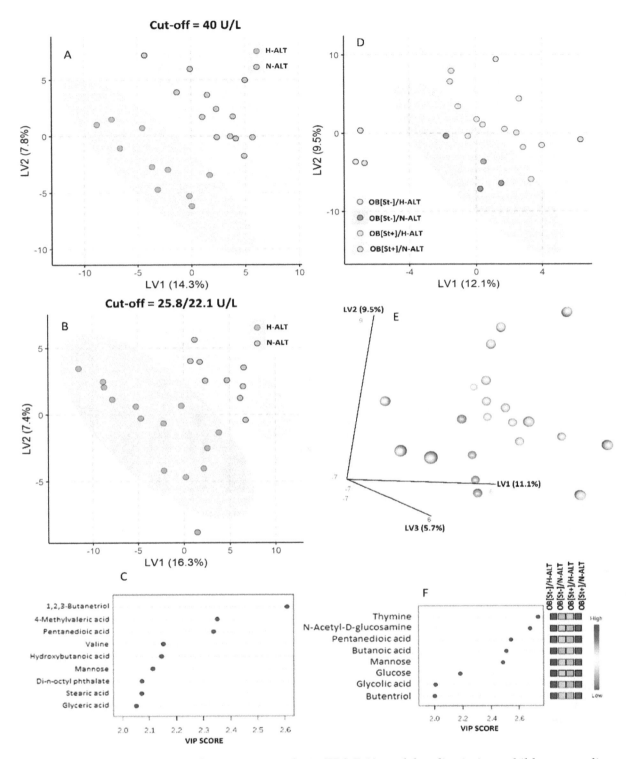

Figure 3. Partial least squares discriminant analysis (PLS-DA) model to discriminate children according to the presence/absence of hypertransaminasemia. Panel **A**: Serum Alanine transaminase (ALT) > 40 U/L was considered as hypertransaminasemia for both boys and girls. The explained variance of each component is shown on the corresponding axis. Panel **B**. Serum ALT > 25.8 U/L for boys and 22.1 U/L for girls was considered as hypertransaminasemia. In panels **A** and **B**, the cyan ellipse contains children with ALT > cut off values, while gray circles represent the children with serum ALT lower than cut off values. The nine metabolites with a VIP-score higher than 2 are shown in Panel **C**. PLS-DA shown in Panels **D/E** cumulates information on the status of both hepatic steatosis and transaminases values with respective variable important in projection scores (VIP-scores) shown in Panel **F**.

When the serum ALT level >25.8U/L for boys and 22.1 U/L for girls were considered hypertransaminasemia [24], the PLS-DA model remained discriminant (panel 3B), and the metabolites showing a VIP score >2 remained unchanged (panel 3C). PLS-DA shown in Panel 3D/E cumulates information on the status of both hepatic steatosis and transaminase values with respective VIP-scores shown in Panel F.

Figure 4 illustrates the UpSet [37] representation summarizing the selected metabolites in several classifications and the relationships between sets.

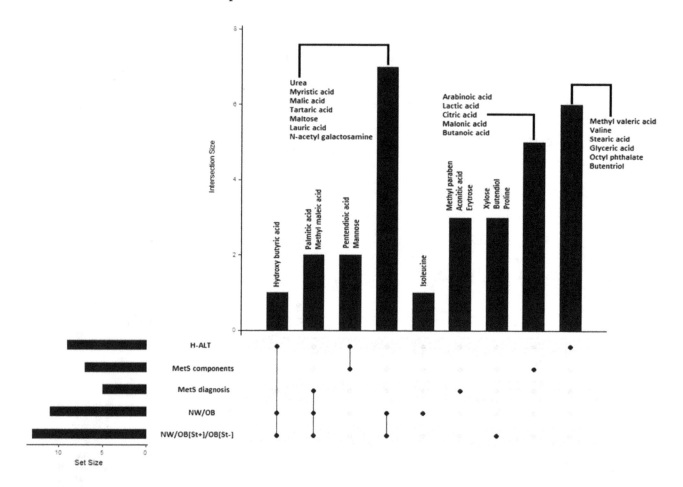

Figure 4. UpSet representation of the metabolites selected in the different classification models. H-ALT: Hypertransaminasemia; MetS: Metabolic Syndrome; NW: normal weight, OB: obese, [St]: hepatic steatosis.

Overall, as shown in the metabolic systemic map (Figure 5), there is a definite interplay of several pathways involving the following processes: de novo fatty acid biosynthesis; saturated fatty acid beta-oxidation; butanoate metabolism; glycolysis and gluconeogenesis; tricarboxylic acid cycle; urea cycle and metabolism of proline, glutamate, aspartate and asparagine; valine, leucine and isoleucine (BCCA) degradation; amino sugar metabolism; purine metabolism; and glycerophospholipid metabolism.

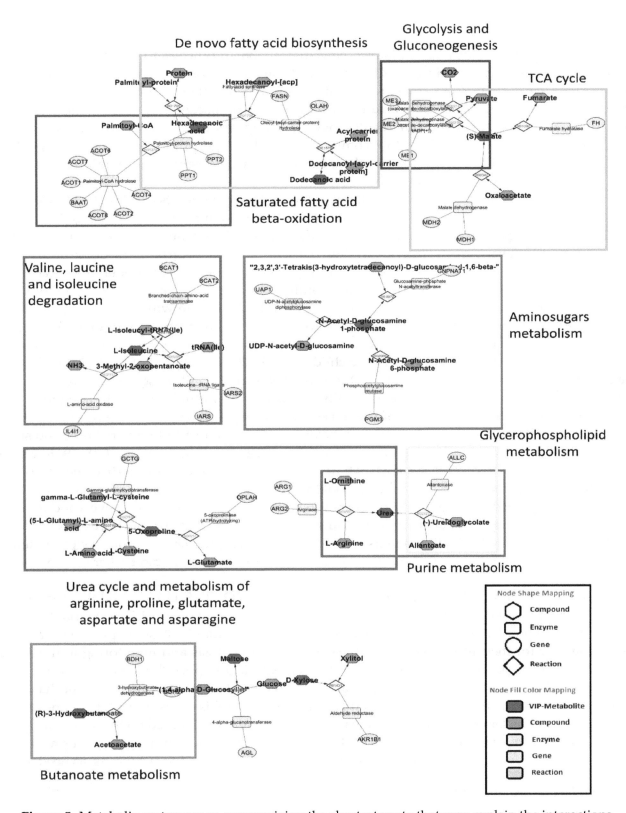

Figure 5. Metabolic systems map summarizing the shortest route that may explain the interactions among the metabolites with a variable important in projection scores higher than 2. There is a clear interplay of several pathways involving: de novo fatty acid biosynthesis; saturated fatty acid beta-oxidation; butanoate metabolism; glycolysis and gluconeogenesis; tricarboxylic acid cycle (TCA); urea cycle and metabolism of proline, glutamate, aspartate and asparagine; valine, and isoleucine (branched chain amino acids) degradation; aminosugars metabolism; purine metabolism; glycerophospholipid metabolism.

4. Discussion

As in a few other conditions (pediatric celiac disease [38], mild cognitive impairment [2], sport performance/fatigue [3,39], T2D [5,40]/T1D [41], and some neurological conditions [42]), our study shows that salivary metabolomics may represent a useful tool to obtain additional pathomechanistic information and serve as a possible clue to individuate novel disease diagnostic biomarkers data also in pediatric obesity. From our results, overall it appears that several salivary metabolites and metabolic pathways contribute to a complex metabolic fingerprint of obesity, obesity-related NAFLD and obesity-related MetS. Some of these metabolites were easily predictable based on obesity pathophysiology whereas others were not.

In line with blood and urinary metabolomic results obtained by others [43–45], the BCAAs valine and isoleucine were among the AAs more prevalently involved in the obesity-deranged pathways, but they did not appear to accurately reflect specific hepatic [43] or metabolic [44,45] involvement. The network of salivary molecules separating the lean and obese groups in obese individuals (independently from having or not MetS/NAFLD comorbidities) was also notably characterized by higher levels of two saturated fatty acids, palmitic acid and myristic acid, which tended to be prevalent in those with steatosis. Interestingly, this finding is in line with recently reported data suggesting that elevated total serum ceramide, as well as specific concentrations of myristic, palmitic, palmitoleic, stearic, oleic, behenic and lignoceric ceramide, with insulin resistance and play a potential role in the development of NAFLD in obese children [46]. The correlation of the lipid profile with glucose and insulin levels has been reported to probably mirror a still preserved ability to adapt to a caloric challenge compared with metabolically unhealthy individuals [47,48], in line with recent suggestions that propose a fatty acid profile is a useful tool to explain part of the heterogeneity between abdominal obesity and MetS [11,48,49]. Others have reported that, in addition to palmitic and stearic acid, other FAs are deranged and that increased activity of C16 Δ9-desaturase and C18 Δ9-desaturase in parallel with decreased Δ5-desaturase activity may be a causative factor in disturbed fatty acid metabolism [50]. In line with recent mouse model studies [51] where chronic oral administration of myristic acid improved hyperglycemia by decreasing insulin-responsive glucose levels and reducing body weight, myristic acid in our enrichment pathway is a fatty acid that appears to be associated with obesity but not with MetS. Finally, patients with fatty liver had higher levels of salivary pyroglutamic acid, a metabolite that has recently been proposed as a possible diagnostic biomarker for more severe liver disease [52].

Even more interestingly, as seen also by others in blood [12], PLS-DA showed that the salivary metabolic profiles could correctly identify children with a fewer number of MetS criteria than those who displayed more. This suggests that metabolic profiles can stratify MetS subpopulations, therefore, paving the way for their utilization for both early disease diagnosis and monitoring in those with MetS. This appears particularly relevant as in a recent Clinical Report, the American Academy of Pediatrics (AAP) Committee on Nutrition [53] acknowledged that although several attempts have been made to define MetS in the pediatric population, the construct at this age is difficult to define and has unclear implications for clinical care. For this reason, the Committee focused on the importance of (a) screening for and treating each individual risk factor component of MetS and (b) increasing awareness of comorbid conditions including NAFLD to be addressed and referred to specialists, as needed.

Study Limitations and Strengths

Our findings should be considered in the context of several study limitations, including a relatively small sample size, methodological flaws, and the lack of liver biopsy and prospective data during follow-up. First, our sample size was somewhat limited, and we may have had insufficient power to detect significant associations, particularly for stratified analyses. Larger series with patient follow-up are needed to confirm the preliminary results of our pilot study. Second, our findings related to VIP metabolites should be interpreted with caution given that these were obtained on only one saliva sample for each of the participant children. Although saliva was revealed to be a reliable biofluid for metabolomics studies [17], neurological disorder [42], and T1D [41], the likely risks of poor reproducibility persist. In fact, possible, differences among unstimulated, stimulated (e.g., obtained with oral movements such as gentle mastication), and pure parotid saliva exist [54,55]. Third, ultrasound may be insensitive compared with biopsy or magnetic resonance imaging (MRI). Nevertheless, it is the reference test for use in pediatric clinical practice. Furthermore, liver biopsy cannot be considered a screening procedure because it is invasive, not riskless and not exempt from possible sampling errors. As a non-invasive alternative to assess hepatic steatosis, US is repeatable because it does not require sedation or the delivery of ionizing radiation [1,56]. Although it is the less robust of the numerous imaging options [57], methodological progress has shown good diagnostic specificity and sensitivity, especially if the steatosis involves at least 20% of the hepatocytes [58]. Overall, these limitations do not allow us to draw definite conclusions but strongly suggest the viability of such an approach. These limitations, however, are balanced by several important strengths, including a full auxological and biochemical characterization of our subjects' cohort that allowed us to build several classification models on the same group of patients and delineate the metabolite/metabolic pathways. Moreover, this represents the first study to show the potential usefulness of saliva to define a metabolomic signature of pediatric obesity and related hepato-metabolic comorbidities.

5. Conclusions

Using the saliva of children affected by obesity, we showed a definite interplay of several metabolic pathways with possible specific patterns capable of sorting fatty liver and MetS. The involved metabolic processes include the following: de novo fatty acid biosynthesis; saturated fatty acid beta-oxidation; butanoate metabolism; glycolysis and gluconeogenesis; tricarboxylic acid cycle; urea cycle; metabolism of proline, glutamate, aspartate and asparagine; valine, leucine and isoleucine (BCAA) degradation; aminosugar metabolism; purine metabolism; and glycerophospholipid metabolism. Overall, this information, along with that of other recent progress regarding the study of salivary simple analytes [4], trace elements [59], major adipocytokines [60,61], and specific microRNAs [62], reinforces the idea that saliva will soon represent a useful tool for deepening pathomechanismistic aspects, noninvasive diagnosis and monitoring of pediatric and adult individuals with obesity. The early and non-invasive detection of incipient MetS/fatty liver in childhood through salivary metabolomics as described here, therefore, appears as a promising helpful tool to prevent further health hepato-metabolic and cardiovascular complications in adulthood, and ultimately serves to minimize their related global socioeconomic burden.

Author Contributions: J.T. and P.V. conceived and designed the experimental study, and contributed equally; F.B., A.B., L.P., C.M., A.D.N., A.G.D.A, L.D.M., A.P.D.B. and S.G.N. characterized clinical/lab features of the patients; J.T., A.C. and G.S. performed GC/MS experiments; P.C., G.S. and J.T. analyzed the data; J.T and G.S. contributed reagents/materials/analysis tools and to the development of the analytical methods; J.T. and P.V. wrote the paper which was integrated and fully agreed by all authors.

References

1. Clemente, M.G.; Mandato, C.; Poeta, M.; Vajro, P. Pediatric non-alcoholic fatty liver disease: Recent solutions, unresolved issues, and future research directions. *World J. Gastroenterol.* **2016**, *22*, 8078–8093. [CrossRef] [PubMed]

2. Zheng, J.; Dixon, R.A.; Li, L. Development of Isotope Labeling LC-MS for Human Salivary Metabolomics and Application to Profiling Metabolome Changes Associated with Mild Cognitive Impairment. *Anal. Chem.* **2012**, *84*, 10802–10811. [CrossRef] [PubMed]

3. Ra, S.-G.; Maeda, S.; Higashino, R.; Imai, T.; Miyakawa, S. Metabolomics of salivary fatigue markers in soccer players after consecutive games. *Appl. Physiol. Nutr. Metab.* **2014**, *39*, 1120–1126. [CrossRef] [PubMed]

4.   Troisi, J.; Belmonte, F.; Bisogno, A.; Lausi, O.; Marciano, F.; Cavallo, P.; Guercio Nuzio, S.; Landolfi, A.; Pierri, L.; Vajro, P. Salivary markers of hepato-metabolic comorbidities in pediatric obesity. *Dig. Liver Dis.* **2018**. [CrossRef] [PubMed]

5.   Martos-Moreno, G.A.; Sackmann-Sala, L.; Barrios, V.; Berrymann, D.E.; Okada, S.; Argente, J.; Kopchick, J.J. Proteomic analysis allows for early detection of potential markers of metabolic impairment in very young obese children. *Int. J. Pediatr. Endocrinol.* **2014**, *2014*, 9. [CrossRef] [PubMed]

6.   Miccheli, A.; Capuani, G.; Marini, F.; Tomassini, A.; Pratico, G.; Ceccarelli, S.; Gnani, D.; Baviera, G.; Alisi, A.; Putignani, L.; et al. Urinary (1)H-NMR-based metabolic profiling of children with NAFLD undergoing VSL#3 treatment. *Int. J. Obes.* **2015**, *39*, 1118–1125.

7.   Wiklund, P.K.; Pekkala, S.; Autio, R.; Munukka, E.; Xu, L.; Saltevo, J.; Cheng, S.; Kujala, U.M.; Alen, M.; Cheng, S. Serum metabolic profiles in overweight and obese women with and without metabolic syndrome. *Diabetol. Metab. Syndr.* **2014**, *6*, 40. [CrossRef]

8.   Wurtz, P.; Makinen, V.-P.; Soininen, P.; Kangas, A.J.; Tukiainen, T.; Kettunen, J.; Savolainen, M.J.; Tammelin, T.; Viikari, J.S.; Ronnemaa, T.; et al. Metabolic signatures of insulin resistance in 7098 young adults. *Diabetes* **2012**, *61*, 1372–1380. [CrossRef]

9.   Jin, T.; Yu, H.; Huang, X.-F. Selective binding modes and allosteric inhibitory effects of lupane triterpenes on protein tyrosine phosphatase 1B. *Sci. Rep.* **2016**, *6*, 20766. [CrossRef]

10. Butte, N.F.; Liu, Y.; Zakeri, I.F.; Mohney, R.P.; Mehta, N.; Voruganti, V.S.; Goring, H.; Cole, S.A.; Comuzzie, A.G. Global metabolomic profiling targeting childhood obesity in the Hispanic population. *Am. J. Clin. Nutr.* **2015**, *102*, 256–267. [CrossRef]

11. Baek, S.H.; Kim, M.; Kim, M.; Kang, M.; Yoo, H.J.; Lee, N.H.; Kim, Y.H.; Song, M.; Lee, J.H. Metabolites distinguishing visceral fat obesity and atherogenic traits in individuals with overweight. *Obesity* **2017**, *25*, 323–331. [CrossRef] [PubMed]

12. Zhong, F.; Xu, M.; Bruno, R.S.; Ballard, K.D.; Zhu, J. Targeted high performance liquid chromatography tandem mass spectrometry-based metabolomics differentiates metabolic syndrome from obesity. *Exp. Biol. Med.* **2017**, *242*, 773–780. [CrossRef]

13. Pujos-Guillot, E.; Brandolini, M.; Pétéra, M.; Grissa, D.; Joly, C.; Lyan, B.; Herquelot, É.; Czernichow, S.; Zins, M.; Goldberg, M. Systems metabolomics for prediction of metabolic syndrome. *J. Proteome Res.* **2017**, *16*, 2262–2272. [CrossRef] [PubMed]

14. Pierri, L.; Saggese, P.; Guercio Nuzio, S.; Troisi, J.; Di Stasi, M.; Poeta, M.; Savastano, R.; Marchese, G.; Tarallo, R.; Massa, G.; et al. Relations of gut liver axis components and gut microbiota in obese children with fatty liver: A pilot study. *Clin. Res. Hepatol. Gastroenterol.* **2018**, *42*, 387–390. [CrossRef]

15. Troisi, J.; Pierri, L.; Landolfi, A.; Marciano, F.; Bisogno, A.; Belmonte, F.; Palladino, C.; Guercio Nuzio, S.; Campiglia, P.; Vajro, P. Urinary Metabolomics in Pediatric Obesity and NAFLD Identifies Metabolic Pathways/Metabolites Related to Dietary Habits and Gut-Liver Axis Perturbations. *Nutrients* **2017**, *9*, E485. [CrossRef] [PubMed]

16. Dame, Z.T.; Aziat, F.; Mandal, R.; Krishnamurthy, R.; Bouatra, S.; Borzouie, S.; Guo, A.C.; Sajed, T.; Deng, L.; Lin, H.; et al. The human saliva metabolome. *Metabolomics* **2015**, *11*, 1864–1883. [CrossRef]

17. Hartman, M.-L.; Goodson, J.M.; Barake, R.; Alsmadi, O.; Al-Mutawa, S.; Ariga, J.; Soparkar, P.; Behbehani, J.; Behbehani, K. Salivary Biomarkers in Pediatric Metabolic Disease Research. *Pediatr. Endocrinol. Rev.* **2016**, *13*, 602–611.

18. Belmonte, F.; Bisogno, A.; Troisi, J.; Landolfi, A.M.; Lausi, O.; Lamberti, R.; Nuzio, S.G.; Pierri, L.; Siano, M.; Viggiano, C.; et al. Salivary levels of uric acid, insulin and HOMA: A promising field of study to non-invasively identify obese children at risk of metabolic syndrome and fatty liver. *Dig. Liver Dis.* **2017**, *49*, e247. [CrossRef]

19. Cho, K.; Moon, J.S.; Kang, J.-H.; Jang, H.B.; Lee, H.-J.; Park, S.I.; Yu, K.-S.; Cho, J.-Y. Combined untargeted and targeted metabolomic profiling reveals urinary biomarkers for discriminating obese from normal-weight adolescents. *Pediatr. Obes.* **2017**, *12*, 93–101. [CrossRef]

20. Ho, J.E.; Larson, M.G.; Ghorbani, A.; Cheng, S.; Chen, M.-H.; Keyes, M.; Rhee, E.P.; Clish, C.B.; Vasan, R.S.; Gerszten, R.E.; et al. Metabolomic Profiles of Body Mass Index in the Framingham Heart Study Reveal Distinct Cardiometabolic Phenotypes. *PLoS ONE* **2016**, *11*, e0148361. [CrossRef]

21. Zheng, H.; Yde, C.C.; Arnberg, K.; Molgaard, C.; Michaelsen, K.F.; Larnkjaer, A.; Bertram, H.C. NMR-based metabolomic profiling of overweight adolescents: An elucidation of the effects of inter-/intraindividual differences, gender, and pubertal development. *Biomed. Res. Int.* **2014**, *2014*, 537157. [CrossRef] [PubMed]

22. Vajro, P.; Lenta, S.; Pignata, C.; Salerno, M.; D'Aniello, R.; De Micco, I.; Paolella, G.; Parenti, G. Therapeutic options in pediatric non alcoholic fatty liver disease: Current status and future directions. *Ital. J. Pediatr.* **2012**, *38*, 55. [CrossRef]

23. Schwenzer, N.F.; Springer, F.; Schraml, C.; Stefan, N.; Machann, J.; Schick, F. Non-invasive assessment and quantification of liver steatosis by ultrasound, computed tomography and magnetic resonance. *J. Hepatol.* **2009**, *51*, 433–445. [CrossRef] [PubMed]

24. Schwimmer, J.B.; Dunn, W.; Norman, G.J.; Pardee, P.E.; Middleton, M.S.; Kerkar, N.; Sirlin, C.B. SAFETY study: Alanine aminotransferase cutoff values are set too high for reliable detection of pediatric chronic liver disease. *Gastroenterology* **2010**, *138*, 1357–1364. [CrossRef] [PubMed]

25. Vajro, P.; Maddaluno, S.; Veropalumbo, C. Persistent hypertransaminasemia in asymptomatic children: A stepwise approach. *World J. Gastroenterol.* **2013**, *19*, 2740–2751. [CrossRef] [PubMed]

26. Zimmet, P.; Alberti, K.G.M.; Kaufman, F.; Tajima, N.; Silink, M.; Arslanian, S.; Wong, G.; Bennett, P.; Shaw, J.; Caprio, S. The metabolic syndrome in children and adolescents—An IDF consensus report. *Pediatr. Diabetes* **2007**, *8*, 299–306. [CrossRef] [PubMed]

27. World Medical Association. World medical association declaration of helsinki: Ethical principles for medical research involving human subjects. *JAMA* **2013**, *310*, 2191–2194. [CrossRef]

28. Kovats, E.S. Gas-chromatographische charakterisierung organischer verbindungen. Teil 1: Retentionsindices aliphatischer halogenide, alkohole, aldehyde und ketone. *Helv. Chim. Acta* **1958**, *41*, 1915–1932. [CrossRef]

29. van den Berg, R.A.; Hoefsloot, H.C.; Westerhuis, J.A.; Smilde, A.K.; van der Werf, M.J. Centering, scaling, and transformations: Improving the biological information content of metabolomics data. *BMC Genom.* **2006**, *7*, 142. [CrossRef]

30. Sumner, L.W.; Amberg, A.; Barrett, D.; Beale, M.H.; Beger, R.; Daykin, C.A.; Fan, T.W.-M.; Fiehn, O.; Goodacre, R.; Griffin, J.L.; et al. Proposed minimum reporting standards for chemical analysis Chemical Analysis Working Group (CAWG) Metabolomics Standards Initiative (MSI). *Metabolomics* **2007**, *3*, 211–221. [CrossRef]

31. Sysi-Aho, M.; Katajamaa, M.; Yetukuri, L.; Oresic, M. Normalization method for metabolomics data using optimal selection of multiple internal standards. *BMC Bioinformatics* **2007**, *8*, 93. [CrossRef] [PubMed]

32. Mevik, B.-H.; Wehrens, R. The pls Package: Principal Component and Partial Least Squares Regression in R. *J. Stat. Softw.* **2007**. [CrossRef]

33. Kuhn, M. Building Predictive Models in R Using the caret Package. *J. Stat. Softw.* **2008**, *28*, 1–26. [CrossRef]

34. Bijlsma, S.; Bobeldijk, I.; Verheij, E.R.; Ramaker, R.; Kochhar, S.; Macdonald, I.A.; van Ommen, B.; Smilde, A.K. Large-scale human metabolomics studies: A strategy for data (pre-) processing and validation. *Anal. Chem.* **2006**, *78*, 567–574. [CrossRef] [PubMed]

35. Karnovsky, A.; Weymouth, T.; Hull, T.; Tarcea, V.G.; Scardoni, G.; Laudanna, C.; Sartor, M.A.; Stringer, K.A.; Jagadish, H.V.; Burant, C.; et al. Metscape 2 bioinformatics tool for the analysis and visualization of metabolomics and gene expression data. *Bioinformatics* **2012**, *28*, 373–380. [CrossRef] [PubMed]

36. Nishida, K.; Ono, K.; Kanaya, S.; Takahashi, K. KEGGscape: A Cytoscape app for pathway data integration. *F1000Research* **2014**, *3*, 144. [CrossRef] [PubMed]

37. Lex, A.; Gehlenborg, N.; Strobelt, H.; Vuillemot, R.; Pfister, H. UpSet: Visualization of Intersecting Sets. *IEEE Trans. Vis. Comput. Gr.* **2014**, *20*, 1983–1992. [CrossRef] [PubMed]

38. Francavilla, R.; Ercolini, D.; Piccolo, M.; Vannini, L.; Siragusa, S.; De Filippis, F.; De Pasquale, I.; Di Cagno, R.; Di Toma, M.; Gozzi, G.; et al. Salivary microbiota and metabolome associated with celiac disease. *Appl. Environ. Microbiol.* **2014**, *80*, 3416–3425. [CrossRef]

39. Santone, C.; Dinallo, V.; Paci, M.; D'Ottavio, S.; Barbato, G.; Bernardini, S. Saliva metabolomics by NMR for the evaluation of sport performance. *J. Pharm. Biomed.* **2014**, *88*, 441–446. [CrossRef]

40. Rao, P.V.; Reddy, A.P.; Lu, X.; Dasari, S.; Krishnaprasad, A.; Biggs, E.; Roberts, C.T.; Nagalla, S.R. Proteomic identification of salivary biomarkers of type-2 diabetes. *J. Proteome Res.* **2009**, *8*, 239–245. [CrossRef]

41. Pappa, E.; Vastardis, H.; Mermelekas, G.; Gerasimidi-Vazeou, A.; Zoidakis, J.; Vougas, K. Saliva Proteomics Analysis Offers Insights on Type 1 Diabetes Pathology in a Pediatric Population. *Front. Physiol.* **2018**, *9*, 444. [CrossRef] [PubMed]

42. Walton, E.L. Saliva biomarkers in neurological disorders: A "spitting image" of brain health? *Biomed. J.* **2018**, *41*, 59–62. [CrossRef] [PubMed]

43. Goffredo, M.; Santoro, N.; Tricò, D.; Giannini, C.; D'Adamo, E.; Zhao, H.; Peng, G.; Yu, X.; Lam, T.T.; Pierpont, B. A branched-chain amino acid-related metabolic signature characterizes obese adolescents with non-alcoholic fatty liver disease. *Nutrients* **2017**, *9*, 642. [CrossRef] [PubMed]

44. Wu, N.; Wang, W.; Yi, M.; Cheng, S.; Wang, D. *Study of the Metabolomics Characteristics of Patients with Metabolic Syndrome Based on Liquid Chromatography Quadrupole Time-Of-Flight Mass Spectrometry*; Elsevier: Amsterdam, The Netherlands, 2018; Volume 79, pp. 37–44.

45. Reddy, P.; Leong, J.; Jialal, I. Amino acid levels in nascent metabolic syndrome: A contributor to the pro-inflammatory burden. *J. Diabetes Complicat.* **2018**, *32*, 465–469. [CrossRef] [PubMed]

46. Wasilewska, N.; Bobrus-Chociej, A.; Harasim-Symbor, E.; Tarasów, E.; Wojtkowska, M.; Chabowski, A.; Lebensztejn, D. Serum concentration of ceramides in obese children with nonalcoholic fatty liver disease. *J. Pediatr. Gastroenterol. Nutr.* **2018**, *66*, S2. [CrossRef] [PubMed]

47. Badoud, F.; Lam, K.P.; Perreault, M.; Zulyniak, M.A.; Britz-McKibbin, P.; Mutch, D.M. Metabolomics reveals metabolically healthy and unhealthy obese individuals differ in their response to a caloric challenge. *PLoS ONE* **2015**, *10*, e0134613. [CrossRef] [PubMed]

48. Aristizabal, J.C.; Barona, J.; Gonzalez-Zapata, L.I.; Deossa, G.C.; Estrada, A. Fatty acid content of plasma triglycerides may contribute to the heterogeneity in the relationship between abdominal obesity and the metabolic syndrome. *Metab. Syndr. Relat. Disord.* **2016**, *14*, 311–317. [CrossRef] [PubMed]

49. Aristizabal, J.C.; González-Zapata, L.I.; Estrada-Restrepo, A.; Monsalve-Alvarez, J.; Restrepo-Mesa, S.L.; Gaitán, D. Concentrations of plasma free palmitoleic and dihomo-gamma linoleic fatty acids are higher in children with abdominal obesity. *Nutrients* **2018**, *10*, 31. [CrossRef]

50. Kang, M.; Lee, A.; Yoo, H.J.; Kim, M.; Kim, M.; Shin, D.Y.; Lee, J.H. Association between increased visceral fat area and alterations in plasma fatty acid profile in overweight subjects: A cross-sectional study. *Lipids Health Dis.* **2017**, *16*, 248. [CrossRef]

51. Takato, T.; Iwata, K.; Murakami, C.; Wada, Y.; Sakane, F. Chronic administration of myristic acid improves hyperglycaemia in the Nagoya–Shibata–Yasuda mouse model of congenital type 2 diabetes. *Diabetologia* **2017**, *60*, 2076–2083. [CrossRef]

52. Qi, S.; Xu, D.; Li, Q.; Xie, N.; Xia, J.; Huo, Q.; Li, P.; Chen, Q.; Huang, S. Metabonomics screening of serum identifies pyroglutamate as a diagnostic biomarker for nonalcoholic steatohepatitis. *Clin. Chim. Acta* **2017**, *473*, 89–95. [CrossRef]

53. Magge, S.N.; Goodman, E.; Armstrong, S.C. The Metabolic Syndrome in Children and Adolescents: Shifting the Focus to Cardiometabolic Risk Factor Clustering. *Pediatrics* **2017**, *24*, e20171603. [CrossRef]

54. Denny, P.; Hagen, F.K.; Hardt, M.; Liao, L.; Yan, W.; Arellanno, M.; Bassilian, S.; Bedi, G.S.; Boontheung, P.; Cociorva, D. The proteomes of human parotid and submandibular/sublingual gland salivas collected as the ductal secretions. *J. Proteome Res.* **2008**, *7*, 1994–2006. [CrossRef]

55. Tiwari, M. Science behind human saliva. *J. Nat. Sci. Biol. Med.* **2011**, *2*, 53–58. [CrossRef]

56. Vajro, P.; Lenta, S.; Socha, P.; Dhawan, A.; McKiernan, P.; Baumann, U.; Durmaz, O.; Lacaille, F.; McLin, V.; Nobili, V. Diagnosis of nonalcoholic fatty liver disease in children and adolescents: Position paper of the ESPGHAN Hepatology Committee. *J. Pediatr. Gastroenterol. Nutr.* **2012**, *54*, 700–713. [CrossRef]

57. Vos, M.B.; Abrams, S.H.; Barlow, S.E.; Caprio, S.; Daniels, S.R.; Kohli, R.; Mouzaki, M.; Sathya, P.; Schwimmer, J.B.; Sundaram, S.S. NASPGHAN clinical practice guideline for the diagnosis and treatment of nonalcoholic fatty liver disease in children: Recommendations from the Expert Committee on NAFLD (ECON) and the North American Society of Pediatric Gastroenterology, Hepatology and Nutrition (NASPGHAN). *J. Pediatr. Gastroenterol. Nutr.* **2017**, *64*, 319–334.

58. Koot, B.G.; van der Baan-Slootweg, O.H.; Bohte, A.E.; Nederveen, A.J.; van Werven, J.R.; Tamminga-Smeulders, C.L.; Merkus, M.P.; Schaap, F.G.; Jansen, P.L.; Stoker, J. Accuracy of prediction scores and novel biomarkers for predicting nonalcoholic fatty liver disease in obese children. *Obesity* **2013**, *21*, 583–590. [CrossRef]

59. Marin Martinez, L.; Molino Pagan, D.; Lopez Jornet, P. Trace Elements in Saliva as Markers of Type 2 Diabetes Mellitus. *Biol. Trace Elem. Res.* **2018**, *186*, 354–360. [CrossRef]

60.   Abdalla, M.M.I.; Soon, S.C. Salivary adiponectin concentration in healthy adult males in relation to anthropometric measures and fat distribution. *Endocr. Regul.* **2017**, *51*, 185–192. [CrossRef]

61.   Ibrahim Abdalla, M.M.; Siew Choo, S. Salivary Leptin Level in Young Adult Males and its Association with Anthropometric Measurements, Fat Distribution and Muscle Mass. *Eur. Endocrinol.* **2018**, *14*, 94–98. [CrossRef]

62.   Vriens, A.; Provost, E.B.; Saenen, N.D.; De Boever, P.; Vrijens, K.; De Wever, O.; Plusquin, M.; Nawrot, T.S. Children's screen time alters the expression of saliva extracellular miR-222 and miR-146a. *Sci. Rep.* **2018**, *8*, 8209. [CrossRef]

13

Sugar-Sweetened Beverages and Cardiometabolic Health

Vasanti S. Malik [1,2,*] **and Frank B. Hu** [2,3,4]

[1] Department of Nutritional Sciences, Faculty of Medicine, University of Toronto, 1 King's College Circle, Toronto, ON M5S 1A8, Canada
[2] Department of Nutrition, Harvard T.H. Chan School of Public Health, 665 Huntington Avenue, Boston, MA 02115, USA
[3] Department of Epidemiology, Harvard T.H. School of Public Health, Boston, MA 02115, USA
[4] Channing Division of Network Medicine, Brigham and Women's Hospital and Harvard Medical School, Boston, MA 02115, USA
* Correspondence: vasanti.malik@utoronto.ca

Abstract: Sugar-sweetened beverages (SSBs) have little nutritional value and a robust body of evidence has linked the intake of SSBs to weight gain and risk of type 2 diabetes (T2D), cardiovascular disease (CVD), and some cancers. Metabolic Syndrome (MetSyn) is a clustering of risk factors that precedes the development of T2D and CVD; however, evidence linking SSBs to MetSyn is not clear. To make informed recommendations about SSBs, new evidence needs to be considered against existing literature. This review provides an update on the evidence linking SSBs and cardiometabolic outcomes including MetSyn. Findings from prospective cohort studies support a strong positive association between SSBs and weight gain and risk of T2D and coronary heart disease (CHD), independent of adiposity. Associations with MetSyn are less consistent, and there appears to be a sex difference with stroke with greater risk in women. Findings from short-term trials on metabolic risk factors provide mechanistic support for associations with T2D and CHD. Conclusive evidence from cohort studies and trials on risk factors support an etiologic role of SSB in relation to weight gain and risk of T2D and CHD. Continued efforts to reduce intake of SSB should be encouraged to improve the cardiometabolic health of individuals and populations.

Keywords: sugar-sweetened beverages; metabolic syndrome; weight gain; type 2 diabetes; cardiovascular disease; cardiometabolic risk

1. Introduction

Metabolic syndrome (MetSyn) is known as a clustering of interrelated risk factors for type 2 diabetes (T2D) and cardiovascular disease (CVD) that occur together more often than by chance alone. Although there is some confusion regarding the clinical definition of MetSyn and whether it is a unique syndrome or a mixture of unrelated phenotypes, the most widespread consensus for a diagnosis is the presence of at least three of five risk factors including hyperglycemia, raised blood pressure, elevated triglyceride levels, low high-density lipoprotein cholesterol levels, and central adiposity [1]. Given the complexity of the definition, the prevalence of MetSyn is difficult to estimate; however, data on individual risk factors suggest that MetSyn is rising across the globe in parallel with obesity trends. It was estimated that 23% of adults in the United States (US) (~50 million) have MetSyn [2,3]. This figure was relatively constant over recent years despite population-level increases in hyperglycemia and waist circumference because of decreases in hypertriglyceridemia and elevated blood pressure corresponding to medication use [4]. However, the burden of MetSyn remains high in the US and is rising in low- and middle-income countries (LMICs) [3]. This is of great concern, since individuals with MetSyn are at twice the risk of developing CVD and have a five-fold higher risk of developing T2D over the next 5–10 years [1]. Preventing or reversing MetSyn could, therefore, be an effective way to stem the rising tide of T2D and CVD.

Sugar-sweetened beverages (SSBs) are the largest source of added sugar in the diet. They include carbonated and non-carbonated soft drinks, fruit drinks, and sports drinks that contain added caloric sweeteners, and they are low in nutritional quality. To date, a large body of evidence supports a strong link between intake of SSBs and weight gain [5] and risk of T2D [6], which is the basis of many dietary guidelines and policies targeting SSBs [7].

Emerging evidence suggests that SSBs are also an important risk factor for cardiovascular diseases and related risk factors [8–12]. However, evidence linking SSBs to MetSyn is not clear. For clinicians and policy-makers to make informed recommendations about SSBs and cardiometabolic health, new evidence needs to be considered alongside existing literature. In this review, we provide an overview of global SSB intake trends and an updated summary on the evidence from prospective cohort studies and trials linking SSBs to weight gain and related cardiometabolic conditions including MetSyn. Findings from cross-sectional or case-control studies were not considered since these designs are more prone to confounding and other biases. Biological mechanisms, alternative beverage options, and policy strategies to limit SSB consumption are also discussed.

2. SSB Intake Trends

Consumption of SSBs has decreased modestly in the US since around 2002 [13]; however, intake levels are still high and, in some groups, nearly exceed the Dietary Guidelines for Americans' [14] and World Health Organization's (WHO) [7] recommendation for no more than 10% of daily calories from all added sugar. National Health and Nutrition Examination Survey (NHANES) data show that US adults consumed an average of 145 kcal/day from SSB, corresponding to 6.5% of total calories, between 2011 and 2014 with higher intake levels reported among younger age groups and among non-Hispanic black and Hispanic men and women [15].

In contrast to the US and other high-income countries where consumption of SSBs is either declining or plateauing, intake of SSBs is increasing in many LMICs as a consequence of widespread urbanization and beverage marketing. A report based on survey data from adults in 187 countries found that SSB consumption was higher in upper–middle-income countries and lower–middle-income countries compared to high-income or low-income countries [16]. Of the 21 world regions evaluated, SSB consumption was highest in the Caribbean and lowest in East Asia [16]. Another study among adolescents in 53 LMICs found that soda intake was most frequent in Central and South America, and least frequent in Southeast Asia. Across all populations surveyed, 54% consumed soda at least once a day, and one in five adolescents in Central and South America consumed soda three or more times per day [17].

These trends are supported by another study that reported that per capita sales of SSB (in daily calories per person) increased in most LMICs, while sales declined in some high-income regions, indicative of consumption patterns [18]. Chile was identified as having the highest per capita sales of SSB in 2014, followed by Mexico, the US, Argentina, and Saudi Arabia [18]. The fastest growth in sales of SSB between 2009 and 2014 was seen in Chile, along with China, Thailand, and Brazil [18](Figure 1). For some regions, disparities in SSB intake tend to track with disparities in obesity and T2D prevalence. For example, in the US, lower socioeconomic status (SES) groups tend to have higher SSB intake levels, and these groups also tend to have a higher risk for developing obesity and T2D.

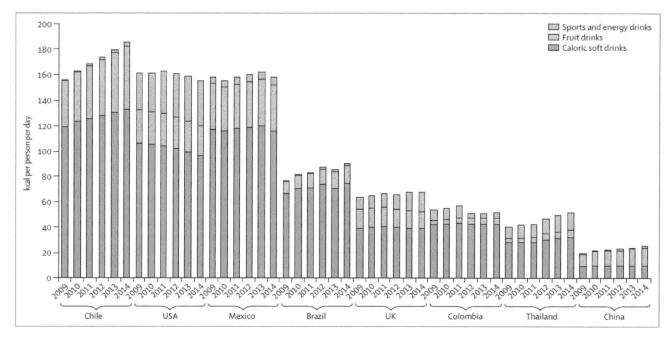

Figure 1. Sales of sugar-sweetened beverages (SSBs) in kcal per person per day by beverage type in 2009–2014 in selected countries. Data from Euromonitor Passport International, which were obtained from nutrition fact panels and websites of sugar-sweetened beverage companies; kcal = kilocalories [18].

3. Weight Gain and Obesity

Many observational studies have evaluated the relationship between consumption of SSBs and weight gain or obesity. The majority [5,19–23] of systematic reviews and meta-analyses on this topic found positive associations between SSBs and weight gain or risk of overweight or obesity. However, others reported null associations [24]. Our previous meta-analysis, the most comprehensive to date, found that a one-serving-per-day increase in SSB was associated with an additional weight gain of 0.12 kg over one year [5]. In this analysis, we included estimates that were not adjusted for total energy intake since the association between SSBs and weight gain is likely mediated through calories. In addition, all of the studies included in the meta-analysis had repeated measurements of diet and weight, and evaluated weight change in relation to change in SSB intake. This type of analysis strategy has some of the features of a quasi-experimental design, although it lacks the element of randomization. An advantage of this design is the generalizability to a real-world setting, because participants are able to change their diet and lifestyle without investigator-driven intervention. Although the results of the meta-analysis seem modest, adult weight gain in the general population is a gradual process, occurring over decades and averaging about one pound (0.45 kg) per year [25]; thus, small gains in weight from SSBs could be substantial over many years.

The association between SSBs and obesity is strengthened by our previous analysis of gene–SSB interactions [26]. Based on data from three large cohorts, we found that individuals who consumed one or more servings of SSB per day had genetic effects on body mass index (BMI) and obesity risk that were twice as large as those who consumed SSBs less than once per month. These data suggest that regular consumers of SSB may be more susceptible to genetic effects on obesity, or that persons with a greater genetic predisposition to obesity may be more susceptible to the deleterious effects of SSBs on BMI.

Compared to observational studies, most trials have evaluated short-term effects on weight change rather than long-term patterns. In our previous meta-analysis of five trials, we found that adding SSBs to the diet significantly increased body weight [5]. Another meta-analysis of seven randomized controlled trials (RCTs) also found a significant increase in body weight when SSBs were added to the diet [24]. However, in their meta-analysis of eight trials attempting to reduce SSB intake, no overall effect on BMI was observed, but a significant benefit on weight loss/less weight gain was observed among individuals who were overweight at baseline [24]. Of note, this meta-analysis included two of the largest and most rigorously conducted RCTs in children and adolescents [27,28] to date.

Another meta-analysis evaluating the effects of dietary sugars on body weight found that, in trials of adults with ad libitum diets, reducing intake of free sugar or SSB was associated with a decrease in body weight, while increasing intake was associated with a comparable weight increase [23]. Because isoenergetic exchange of dietary sugars with other carbohydrates showed no change in body weight, it seems likely that the change in body weight that occurs with modifying intakes of SSBs is mediated via changes in calories [23]. The majority of studies on SSBs and body weight focused on prevention of weight gain rather than weight loss, which is an important distinguishing factor. From a public health point of view, identifying determinants of weight gain is more impactful than short-term weight loss in reducing obesity prevalence [29]. This is because, once an individual develops obesity, it is difficult to achieve and maintain weight loss. For this reason, fewer studies have evaluated the impact of SSB restriction on weight loss.

4. Metabolic Syndrome and Risk Factors

Few prospective studies have examined intake of SSBs in relation to the development of MetSyn, most likely due to challenges in outcome assessment. However, these along with studies of individual risk factors generally show adverse associations that are consistent with studies linking SSBs to weight gain and risk of T2D. Our previous meta-analysis of three cohort studies found a higher risk of about 20% (relative risk (RR), 1.20; 95% confidence interval (CI), 1.02–1.42) comparing highest to lowest categories of SSB intake [6]. However, a recent meta-analysis of three cohort studies by Narain et al. found a marginal positive association between intake of SSB and risk of MetSyn [30]. The discrepancy may be due to inclusion of different studies. The more recent meta-analysis included a new study among children and adolescents [31], which was combined with studies in adults and excluded a study from the Multi-Ethnic Study of Atherosclerosis (MESA) cohort [32], which we included. We also included the cohort-wide estimate from the Framingham Heart study that combined diet and regular soft drinks, while Narain et al. used an estimate from a sub-group with regular soft drink consumption but limited power [33]. Recent studies not included in these meta-analyses have also found positive associations. A study in the Prevención con Dieta Mediterránea (PREDIMED) trial found a positive association between SSBs and fruit juice with MetSyn among participants at high risk for CVD, but cautioned that associations should be interpreted conservatively due to low intake levels [34]. In a cohort of healthy Korean adults, a positive association between SSB and MetSyn was observed in women but not men [35]. According to the authors, the sex difference could be due to the action of sex hormones. Some studies of MetSyn found marginal associations with SSBs; however, because they adjusted for total energy intake, the results may have been underestimated [32,36].

Studies examining individual risk factors rather than MetSyn tend to be more consistent. In the Coronary Artery Risk Development in Young Adults (CARDIA) study, higher SSB consumption was associated with a number of cardiometabolic outcomes: high waist circumference (RR: 1.09; 95% CI 1.04, 1.14), high low-density lipoprotein (LDL) cholesterol (RR: 1.18; 95% CI 1.02, 1.35), high triglycerides (RR: 1.06; 95% CI 1.01, 1.13), and hypertension (RR: 1.06; 95% CI 1.01, 1.12) [37]. Although central adiposity is a risk factor for CVD independent of body weight, few cohort studies have examined this relationship with SSBs, likely due to challenges in measurement. In the Mexican Teacher's cohort, compared to no change, increasing soda consumption by one serving per day was associated with a ~1-cm increase in waist circumference (0.9 cm; 95% CI = 0.5, 1.4) over two years [38]. Similar findings were observed in a Spanish cohort [39]. Both of these studies used waist circumference as a proxy for central adiposity. However, waist circumference does not distinguish between different types of abdominal fat accumulation, e.g., visceral vs. subcutaneous adipose tissues, which may be differently associated with cardiometabolic risk. In the Framingham Third Generation cohort, Ma and colleagues found that SSB intake was associated with a long-term adverse change in visceral adiposity as measured by abdominal computed tomography scan (i.e., increased visceral adipose tissue (VAT) volume and decrease in VAT attenuation), independent of weight gain [40].

In a systematic review including five prospective cohort studies examining SSB intake in relation to vascular risk factors, positive associations were observed for blood pressure, triglycerides, LDL cholesterol, and blood glucose, and an inverse association was observed for high-density lipoprotein (HDL) cholesterol [12]. These findings were supported by cross-sectional analyses in the Health Professionals Follow-up Study (HPFS) and Nurses' Health Study (NHS) cohorts that found associations between SSB and higher plasma triglycerides, along with inflammatory cytokines and other cardiometabolic risk factors [9,41]. Accumulating evidence also suggests a role of SSBs in the development of hypertension [42–44]. A meta-analysis of six cohort studies found that a one serving/day increase in SSB intake was associated with ~8% higher risk of hypertension (RR: 1.08, 95% CI: 1.06, 1.11) [42]. Similar results were reported in two previous meta-analyses [43,44]. Regular consumption of SSBs was also associated with hyperuricemia and with gout [45,46].

Findings from short-term trials and experimental studies also provide important evidence linking SSBs with cardiometabolic risk factors, and they provide mechanistic support for the epidemiologic evidence linking intake of SSBs to higher risk of T2D and coronary heart disease (CHD). Many of these studies explored the effects of sugars used to flavor SSBs such as high-fructose corn syrup (HFCS) (~42–55% fructose, glucose and water) or sucrose (50% fructose and glucose) in liquid form. A meta-analysis of 39 RCTs found that higher compared to lower intakes of dietary sugars or SSB significantly raised triglyceride concentrations (mean difference (MD): 0.11 mmol/L; 95% CI: 0.07, 0.15), total cholesterol (MD: 0.16 mmol/L; 95% CI: 0.10, 0.24), LDL cholesterol (MD: 0.12 mmol/L; 95% CI: 0.05, 0.19), and HDL cholesterol (MD: 0.02 mmol/L; 95% CI: 0.00, 0.03) [47]. The most pronounced effects were noted in studies that ensured energy balance and when no difference in weight change was reported, suggesting that the effects of SSBs on lipids are independent of body weight [47]. This meta-analysis also found a significant blood-pressure-raising effect of sugars, particularly in studies ≥8 weeks in duration (MD 6.9 mm Hg (95% CI: 3.4, 10.3) for systolic blood pressure, and 5.6 mm Hg (95% CI: 2.5, 8.8) for diastolic blood pressure) [47].

In a two-week parallel-arm trial, Stanhope and colleagues showed that consuming beverages containing 10%, 17.5%, or 25% of energy requirements from HFCS produced a significant linear dose–response increase in postprandial triglycerides, fasting LDL cholesterol, and 24-h mean uric acid concentrations [48]. In another study, uric acid was found to increase after six months of consuming 1 L/day of sucrose-sweetened cola compared to isocaloric consumption of milk, water, or diet beverages [49]. The change in uric acid correlated with changes in liver fat ($p = 0.005$), triglycerides ($p = 0.02$), and insulin ($p = 0.002$) [49] In a 10-week trial among overweight healthy participants, consuming a sucrose-rich diet compared to a diet rich in artificial sweeteners, significant increases in postprandial glycemia, insulinemia, and lipidemia were observed [50]. A randomized crossover trial among normal-weight healthy men found that, after three weeks, SSBs consumed in small to moderate quantities resulted in impaired glucose and lipid metabolism and promoted inflammation [51]. Other trials have found inconsistent results on markers of inflammation, which may be due to differences in study duration. [52,53].

5. Diabetes and CVD

Although experimental evidence from RCTs is lacking due to high cost and other feasibility considerations, findings from prospective cohort studies have shown strong and consistent associations in well-powered studies. A meta-analysis of 17 prospective cohort studies evaluating SSB consumption and risk of T2D found that a one-serving-per-day increment in SSB was associated with an 18% higher risk of T2D (95% CI: 9% to 28%) among studies that did not adjust for adiposity [54] (Figure 2). Among studies that adjusted for adiposity, the estimate was attenuated to 13% (6% to 21%), suggesting a partial mediating role of adiposity in this association. Positive yet weaker associations were also noted for juice and artificially sweetened beverages (ASB). This study also estimated the population attributable fraction for T2D from consumption of SSB in the US and United Kingdom (UK). Based on their estimates, 8.7% (95% CI, 3.9% to 12.9%) of T2D cases in the US and 3.6% (95% CI, 1.7% to 5.6%) in the UK would be attributable to the consumption of SSBs [54]. These results, which are consistent with previous meta-analyses [6,55,56], confirm that the consumption of SSBs is associated with increased risk of T2D independently of adiposity and suggests that the consumption of SSBs over many years could be related to a substantial number of new cases. Recent studies in the Mexican Teacher's cohort [57] and Northern Manhattan study [58], a multi ethnic urban cohort in New York City, provide additional support linking intake of SSBs to risk of T2D, and have expanded the generalizability of the findings across different populations.

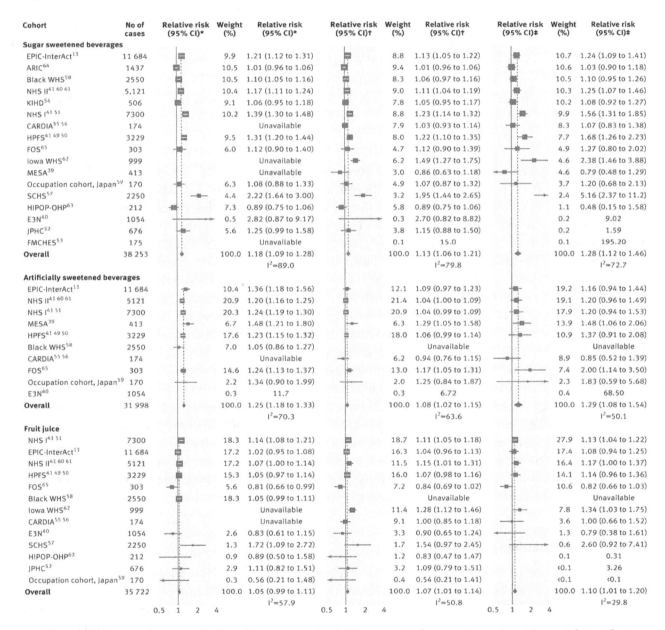

Cohort	No of cases	Weight (%)	Relative risk (95% CI)*	Weight (%)	Relative risk (95% CI)†	Weight (%)	Relative risk (95% CI)‡
Sugar sweetened beverages							
EPIC-InterAct[11]	11 684	9.9	1.21 (1.12 to 1.31)	8.8	1.13 (1.05 to 1.22)	10.7	1.24 (1.09 to 1.41)
ARIC[64]	1437	10.5	1.01 (0.96 to 1.06)	9.4	1.01 (0.96 to 1.06)	10.6	1.03 (0.90 to 1.18)
Black WHS[58]	2550	10.5	1.10 (1.05 to 1.16)	8.3	1.06 (0.97 to 1.16)	10.5	1.10 (0.95 to 1.26)
NHS II[41 60 61]	5,121	10.4	1.17 (1.11 to 1.24)	9.0	1.11 (1.04 to 1.19)	10.3	1.25 (1.07 to 1.46)
KIHD[54]	506	9.1	1.06 (0.95 to 1.18)	7.8	1.05 (0.95 to 1.17)	10.2	1.08 (0.92 to 1.27)
NHS I[41 51]	7300	10.2	1.39 (1.30 to 1.48)	8.8	1.23 (1.14 to 1.32)	9.9	1.56 (1.31 to 1.85)
CARDIA[55 56]	174		Unavailable	7.9	1.03 (0.93 to 1.14)	8.3	1.07 (0.83 to 1.38)
HPFS[41 49 50]	3229	9.5	1.31 (1.20 to 1.44)	8.0	1.22 (1.10 to 1.35)	7.7	1.68 (1.26 to 2.23)
FOS[65]	303	6.0	1.12 (0.90 to 1.40)	4.7	1.12 (0.90 to 1.39)	4.9	1.27 (0.80 to 2.02)
Iowa WHS[62]	999		Unavailable	6.2	1.49 (1.27 to 1.75)	4.6	2.38 (1.46 to 3.88)
MESA[39]	413		Unavailable	3.0	0.86 (0.63 to 1.18)	4.6	0.79 (0.48 to 1.29)
Occupation cohort, Japan[59]	170	6.3	1.08 (0.88 to 1.33)	4.9	1.07 (0.87 to 1.32)	3.7	1.20 (0.68 to 2.13)
SCHS[57]	2250	4.4	2.22 (1.64 to 3.00)	3.2	1.95 (1.44 to 2.65)	2.4	5.16 (2.37 to 11.2)
HIPOP-OHP[63]	212	7.3	0.89 (0.75 to 1.06)	5.8	0.89 (0.75 to 1.06)	1.1	0.48 (0.15 to 1.58)
E3N[40]	1054	0.5	2.82 (0.87 to 9.17)	0.3	2.70 (0.82 to 8.82)	0.2	9.02
JPHC[52]	676	5.6	1.25 (0.99 to 1.58)	3.8	1.15 (0.88 to 1.50)	0.2	1.59
FMCHES[53]	175		Unavailable	0.1	15.0	0.1	195.20
Overall	38 253	100.0	1.18 (1.09 to 1.28) $I^2=89.0$	100.0	1.13 (1.06 to 1.21) $I^2=79.8$	100.0	1.28 (1.12 to 1.46) $I^2=72.7$
Artificially sweetened beverages							
EPIC-InterAct[11]	11 684	10.4	1.36 (1.18 to 1.56)	12.1	1.09 (0.97 to 1.23)	19.2	1.16 (0.94 to 1.44)
NHS II[41 60 61]	5121	20.9	1.20 (1.16 to 1.25)	21.4	1.04 (1.00 to 1.09)	19.1	1.20 (0.96 to 1.49)
NHS I[41 51]	7300	20.3	1.24 (1.19 to 1.30)	20.9	1.04 (0.99 to 1.09)	17.9	1.20 (0.94 to 1.53)
MESA[39]	413	6.7	1.48 (1.21 to 1.80)	6.3	1.29 (1.05 to 1.58)	13.9	1.48 (1.06 to 2.06)
HPFS[41 49 50]	3229	17.6	1.23 (1.15 to 1.32)	18.0	1.06 (0.99 to 1.14)	10.9	1.37 (0.91 to 2.08)
Black WHS[58]	2550	7.0	1.05 (0.86 to 1.27)		Unavailable		Unavailable
CARDIA[55 56]	174		Unavailable	6.2	0.94 (0.76 to 1.15)	8.9	0.85 (0.52 to 1.39)
FOS[65]	303	14.6	1.24 (1.13 to 1.37)	13.0	1.17 (1.05 to 1.31)	7.4	2.00 (1.14 to 3.50)
Occupation cohort, Japan[59]	170	2.2	1.34 (0.90 to 1.99)	2.0	1.25 (0.84 to 1.87)	2.3	1.83 (0.59 to 5.68)
E3N[40]	1054	0.3	11.7	0.3	6.72	0.4	68.50
Overall	31 998	100.0	1.25 (1.18 to 1.33) $I^2=70.3$	100.0	1.08 (1.02 to 1.15) $I^2=63.6$	100.0	1.29 (1.08 to 1.54) $I^2=50.1$
Fruit juice							
NHS I[41 51]	7300	18.3	1.14 (1.08 to 1.21)	18.7	1.11 (1.05 to 1.18)	27.9	1.13 (1.04 to 1.22)
EPIC-InterAct[11]	11 684	17.2	1.02 (0.95 to 1.08)	16.3	1.04 (0.96 to 1.13)	17.4	1.08 (0.94 to 1.25)
NHS II[41 60 61]	5121	17.2	1.07 (1.00 to 1.14)	11.5	1.15 (1.01 to 1.31)	16.4	1.17 (1.00 to 1.37)
HPFS[41 49 50]	3229	15.3	1.05 (0.97 to 1.14)	16.0	1.07 (0.98 to 1.16)	14.1	1.14 (0.96 to 1.36)
FOS[65]	303	5.6	0.81 (0.66 to 0.99)	7.2	0.84 (0.69 to 1.02)	10.6	0.82 (0.66 to 1.03)
Black WHS[58]	2550	18.3	1.05 (0.99 to 1.11)		Unavailable		Unavailable
Iowa WHS[62]	999		Unavailable	11.4	1.28 (1.12 to 1.46)	7.8	1.34 (1.03 to 1.75)
CARDIA[55 56]	174		Unavailable	9.1	1.00 (0.85 to 1.18)	3.6	1.00 (0.66 to 1.52)
E3N[40]	1054	2.6	0.83 (0.61 to 1.15)	3.3	0.90 (0.65 to 1.24)	1.3	0.79 (0.38 to 1.61)
SCHS[57]	2250	1.3	1.72 (1.09 to 2.72)	1.7	1.54 (0.97 to 2.45)	0.6	2.60 (0.92 to 7.41)
HIPOP-OHP[63]	212	0.9	0.89 (0.50 to 1.58)	1.2	0.83 (0.47 to 1.47)	0.1	0.31
JPHC[52]	676	2.9	1.11 (0.82 to 1.51)	3.2	1.09 (0.79 to 1.51)	<0.1	3.26
Occupation cohort, Japan[59]	170	0.3	0.56 (0.21 to 1.48)	0.4	0.54 (0.21 to 1.41)	<0.1	<0.1
Overall	35 722	100.0	1.05 (0.99 to 1.11) $I^2=57.9$	100.0	1.07 (1.01 to 1.14) $I^2=50.8$	100.0	1.10 (1.01 to 1.20) $I^2=29.8$

Figure 2. Prospective associations for an incremental increase in beverage consumption with incident type 2 diabetes (T2D): random effects meta-analysis. * Unadjusted for adiposity; † adjusted for adiposity; ‡ adjusted for adiposity and within person variation [54].

Emerging evidence linking intake of SSBs to CVD is strengthened by consistent associations of SSBs with cardiometabolic risk factors, in addition to weight gain and risk of T2D. A meta-analysis of nine prospective cohort studies found that a one-serving-per-day increase in SSB was associated with a 13% higher risk of stroke (RR: 1.13, 95% CI: 1.02, 1.24) based on one study, and 22% higher risk of myocardial infarction (MI) (RR: 1.22, 95% CI: 1.14, 1.30) based on two studies [10]. In the categorical analysis comparing high vs. low SSB intake, there was a 19% higher risk of MI (RR: 1.19, 95% CI: 1.09, 1.31) based on three studies, but no significant association was observed for stroke (three studies) [10]. For the association with stroke, moderate heterogeneity was evident. After stratification by sex and stroke type, the pooled results suggested that women who consume SSBs have a higher risk of ischemic stroke (RR: 1.33, 95% CI: 1.07, 1.66), while no differences were noted for men or for men and women with hemorrhagic stroke [10]. These findings are consistent with a previous meta-analysis of four prospective cohort studies, which found a 17% higher risk of CHD (95% CI: 7% to 28%) comparing extreme SSB intake categories and a 16% higher risk of CHD per one-serving-per-day increment (10% to 23%) [11]. Similar to studies of T2D, when estimates that did not adjust for BMI or energy intake were included in the meta-analysis, the magnitude of the association increased (RR: 1.26, 95% CI: 1.16, 1.37), suggesting these factors as partial mediators of the association. A systematic review by Keller et al. also reported positive associations between SSB and CHD but noted that associations were only apparent in large studies with long durations of follow-up [12]. This review also found that, among studies that evaluated SSB intake in relation to risk of stroke, positive associations were observed only among women.

Building on the clinical evidence, a few studies have also shown a link between SSB intake and risk of all-cause or CVD mortality. We recently found that, among over 118,000 women and men from the NHS and HPFS, intake of SSBs was positively associated with risk of death from any cause in a dose-dependent manner [59]. Compared with drinking SSBs less than once per month, drinking one to four per month was linked with a 1% higher risk, two to six per week with a 6% higher risk, one to two per day with a 14% higher risk, and two or more per day with a 21% higher risk [59]. The higher risk of death associated with SSBs was more pronounced among women than men and was driven by CVD mortality. Compared with infrequent SSB consumers, those who consumed two or more per day had a 31% higher risk of death from CVD [59]. These findings are consistent with a previous study conducted in a prospective analysis of NHANES, which found a 29% higher risk of CVD mortality (RR: 1.29, 95% CI: 1.04, 1.60) comparing participants who consumed seven or more servings of SSBs per week to those who consumed one serving per week or less [60]. It was also estimated in NHANES that 7.4% of all cardiometabolic deaths in the US could be attributed to intake of SSBs in 2012 [61]. More recently, in the US-based Reasons for Geographic and Racial Differences in Stroke (REGARDS) study, each additional 12-oz serving/day of SSBs was associated with an 11% higher risk of all-cause mortality [62]. However, no association was observed for risk of death from CHD, which may have been due to a limited number of cases. In contrast, results from a cohort of Chinese adults in Singapore [63] and an elderly population in the US [64], both with very low intake levels, found no significant association between SSBs and mortality.

6. Biological Mechanisms

SSBs contribute to weight gain through decreased satiety and an incomplete compensatory reduction in energy intake at subsequent meals following ingestion of liquid calories [20]. A typical 12-oz (360 mL) serving of soda contains ~140–150 calories and ~35–37.5 g of sugar. If these calories are added to the diet without compensating for the additional calories, one can of soda per day could in theory lead to a weight gain of five pounds in one year [65]. Short-term feeding trials that show greater energy intake [66] and weight gain [50,66–69] from consuming SSBs compared to ASBs indirectly illustrate this point. While few studies have evaluated this mechanism, some evidence supporting incomplete compensation for liquid calories has been provided by studies showing greater energy intake and weight gain after isocaloric consumption of beverages compared to solid food [70–72]. These studies suggest that calories from sugar in liquid beverages may not suppress intake of solid foods to the level needed to maintain energy balance; however, the mechanisms responsible for this response are largely unknown.

SSBs contribute to the development of T2D and cardiometabolic risk in part through their ability to induce weight gain, but also independently through metabolic effects of constituent sugars (Figure 3). Consumption of SSBs has been shown to induce rapid spikes in blood glucose and insulin levels [73,74].

As such, these beverages have moderate-to-high glycemic index (GI) values [75], which, in combination with the large quantities consumed, contribute to a high dietary glycemic load (GL). High-GL diets can promote insulin resistance [76], exacerbate inflammatory biomarkers [77], and are associated with higher risk of T2D [78,79] and CHD [80]. Consuming fructose from SSBs as a component of sucrose or HFCS may further impact cardiometabolic risk. Fructose alone is poorly absorbed but is enhanced by glucose in the gut, thus accounting for the rapid and complete absorption of both fructose and glucose when ingested as sucrose or HFCS. Fructose, when consumed in moderate amounts, is metabolized in the liver where it is converted to glucose, lactate, and fatty acids to serve as metabolic substrates for other cells in the body [81]. When consumed in excess, this can lead to increased hepatic de novo lipogenesis, atherogenic dyslipidemia, and insulin resistance. The increase in hepatic lipid promotes production and secretion of very-low-density lipoproteins (VLDLs) leading to increased concentrations of postprandial triglycerides. Consumption of fructose-containing sugars is associated with production of small dense LDL cholesterol, which may be due to increased levels of VLDL-induced lipoprotein remodeling [48,82]. Fructose was also shown to promote the accumulation of VAT and the deposition of ectopic fat [83–86], processes indicative of cardiometabolic risk. Accumulating evidence suggests that the metabolic effects of fructose may be modified by physical activity level with more adverse effects observed under conditions of high fructose intake and low levels of physical activity [87].

According to this model, the adverse metabolic effects of fructose would occur when fructose intake chronically exceeds the capacity of the liver to release lactate and glucose for muscle, i.e., when there is a mismatch between fructose intake and energy output in the muscle. Fructose is the only sugar known to increase production of uric acid [87]. The production of uric acid in the liver has been shown to reduce endothelial nitric oxide, which may be implicated in the association between SSBs and CHD [88]. Hyperuricemia often precedes development of obesity and T2D, and clinical evidence suggests that hyperuricemia may mediate the association between SSB consumption and hypertension through the development of renal disease, endothelial dysfunction, and activation of the renin–angiotensin system [88]. In addition, hyperuricemia is associated with the development of gout [45,46], and gout and hyperuricemia are associated with hypertension, T2D, MetSyn, kidney disease, and CVD [88,89].

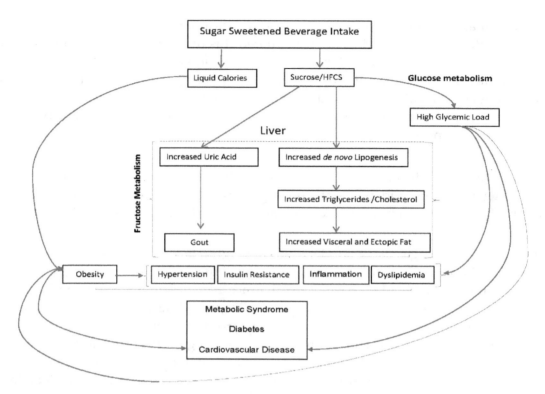

Figure 3. Biological mechanisms linking intake of sugar-sweetened beverages (SSB) to the development of obesity, metabolic syndrome (Met Syn), diabetes, and cardiovascular disease (CVD). Incomplete compensation for liquid calories leads to obesity, which is a risk factor for cardiometabolic outcomes. Increased diabetes, MetSyn, and CVD risk also occur independent of weight through development of risk factors precipitated by adverse glycemic effects and increased fructose metabolism in the liver. Excess fructose ingestion promotes hepatic uric acid production, de novo lipogenesis, and accumulation of visceral and ectopic fat, and also leads to gout. HFCS = high-fructose corn syrup.

7. Alternative Beverages

Several beverages have been suggested as alternatives to SSBs including water, 100% fruit juice, coffee, tea, and ASBs. Unlike SSBs, water does not contain liquid calories and, for most people with access to safe drinking water, it is the optimal calorie-free beverage. We found that replacement of one serving per day of SSBs with one serving of water was associated with less weight gain [90] and a lower risk of T2D [91]. With more consumers opting for water, several types of sparkling and flavored waters have emerged on the market, which may make switching to water more feasible for habitual SSB consumers.

Although 100% fruit juice might be perceived as a healthy choice since juice contains some vitamins and nutrients, they also contain a relatively high number of calories from natural sugars. Previous cohort studies have found positive associations between consumption of fruit juice and weight gain [92] and T2D [93], while the opposite has been shown for whole fruit [25,94]. Sugars in juice are absorbed more quickly than those in fruit and vegetables, which are absorbed more slowly due in part to their fiber content [95,96]. The rapid absorption of liquid fructose (from juice) compared to solid forms is more likely to result in higher concentrations of fructose in the liver and increase the rate of hepatic extraction of fructose, de novo lipogenesis, and production of lipids [97,98]. A recent study in the REGARDS cohort found that fruit juice intake was associated with a higher risk of all-cause mortality [62]. However, other studies have shown benefits of juice on cardiometabolic markers [92,99]. This suggests a need for further research that can evaluate different types of juice, since the nutrient profile and sugar content across various juices may differ. Nonetheless, based on the current evidence, it is recommended that daily intake of fruit juice be limited to 8 oz for adults.

Numerous studies have shown that regular consumption of coffee (decaffeinated or regular) and tea can have favorable effects on T2D and CVD risk [100,101], possibly due to their high polyphenol content. These beverages can thus be considered healthful alternatives to SSBs for individuals without contraindications, provided that caloric sweeteners and creamers are used sparingly, and that intake does not exceed the guidelines for caffeine. We found that substituting one serving per day of SSBs with one cup of coffee was associated with a 17% lower risk of T2D [102].

ASBs provide few to no calories but retain a sweet flavor, making them an attractive alternative to SSBs. Paradoxically, some cohort studies have reported positive associations between ASB consumption and weight gain and risk of T2D and CVD [32,36]. These findings may be due in part to residual confounding by unmeasured or poorly measured lifestyle factors or reverse causation, since individuals with obesity or metabolic risk may switch to ASBs for health reasons, which can result in spurious associations between ASBs and cardiometabolic outcomes. Studies with repeated measurements of diet, which are less prone to reverse causation, have shown only marginal nonsignificant associations with ASBs [8,9,25,59,102]. Cohort-based substitution analysis has also shown inverse associations with weight gain, T2D and mortality with replacement of SSBs with ASBs [59,90,91]. In addition, short-term trials that assessed ASBs as a replacement for SSBs reported modest benefits on body weight and metabolic risk factors [5,103]. On the other hand, some mechanisms have been proposed linking ASBs to adverse cardiometabolic health such as the intense sweetness of artificial sweeteners conditioning toward a preference for sweets or stimulating a cephalic insulin response, and more recently through alterations in gut microflora linked to insulin resistance [104]. However, these mechanisms are not well understood, and different types of artificial sweeteners may have different metabolic effects.

Consumption of ASBs in place of SSBs could be a helpful strategy to reduce cardiometabolic risk among heavy SSB consumers with the ultimate goal of switching to water or other healthful beverages. Further studies are needed to evaluate potential metabolic consequences of consuming ASBs over the life course and better understand underlying biological mechanisms. Understanding potential health impacts of ASB consumption is especially important in the context of sugar reduction policies such as taxation and labeling, which may lead to product reformulation and more ASBs in the food supply.

8. Policy Considerations

In response to the strong evidence linking consumption of SSBs to weight gain and risk of T2D and CVD, national and international organizations are already calling for reductions in intake of these beverages to help curb obesity and improve cardiometabolic health [105]. Both the WHO and 2015–2020 US Dietary Guidelines recommend an upper limit of 10% of total energy from added sugar, and numerous associations specifically recommend limiting intake of SSBs. In addition to widespread public health recommendations, public policies are needed to change consumption pattern at the population level (Box 1). The most common actions implemented to reduce SSB consumption include taxation, reduction of availability in schools, restrictions on marketing to children, public awareness campaigns, and front-of-package labelling [18,106]. Several cities in the US and globally have implemented excise taxes on SSBs as a strategy to reduce intake levels and generate revenue to support various public efforts. The most rigorously evaluated SSB tax to date is in Mexico, where a nationwide excise tax of 10% (one peso per liter) was implemented in 2014. Two years after the tax was implemented, a net decrease of 7.6% in sales of sugary drinks was observed, while sales of untaxed beverages such as water increased by 2.1% [107]. It was estimated that, between 2013 to 2022, the tax alone will prevent nearly 200,000 cases of obesity and save $980 million in direct healthcare costs, with the majority of benefits in young adults [108]. In Berkeley, California, the first US city to levy a penny-per-ounce excise tax on SSBs, sales of SSBs fell 9.6%, while sales of untaxed beverages, such as water and milk, increased 3.5%, comparing pre-tax to one-year-post-implementation trends [109]. Whether these early benefits of the tax will continue over the long term and translate into improvements in health will be important factors to monitor over time. In the US, the recently revised nutrition facts label will now require manufacturers (compliance by 1 January2020 to 1 July

2021, depending on annual food sales) to disclose the added sugar content of products, and will be accompanied by a percent daily value, with a goal of helping consumers make healthier choices. To achieve meaningful changes in beverage consumption patterns, a combination of multiple strategies will be needed, together with consumer education, and will serve as important steps in changing social norms surrounding beverage habits. Implementing and evaluating these policy actions in relation to behavior changes in the short term and clinical outcomes in the long term should remain a priority for scientists and policy-makers.

Box 1. Policy strategies to reduce consumption of sugar-sweetened beverages (SSBs).

- Governments should impose financial incentives such as taxation of SSBs of at least a 10% price increase, and implement limits for use of Supplemental Nutrition Assistance Program (SNAP) benefits for SSBs or subsidizing SNAP purchases of healthier foods, to encourage healthier beverages choices.
- Regulations are needed to reduce exposure to marketing of unhealthy foods and beverages in the media and at sports events or other activities, particularly in relation to children.
- Front-of-package labelling or other nutrition labeling strategies should be implemented to help guide consumers to make healthy food and beverage choices. These changes should be accompanied by concurrent public health awareness campaigns.
- Policies should be adopted to reduce the availability of SSBs in the workplace, healthcare facilities, government institutions, and other public spaces, and ensure access to safe water and healthy alternatives. Policies that make healthful beverages the default choice should also be adopted.
- Educational campaigns about the health risks associated with overconsumption of SSBs should be aimed at healthcare professionals and clinical populations.
- National and international campaigns targeting obesity and chronic disease prevention should include the health risks associated with overconsumption of SSBs.
- National and international dietary recommendations should include specific guidelines for healthy beverage consumption.

9. Conclusions

Intake of SSBs remains high in the US and is rising in many parts of the world. Based on findings from prospective cohort studies and short-term experimental trials of cardiometabolic risk factors, there is strong evidence for an etiological relationship between intake of SSBs and weight gain and risk of T2D and CHD. The evidence for a link with stroke is less clear and warrants further research, including the potential sex difference. Few studies have investigated intake of SSBs in relation to MetSyn, and this may be due to challenges in assessment and controversy about its clinical utility. However, findings on individual risk factors suggest a link. Since development of MetSyn often precedes onset of T2D and CHD, preventing or reversing MetSyn could be an effective way to curtail rising T2D and CHD rates.

SSBs are thought to promote weight gain through incomplete compensation for liquid calories at subsequent meals. These beverages may increase T2D and CHD in part through weight gain and independently through metabolic effects of constituent sugars. A mechanistic area that warrants future research is exploring the health effects of sugar consumed in solid form compared to SSB, and further elucidating compensatory effects of liquid vs. solid sugars. With the strength of evidence sufficient to call for reductions in intake of SSB for optimal cardiometabolic health, important research gaps exist regarding suitable alternative beverages, including the long-term health effects of consuming ASBs. Continued evaluation of SSB policies that are already in place is needed, as are more and higher-quality RCTs to identify effective strategies to reduce intake of SSBs at the individual and population level. SSBs present a clear target for health policy; however, chronic disease prevention should focus on improving overall diet quality by consuming more healthful foods and limiting unhealthy ones. Given the high levels of intake across the globe, reducing consumption of SSBs is an important step in improving diet quality that could have a measurable impact on weight control and improving cardiometabolic health.

Author Contributions: Original draft preparation, V.S.M.; critical review and editing, F.B.H. Both authors approved the submitted version and take responsibility for the accuracy and integrity of the work.

Acknowledgments: This research was supported by NIH grants P30 DK46200 and HL607.

References

1. Alberti, K.G.; Eckel, R.H.; Grundy, S.M.; Zimmet, P.Z.; Cleeman, J.I.; Donato, K.A.; Fruchart, J.C.; James, W.P.; Loria, C.M.; Smith, S.C., Jr.; et al. Harmonizing the metabolic syndrome: A joint interim statement of the International Diabetes Federation Task Force on Epidemiology and Prevention; National Heart, Lung, and Blood Institute; American Heart Association; World Heart Federation; International Atherosclerosis Society; and International Association for the Study of Obesity. *Circulation* **2009**, *120*, 1640–1645. [PubMed]
2. Beltran-Sanchez, H.; Harhay, M.O.; Harhay, M.M.; McElligott, S. Prevalence and trends of metabolic syndrome in the adult U.S. population, 1999–2010. *J. Am. Coll. Cardiol.* **2013**, *62*, 697–703. [CrossRef] [PubMed]
3. Saklayen, M.G. The Global Epidemic of the Metabolic Syndrome. *Curr. Hypertens. Rep.* **2018**, *20*, 12. [CrossRef] [PubMed]
4. Palmer, M.K.; Toth, P.P. Trends in Lipids, Obesity, Metabolic Syndrome, and Diabetes Mellitus in the United States: An NHANES Analysis (2003–2004 to 2013–2014). *Obesity* **2019**, *27*, 309–314. [CrossRef] [PubMed]
5. Malik, V.S.; Pan, A.; Willett, W.C.; Hu, F.B. Sugar-sweetened beverages and weight gain in children and adults: A systematic review and meta-analysis. *Am. J. Clin. Nutr.* **2013**, *98*, 1084–1102. [CrossRef] [PubMed]
6. Malik, V.S.; Popkin, B.M.; Bray, G.A.; Despres, J.P.; Willett, W.C.; Hu, F.B. Sugar-sweetened beverages and risk of metabolic syndrome and type 2 diabetes: A meta-analysis. *Diabetes Care* **2010**, *33*, 2477–2483. [CrossRef] [PubMed]
7. *Guideline: Sugar Intake for Adults and Children*; World Health Organization: Geneva, Switzerland, 2015.
8. Fung, T.T.; Malik, V.; Rexrode, K.M.; Manson, J.E.; Willett, W.C.; Hu, F.B. Sweetened beverage consumption and risk of coronary heart disease in women. *Am. J. Clin. Nutr.* **2009**, *89*, 1037–1042. [CrossRef]
9. De Koning, L.; Malik, V.S.; Kellogg, M.D.; Rimm, E.B.; Willett, W.C.; Hu, F.B. Sweetened beverage consumption, incident coronary heart disease, and biomarkers of risk in men. *Circulation* **2012**, *125*, 1735–1741. [CrossRef]
10. Narain, A.; Kwok, C.S.; Mamas, M.A. Soft drinks and sweetened beverages and the risk of cardiovascular disease and mortality: A systematic review and meta-analysis. *Int. J. Clin. Pract.* **2016**, *70*, 791–805. [CrossRef]
11. Huang, C.; Huang, J.; Tian, Y.; Yang, X.; Gu, D. Sugar sweetened beverages consumption and risk of coronary heart disease: A meta-analysis of prospective studies. *Atherosclerosis* **2014**, *234*, 11–16. [CrossRef]
12. Keller, A.; Heitmann, B.L.; Olsen, N. Sugar-sweetened beverages, vascular risk factors and events: A systematic literature review. *Public Health Nutr.* **2015**, *18*, 1145–1154. [CrossRef] [PubMed]
13. Welsh, J.A.; Sharma, A.J.; Grellinger, L.; Vos, M.B. Consumption of added sugars is decreasing in the United States. *Am. J. Clin. Nutr.* **2011**, *94*, 726–734. [CrossRef] [PubMed]
14. Dietary Guidelines for Americans 2015–2020. Available online: http://health.gov/dietaryguidelines/2015/guidelines/ (accessed on 7 August 2019).
15. Rosinger, A.; Herrick, K.; Gahche, J.; Park, S. Sugar-sweetened Beverage Consumption Among U.S. Adults, 2011–2014. *NCHS Data Brief* **2017**, *270*, 1–8.
16. Singh, G.M.; Micha, R.; Khatibzadeh, S.; Shi, P.; Lim, S.; Andrews, K.G.; Engell, R.E.; Ezzati, M.; Mozaffarian, D.; Global Burden of Diseases Nutrition and Chronic Diseases Expert Group (NutriCoDE). Global, Regional, and National Consumption of Sugar-Sweetened Beverages, Fruit Juices, and Milk: A Systematic Assessment of Beverage Intake in 187 Countries. *PLoS ONE* **2015**, *10*, e0124845. [CrossRef] [PubMed]
17. Yang, L.; Bovet, P.; Liu, Y.; Zhao, M.; Ma, C.; Liang, Y.; Xi, B. Consumption of Carbonated Soft Drinks Among Young Adolescents Aged 12 to 15 Years in 53 Low- and Middle-Income Countries. *Am. J. Public Health* **2017**, *107*, 1095–1100. [CrossRef] [PubMed]

18. Popkin, B.M.; Hawkes, C. Sweetening of the global diet, particularly beverages: Patterns, trends, and policy responses. *Lancet Diabetes Endocrinol.* **2016**, *4*, 174–186. [CrossRef]

19. Hu, F.B.; Malik, V.S. Sugar-sweetened beverages and risk of obesity and type 2 diabetes: Epidemiologic evidence. *Physiol. Behav.* **2010**, *100*, 47–54. [CrossRef]

20. Malik, V.S.; Popkin, B.M.; Bray, G.A.; Despres, J.P.; Hu, F.B. Sugar-sweetened beverages, obesity, type 2 diabetes mellitus, and cardiovascular disease risk. *Circulation* **2010**, *121*, 1356–1364. [CrossRef]

21. Malik, V.S.; Schulze, M.B.; Hu, F.B. Intake of sugar-sweetened beverages and weight gain: A systematic review. *Am. J. Clin. Nutr.* **2006**, *84*, 274–288. [CrossRef]

22. Vartanian, L.R.; Schwartz, M.B.; Brownell, K.D. Effects of soft drink consumption on nutrition and health: A systematic review and meta-analysis. *Am. J. Public Health* **2007**, *97*, 667–675. [CrossRef]

23. Te Morenga, L.; Mallard, S.; Mann, J. Dietary sugars and body weight: Systematic review and meta-analyses of randomised controlled trials and cohort studies. *BMJ* **2013**, *346*, e7492. [CrossRef] [PubMed]

24. Kaiser, K.A.; Shikany, J.M.; Keating, K.D.; Allison, D.B. Will reducing sugar-sweetened beverage consumption reduce obesity? Evidence supporting conjecture is strong, but evidence when testing effect is weak. *Obes. Rev.* **2013**, *14*, 620–633. [CrossRef] [PubMed]

25. Mozaffarian, D.; Hao, T.; Rimm, E.B.; Willett, W.C.; Hu, F.B. Changes in diet and lifestyle and long-term weight gain in women and men. *N. Engl. J. Med.* **2011**, *364*, 2392–2404. [CrossRef] [PubMed]

26. Qi, Q.; Chu, A.Y.; Kang, J.H.; Jensen, M.K.; Curhan, G.C.; Pasquale, L.R.; Ridker, P.M.; Hunter, D.J.; Willett, W.C.; Rimm, E.B.; et al. Sugar-sweetened beverages and genetic risk of obesity. *N. Engl. J. Med.* **2012**, *367*, 1387–1396. [CrossRef] [PubMed]

27. Ebbeling, C.B.; Feldman, H.A.; Chomitz, V.R.; Antonelli, T.A.; Gortmaker, S.L.; Osganian, S.K.; Ludwig, D. A randomized trial of sugar-sweetened beverages and adolescent body weight. *N. Engl. J. Med.* **2012**, *367*, 1407–1416. [CrossRef] [PubMed]

28. De Ruyter, J.C.; Olthof, M.R.; Seidell, J.C.; Katan, M.B. A trial of sugar-free or sugar-sweetened beverages and body weight in children. *N. Engl. J. Med.* **2012**, *367*, 1397–1406. [CrossRef] [PubMed]

29. Hu, F.B. Resolved: There is sufficient scientific evidence that decreasing sugar-sweetened beverage consumption will reduce the prevalence of obesity and obesity-related diseases. *Obes. Rev.* **2013**, *14*, 606–619. [CrossRef]

30. Narain, A.; Kwok, C.S.; Mamas, M.A. Soft drink intake and the risk of metabolic syndrome: A systematic review and meta-analysis. *Int. J. Clin. Pract.* **2017**, *71*, e12927. [CrossRef]

31. Mirmiran, P.; Yuzbashian, E.; Asghari, G.; Hosseinpour-Niazi, S.; Azizi, F. Consumption of sugar sweetened beverage is associated with incidence of metabolic syndrome in Tehranian children and adolescents. *Nutr. Metab.* **2015**, *12*, 25. [CrossRef]

32. Nettleton, J.A.; Lutsey, P.L.; Wang, Y.; Lima, J.A.; Michos, E.D.; Jacobs, D.R., Jr. Diet soda intake and risk of incident metabolic syndrome and type 2 diabetes in the Multi-Ethnic Study of Atherosclerosis (MESA). *Diabetes Care* **2009**, *32*, 688–694. [CrossRef]

33. Dhingra, R.; Sullivan, L.; Jacques, P.F.; Wang, T.J.; Fox, C.S.; Meigs, J.B.; D'Agostino, R.B.; Gaziano, J.M.; Vasan, R.S. Soft drink consumption and risk of developing cardiometabolic risk factors and the metabolic syndrome in middle-aged adults in the community. *Circulation* **2007**, *116*, 480–488. [CrossRef] [PubMed]

34. Ferreira-Pego, C.; Babio, N.; Bes-Rastrollo, M.; Corella, D.; Estruch, R.; Ros, E.; Fitó, M.; Serra-Majem, L.; Arós, F.; Fiol, M.; et al. Frequent Consumption of Sugar- and Artificially Sweetened Beverages and Natural and Bottled Fruit Juices Is Associated with an Increased Risk of Metabolic Syndrome in a Mediterranean Population at High Cardiovascular Disease Risk. *J. Nutr.* **2016**, *146*, 1528–1536. [PubMed]

35. Kang, Y.; Kim, J. Soft drink consumption is associated with increased incidence of the metabolic syndrome only in women. *Br. J. Nutr.* **2017**, *117*, 315–324. [CrossRef] [PubMed]

36. Lutsey, P.L.; Steffen, L.M.; Stevens, J. Dietary intake and the development of the metabolic syndrome: The Atherosclerosis Risk in Communities study. *Circulation* **2008**, *117*, 754–761. [CrossRef] [PubMed]

37. Duffey, K.J.; Gordon-Larsen, P.; Steffen, L.M.; Jacobs, D.R., Jr.; Popkin, B.M. Drinking caloric beverages increases the risk of adverse cardiometabolic outcomes in the Coronary Artery Risk Development in Young Adults (CARDIA) Study. *Am. J. Clin. Nutr.* **2010**, *92*, 954–959. [CrossRef] [PubMed]

38. Stern, D.; Middaugh, N.; Rice, M.S.; Laden, F.; Lopez-Ridaura, R.; Rosner, B.; Willett, W.; Lajous, M. Changes in Sugar-Sweetened Soda Consumption, Weight, and Waist Circumference: 2-Year Cohort of Mexican Women. *Am. J. Public Health* **2017**, *107*, 1801–1808. [CrossRef]

39. Funtikova, A.N.; Subirana, I.; Gomez, S.F.; Fito, M.; Elosua, R.; Benitez-Arciniega, A.A.; Schröder, H. Soft drink consumption is positively associated with increased waist circumference and 10-year incidence of abdominal obesity in Spanish adults. *J. Nutr.* **2015**, *145*, 328–334. [CrossRef]

40. Ma, J.; McKeown, N.M.; Hwang, S.J.; Hoffmann, U.; Jacques, P.F.; Fox, C.S. Sugar-Sweetened Beverage Consumption Is Associated With Change of Visceral Adipose Tissue Over 6 Years of Follow-Up. *Circulation* **2016**, *133*, 370–377. [CrossRef]

41. Yu, Z.; Ley, S.H.; Sun, Q.; Hu, F.B.; Malik, V.S. Cross-sectional association between sugar-sweetened beverage intake and cardiometabolic biomarkers in US women. *Br. J. Nutr.* **2018**, *119*, 570–580. [CrossRef]

42. Kim, Y.; Je, Y. Prospective association of sugar-sweetened and artificially sweetened beverage intake with risk of hypertension. *Arch. Cardiovasc. Dis.* **2016**, *109*, 242–253. [CrossRef]

43. Jayalath, V.H.; de Souza, R.J.; Ha, V.; Mirrahimi, A.; Blanco-Mejia, S.; Di Buono, M.; Jenkins, A.L.; Leiter, L.A.; Wolever, T.; Beyene, J.; et al. Sugar-sweetened beverage consumption and incident hypertension: A systematic review and meta-analysis of prospective cohorts. *Am. J. Clin. Nutr.* **2015**, *102*, 914–921. [CrossRef] [PubMed]

44. Xi, B.; Huang, Y.; Reilly, K.H.; Li, S.; Zheng, R.; Barrio-Lopez, M.T.; Martinez-Gonzalez, M.A.; Zhou, D. Sugar-sweetened beverages and risk of hypertension and CVD: A dose-response meta-analysis. *Br. J. Nutr.* **2015**, *113*, 709–717. [CrossRef] [PubMed]

45. Choi, H.K.; Curhan, G. Soft drinks, fructose consumption, and the risk of gout in men: Prospective cohort study. *BMJ* **2008**, *336*, 309–312. [CrossRef] [PubMed]

46. Choi, H.K.; Willett, W.; Curhan, G. Fructose-rich beverages and risk of gout in women. *JAMA* **2010**, *304*, 2270–2278. [CrossRef] [PubMed]

47. Te Morenga, L.A.; Howatson, A.J.; Jones, R.M.; Mann, J. Dietary sugars and cardiometabolic risk: Systematic review and meta-analyses of randomized controlled trials of the effects on blood pressure and lipids. *Am. J. Clin. Nutr.* **2014**, *100*, 65–79. [CrossRef] [PubMed]

48. Stanhope, K.L.; Medici, V.; Bremer, A.A.; Lee, V.; Lam, H.D.; Nunez, M.V.; Chen, G.X.; Keim, N.L.; Havel, P.J. A dose-response study of consuming high-fructose corn syrup-sweetened beverages on lipid/lipoprotein risk factors for cardiovascular disease in young adults. *Am. J. Clin. Nutr.* **2015**, *101*, 1144–1154. [CrossRef]

49. Bruun, J.M.; Maersk, M.; Belza, A.; Astrup, A.; Richelsen, B. Consumption of sucrose-sweetened soft drinks increases plasma levels of uric acid in overweight and obese subjects: A 6-month randomised controlled trial. *Eur. J. Clin. Nutr.* **2015**, *69*, 949–953. [CrossRef]

50. Raben, A.; Moller, B.K.; Flint, A.; Vasilaris, T.H.; Christina Moller, A.; Juul Holst, J.; Astrup, A. Increased postprandial glycaemia, insulinemia, and lipidemia after 10 weeks' sucrose-rich diet compared to an artificially sweetened diet: A Randomised controlled trial. *Food Nutr. Res.* **2011**, *55*, 5961. [CrossRef]

51. Aeberli, I.; Gerber, P.A.; Hochuli, M.; Kohler, S.; Haile, S.R.; Gouni-Berthold, I.; Berthold, H.K.; Spinas, G.A.; Berneis, K. Low to moderate sugar-sweetened beverage consumption impairs glucose and lipid metabolism and promotes inflammation in healthy young men: A randomized controlled trial. *Am. J. Clin. Nutr.* **2011**, *94*, 479–485. [CrossRef]

52. Sorensen, L.B.; Raben, A.; Stender, S.; Astrup, A. Effect of sucrose on inflammatory markers in overweight humans. *Am. J. Clin. Nutr.* **2005**, *82*, 421–427. [CrossRef]

53. Kuzma, J.N.; Cromer, G.; Hagman, D.K.; Breymeyer, K.L.; Roth, C.L.; Foster-Schubert, K.E.; Holte, S.E.; Weigle, D.S.; Kratz, M. No differential effect of beverages sweetened with fructose, high-fructose corn syrup, or glucose on systemic or adipose tissue inflammation in normal-weight to obese adults: A randomized controlled trial. *Am. J. Clin. Nutr.* **2016**, *104*, 306–314. [CrossRef] [PubMed]

54. Imamura, F.; O'Connor, L.; Ye, Z.; Mursu, J.; Hayashino, Y.; Bhupathiraju, S.N.; Forouhi, N.G. Consumption of sugar sweetened beverages, artificially sweetened beverages, and fruit juice and incidence of type 2 diabetes: Systematic review, meta-analysis, and estimation of population attributable fraction. *Br. J. Sports Med.* **2016**, *50*, 496–504. [CrossRef] [PubMed]

55. Fagherazzi, G.; Vilier, A.; Saes Sartorelli, D.; Lajous, M.; Balkau, B.; Clavel-Chapelon, F. Consumption of artificially and sugar-sweetened beverages and incident type 2 diabetes in the Etude Epidemiologique aupres des femmes de la Mutuelle Generale de l'Education Nationale-European Prospective Investigation into Cancer and Nutrition cohort. *Am. J. Clin. Nutr.* **2013**, *97*, 517–523. [PubMed]

56. Consumption of sweet beverages and type 2 diabetes incidence in European adults: Results from EPIC-InterAct. *Diabetologia* **2013**, *56*, 1520–1530. [CrossRef] [PubMed]

57. Stern, D.; Mazariegos, M.; Ortiz-Panozo, E.; Campos, H.; Malik, V.S.; Lajous, M.; López-Ridaura, R. Sugar-Sweetened Soda Consumption Increases Diabetes Risk Among Mexican Women. *J. Nutr.* **2019**, *149*, 795–803. [CrossRef] [PubMed]

58. Gardener, H.; Moon, Y.P.; Rundek, T.; Elkind, M.S.V.; Sacco, R.L. Diet Soda and Sugar-Sweetened Soda Consumption in Relation to Incident Diabetes in the Northern Manhattan Study. *Curr. Dev. Nutr.* **2018**, *2*, nzy008. [CrossRef] [PubMed]

59. Malik, V.S.; Li, Y.; Pan, A.; De Koning, L.; Schernhammer, E.; Willett, W.C.; Hu, F.B. Long-Term Consumption of Sugar-Sweetened and Artificially Sweetened Beverages and Risk of Mortality in US Adults. *Circulation* **2019**, *139*, 2113–2125. [CrossRef] [PubMed]

60. Yang, Q.; Zhang, Z.; Gregg, E.W.; Flanders, W.D.; Merritt, R.; Hu, F.B. Added Sugar Intake and Cardiovascular Diseases Mortality Among US Adults. *JAMA Intern Med.* **2014**, *174*, 516–524. [CrossRef] [PubMed]

61. Micha, R.; Penalvo, J.L.; Cudhea, F.; Imamura, F.; Rehm, C.D.; Mozaffarian, D. Association Between Dietary Factors and Mortality From Heart Disease, Stroke, and Type 2 Diabetes in the United States. *JAMA* **2017**, *317*, 912–924. [CrossRef] [PubMed]

62. Collin, L.J.; Judd, S.; Safford, M.; Vaccarino, V.; Welsh, J.A. Association of Sugary Beverage Consumption With Mortality Risk in US Adults: A Secondary Analysis of Data from the REGARDS Study. *JAMA Netw. Open* **2019**, *2*, e193121. [CrossRef] [PubMed]

63. Odegaard, A.O.; Koh, W.P.; Yuan, J.M.; Pereira, M.A. Beverage habits and mortality in Chinese adults. *J. Nutr.* **2015**, *145*, 595–604. [CrossRef] [PubMed]

64. Paganini-Hill, A.; Kawas, C.H.; Corrada, M.M. Non-alcoholic beverage and caffeine consumption and mortality: The Leisure World Cohort Study. *Prev. Med.* **2007**, *44*, 305–310. [CrossRef] [PubMed]

65. Malik, V.S.; Hu, F.B. Sweeteners and Risk of Obesity and Type 2 Diabetes: The Role of Sugar-Sweetened Beverages. *Curr. Diab. Rep.* **2012**, *12*, 195–203. [CrossRef] [PubMed]

66. DellaValle, D.M.; Roe, L.S.; Rolls, B.J. Does the consumption of caloric and non-caloric beverages with a meal affect energy intake? *Appetite* **2005**, *44*, 187–193. [CrossRef] [PubMed]

67. Raben, A.; Vasilaras, T.H.; Moller, A.C.; Astrup, A. Sucrose compared with artificial sweeteners: Different effects on ad libitum food intake and body weight after 10 wk of supplementation in overweight subjects. *Am. J. Clin. Nutr.* **2002**, *76*, 721–729. [CrossRef] [PubMed]

68. Tordoff, M.G.; Alleva, A.M. Effect of drinking soda sweetened with aspartame or high-fructose corn syrup on food intake and body weight. *Am. J. Clin. Nutr.* **1990**, *51*, 963–969. [CrossRef] [PubMed]

69. Reid, M.; Hammersley, R.; Hill, A.J.; Skidmore, P. Long-term dietary compensation for added sugar: Effects of supplementary sucrose drinks over a 4-week period. *Br. J. Nutr.* **2007**, *97*, 193–203. [CrossRef]

70. DiMeglio, D.P.; Mattes, R.D. Liquid versus solid carbohydrate: Effects on food intake and body weight. *Int. J. Obes. Relat. Metab. Disord.* **2000**, *24*, 794–800. [CrossRef]

71. Pan, A.; Hu, F.B. Effects of carbohydrates on satiety: Differences between liquid and solid food. *Curr. Opin. Clin. Nutr. Metab. Care* **2011**, *14*, 385–390. [CrossRef]

72. Mourao, D.M.; Bressan, J.; Campbell, W.W.; Mattes, R.D. Effects of food form on appetite and energy intake in lean and obese young adults. *Int. J. Obes.* **2007**, *31*, 1688–1695. [CrossRef]

73. Tey, S.L.; Salleh, N.B.; Henry, J.; Forde, C.G. Effects of aspartame-, monk fruit-, stevia- and sucrose-sweetened beverages on postprandial glucose, insulin and energy intake. *Int. J. Obes.* **2017**, *41*, 450–457. [CrossRef] [PubMed]

74. Solomi, L.; Rees, G.A.; Redfern, K.M. The acute effects of the non-nutritive sweeteners aspartame and acesulfame-K in UK diet cola on glycaemic response. *Int. J. Food Sci. Nutr.* **2019**, 1–7. [CrossRef] [PubMed]

75. Atkinson, F.S.; Foster-Powell, K.; Brand-Miller, J.C. International tables of glycemic index and glycemic load values: 2008. *Diabetes Care* **2008**, *31*, 2281–2283. [CrossRef] [PubMed]

76. Ludwig, D.S. The glycemic index: Physiological mechanisms relating to obesity, diabetes, and cardiovascular disease. *JAMA* **2002**, *287*, 2414–2423. [CrossRef] [PubMed]

77. Liu, S.; Manson, J.E.; Buring, J.E.; Stampfer, M.J.; Willett, W.C.; Ridker, P.M. Relation between a diet with a high glycemic load and plasma concentrations of high-sensitivity C-reactive protein in middle-aged women. *Am. J. Clin. Nutr.* **2002**, *75*, 492–498. [CrossRef] [PubMed]

78. Bhupathiraju, S.N.; Tobias, D.K.; Malik, V.S.; Pan, A.; Hruby, A.; Manson, J.E.; Willett, W.C.; Hu, F.B. Glycemic index, glycemic load, and risk of type 2 diabetes: Results from 3 large US cohorts and an updated meta-analysis. *Am. J. Clin. Nutr.* **2014**, *100*, 218–232. [CrossRef] [PubMed]

79. Livesey, G.; Taylor, R.; Livesey, H.F.; Buyken, A.E.; Jenkins, D.J.A.; Augustin, L.S.A.; Sievenpiper, J.L.; Barclay, A.W.; Liu, S.; Wolever, T.M.S.; et al. Dietary Glycemic Index and Load and the Risk of Type 2 Diabetes: A Systematic Review and Updated Meta-Analyses of Prospective Cohort Studies. *Nutrients* **2019**, *11*, 1280. [CrossRef]

80. Livesey, G.; Livesey, H. Coronary Heart Disease and Dietary Carbohydrate, Glycemic Index, and Glycemic Load: Dose-Response Meta-analyses of Prospective Cohort Studies. *Mayo Clin. Proc. Innov. Qual. Outcomes* **2019**, *3*, 52–69. [CrossRef]

81. Sun, S.Z.; Empie, M.W. Fructose metabolism in humans—What isotopic tracer studies tell us. *Nutr. Metab. (London)* **2012**, *9*, 89. [CrossRef]

82. Goran, M.I.; Tappy, L.; Lê, K.A. *Dietary Sugars and Health*; CRC Press, Taylor & Francis Group: Boca Raton, FL, USA, 2015.

83. Teff, K.L.; Grudziak, J.; Townsend, R.R.; Dunn, T.N.; Grant, R.W.; Adams, S.H.; Keim, N.L.; Cummings, B.P.; Stanhope, K.L.; Havel, P.J. Endocrine and metabolic effects of consuming fructose- and glucose-sweetened beverages with meals in obese men and women: Influence of insulin resistance on plasma triglyceride responses. *J. Clin. Endocrinol. Metab.* **2009**, *94*, 1562–1569. [CrossRef]

84. Stanhope, K.L.; Schwarz, J.M.; Keim, N.L.; Griffen, S.C.; Bremer, A.A.; Graham, J.L.; Hatcher, B.; Cox, C.L.; Dyachenko, A.; Zhang, W.; et al. Consuming fructose-sweetened, not glucose-sweetened, beverages increases visceral adiposity and lipids and decreases insulin sensitivity in overweight/obese humans. *J. Clin. Investig.* **2009**, *119*, 1322–1334. [CrossRef] [PubMed]

85. Stanhope, K.L.; Griffen, S.C.; Bair, B.R.; Swarbrick, M.M.; Keim, N.L.; Havel, P.J. Twenty-four-hour endocrine and metabolic profiles following consumption of high-fructose corn syrup-, sucrose-, fructose-, and glucose-sweetened beverages with meals. *Am. J. Clin. Nutr.* **2008**, *87*, 1194–1203. [CrossRef] [PubMed]

86. Stanhope, K.L.; Havel, P.J. Endocrine and metabolic effects of consuming beverages sweetened with fructose, glucose, sucrose, or high-fructose corn syrup. *Am. J. Clin. Nutr.* **2008**, *88*, 1733S–1737S. [CrossRef] [PubMed]

87. Tappy, L.; Rosset, R. Health outcomes of a high fructose intake: The importance of physical activity. *J. Physiol.* **2019**, *597*, 3561–3571. [CrossRef] [PubMed]

88. Richette, P.; Bardin, T. Gout. *Lancet* **2009**. [CrossRef]

89. Nakagawa, T.; Tuttle, K.R.; Short, R.A.; Johnson, R.J. Hypothesis: Fructose-induced hyperuricemia as a causal mechanism for the epidemic of the metabolic syndrome. *Nat. Clin. Pract. Nephrol.* **2005**, *1*, 80–86. [CrossRef] [PubMed]

90. Pan, A.; Malik, V.S.; Hao, T.; Willett, W.C.; Mozaffarian, D.; Hu, F.B. Changes in water and beverage intake and long-term weight changes: Results from three prospective cohort studies. *Int. J. Obes.* **2013**, *37*, 1378. [CrossRef] [PubMed]

91. Pan, A.; Malik, V.S.; Schulze, M.B.; Manson, J.E.; Willett, W.C.; Hu, F.B. Plain-water intake and risk of type 2 diabetes in young and middle-aged women. *Am. J. Clin. Nutr.* **2012**, *95*, 1454–1460. [CrossRef] [PubMed]

92. Schulze, M.B.; Manson, J.E.; Ludwig, D.S.; Colditz, G.A.; Stampfer, M.J.; Willett, W.C.; Hu, F.B. Sugar-sweetened beverages, weight gain, and incidence of type 2 diabetes in young and middle-aged women. *JAMA* **2004**, *292*, 927–934. [CrossRef]

93. Bazzano, L.A.; Li, T.Y.; Joshipura, K.J.; Hu, F.B. Intake of fruit, vegetables, and fruit juices and risk of diabetes in women. *Diabetes Care* **2008**, *31*, 1311–1317. [CrossRef]

94. Muraki, I.; Imamura, F.; Manson, J.E.; Hu, F.B.; Willett, W.C.; van Dam, R.M.; Sun, Q. Fruit consumption and risk of type 2 diabetes: Results from three prospective longitudinal cohort studies. *BMJ* **2013**, *347*, f5001. [CrossRef] [PubMed]

95. Ravn-Haren, G.; Dragsted, L.O.; Buch-Andersen, T.; Jensen, E.N.; Jensen, R.I.; Nemeth-Balogh, M.; Paulovicsová, B.; Bergström, A.; Wilcks, A.; Licht, T.R.; et al. Intake of whole apples or clear apple juice has contrasting effects on plasma lipids in healthy volunteers. *Eur. J. Nutr.* **2013**, *52*, 1875–1889. [CrossRef] [PubMed]

96. Pepin, A.; Stanhope, K.L.; Imbeault, P. Are Fruit Juices Healthier Than Sugar-Sweetened Beverages? A Review. *Nutrients* **2019**, *11*, 1006. [CrossRef] [PubMed]

97. Sundborn, G.; Thornley, S.; Merriman, T.R.; Lang, B.; King, C.; Lanaspa, M.A.; Johnson, R.J. Are Liquid Sugars Different from Solid Sugar in Their Ability to Cause Metabolic Syndrome? *Obesity* **2019**, *27*, 879–887. [CrossRef] [PubMed]

98. Lanaspa, M.A.; Sanchez-Lozada, L.G.; Choi, Y.J.; Cicerchi, C.; Kanbay, M.; Roncal-Jimenez, C.A.; Schreiner, G. Uric acid induces hepatic steatosis by generation of mitochondrial oxidative stress: Potential role in fructose-dependent and -independent fatty liver. *J. Biol. Chem.* **2012**, *287*, 40732–40744. [CrossRef] [PubMed]

99. Ghanim, H.; Mohanty, P.; Pathak, R.; Chaudhuri, A.; Sia, C.L.; Dandona, P. Orange juice or fructose intake does not induce oxidative and inflammatory response. *Diabetes Care* **2007**, *30*, 1406–1411. [CrossRef] [PubMed]

100. Van Dam, R.M. Coffee consumption and risk of type 2 diabetes, cardiovascular diseases, and cancer. *Appl. Physiol. Nutr. Metab.* **2008**, *33*, 1269–1283. [CrossRef]

101. Bhupathiraju, S.N.; Pan, A.; Malik, V.S.; Manson, J.E.; Willett, W.C.; van Dam, R.M.; Hu, F.B. Caffeinated and caffeine-free beverages and risk of type 2 diabetes. *Am. J. Clin. Nutr.* **2013**, *97*, 155–166. [CrossRef]

102. De Koning, L.; Malik, V.S.; Rimm, E.B.; Willett, W.C.; Hu, F.B. Sugar-sweetened and artificially sweetened beverage consumption and risk of type 2 diabetes in men. *Am. J. Clin. Nutr.* **2011**, *93*, 1321–1327. [CrossRef]

103. Malik, V.S. Non-sugar sweeteners and health. *BMJ* **2019**, *364*, k5005. [CrossRef]

104. Swithers, S.E. Not so Sweet Revenge: Unanticipated Consequences of High-Intensity Sweeteners. *Behav. Anal.* **2015**, *38*, 1–17. [CrossRef] [PubMed]

105. Yale Rudd Center for Food Policy and Obesity. SUgar-Sweetened Beverage Taxes and Sugar Intake: Policy Statements, Endorsements, and Recommendations. Available online: http://www.yaleruddcenter.org/resources/upload/docs/what/policy/SSBtaxes/SSBTaxStatements.pdf (accessed on 10 January 2013).

106. Muth, N.D.; Dietz, W.H.; Magge, S.N.; Johnson, R.K.; American Academy Of Pediatrics; Section On Obesity; Committee On Nutrition; American Heart Association. Public Policies to Reduce Sugary Drink Consumption in Children and Adolescents. *Pediatrics* **2019**, *143*, e20190282. [CrossRef] [PubMed]

107. Colchero, M.A.; Rivera-Dommarco, J.; Popkin, B.M.; Ng, S.W. In Mexico, Evidence Of Sustained Consumer Response Two Years After Implementing A Sugar-Sweetened Beverage Tax. *Health Aff.* **2017**, *36*, 564–571. [CrossRef] [PubMed]

108. Sanchez-Romero, L.M.; Penko, J.; Coxson, P.G.; Fernandez, A.; Mason, A.; Moran, A.E.; Ávila-Burgos, L.; Odden, M.; Barquera, S.; Bibbins-Domingo, K. Projected Impact of Mexico's Sugar-Sweetened Beverage Tax Policy on Diabetes and Cardiovascular Disease: A Modeling Study. *PLoS Med.* **2016**, *13*, e1002158. [CrossRef] [PubMed]

109. Silver, L.D.; Ng, S.W.; Ryan-Ibarra, S.; Taillie, L.S.; Induni, M.; Miles, D.R.; Poti, J.M.; Popkin, B.M. Changes in prices, sales, consumer spending, and beverage consumption one year after a tax on sugar-sweetened beverages in Berkeley, California, US: A before-and-after study. *PLoS Med.* **2017**, *14*, e1002283. [CrossRef] [PubMed]

14

Physical Activity, Cardiorespiratory Fitness and the Metabolic Syndrome

Jonathan Myers [1,*], Peter Kokkinos [2] and Eric Nyelin [3]

[1] Cardiology Division, Veterans Affairs Palo Alto Health Care System and Stanford University, Stanford, CA 94304, USA
[2] Cardiology Division, Washington DC Veterans Affairs Medical Center and Rutgers University, Washington, DC 20422, USA
[3] Endocrinology Division, Washington DC Veterans Affairs Medical Center, Washington, DC 20422, USA
* Correspondence: drj993@aol.com

Abstract: Both observational and interventional studies suggest an important role for physical activity and higher fitness in mitigating the metabolic syndrome. Each component of the metabolic syndrome is, to a certain extent, favorably influenced by interventions that include physical activity. Given that the prevalence of the metabolic syndrome and its individual components (particularly obesity and insulin resistance) has increased significantly in recent decades, guidelines from various professional organizations have called for greater efforts to reduce the incidence of this condition and its components. While physical activity interventions that lead to improved fitness cannot be expected to normalize insulin resistance, lipid disorders, or obesity, the combined effect of increasing activity on these risk markers, an improvement in fitness, or both, has been shown to have a major impact on health outcomes related to the metabolic syndrome. Exercise therapy is a cost-effective intervention to both prevent and mitigate the impact of the metabolic syndrome, but it remains underutilized. In the current article, an overview of the effects of physical activity and higher fitness on the metabolic syndrome is provided, along with a discussion of the mechanisms underlying the benefits of being more fit or more physically active in the prevention and treatment of the metabolic syndrome.

Keywords: metabolic syndrome; cardiorespiratory fitness; insulin resistance; cardiovascular disease; exercise training

1. Overview

Chronic, non-communicable diseases currently represent the predominant challenge to global health. In a recent global status report on chronic disease, the World Health Organization stated that non-communicable conditions, including cardiovascular disease (CVD), diabetes and obesity, now account for roughly two-thirds of deaths worldwide [1]. The prevalence of many of the components of the "metabolic syndrome", particularly obesity and diabetes, has grown considerably throughout the Western World since this term was initially suggested by Haller in 1977 [2]. Given that the metabolic syndrome is an important precursor to CVD and other chronic conditions [3–7], guidelines from various professional organizations have called for greater efforts to reduce the incidence of this condition and its components [3,4]. A notable parallel over the last 4 decades is the fact that numerous surveys and cohort studies have consistently reported that Western societies are significantly less physically active than past generations [7–11]. Moreover, a growing number of studies has reported that higher cardiorespiratory fitness (CRF; which is defined as the maximal capacity of the cardiovascular and respiratory systems to supply oxygen to the skeletal muscles during exercise) is inversely related to the development of the metabolic syndrome [12,13]. These studies, along with recent intervention trials [14,15], suggest a compelling link between impaired CRF, low physical activity patterns (defined as movement that requires energy), exercise (defined as planned, structured, repetitive, intentional movement intended to improve CRF), and the metabolic syndrome.

Although the metabolic syndrome is complex and has been defined differently by different organizations, the clustering of risk factors that define it (high waist circumference, dyslipidemia, hypertension, and insulin resistance) are, to a certain extent, commonly associated with sedentary lifestyles. Indeed, numerous studies in recent decades have shown that increasing amounts of physical activity and higher CRF have a favorable impact on each of the components of the metabolic syndrome [12–16]. While physical activity interventions alone cannot be expected to normalize insulin resistance, lipid disorders, or obesity, the combined effect of increasing activity on these risk markers, an improvement in CRF, or both, can have a major impact on health outcomes related to the metabolic syndrome. However, physical activity as a treatment for metabolic disease remains underutilized. In fact, physical activity interventions are often dismissed in favor of pharmacologic treatments or other interventions that tend to be more economically driven [8,17–19]. Although physical activity counseling is now mandated by many health care systems, the fact remains that activity counseling rarely occurs as part of clinical encounters [20,21]. The lack of attention paid to physical activity is unfortunate given the strength of exercise interventions on health outcomes among individuals with metabolic disorders [12–16].

In the following, an overview of the effects of physical activity and CRF on the metabolic syndrome is provided, along with a discussion of the mechanisms underlying the benefits of being more fit or more physically active in the prevention and treatment of the metabolic syndrome.

2. Physical Activity and the Metabolic Syndrome

Collectively, studies on the impact of being more physically active, whether studied in a cross-sectional cohort or as a result of a structured exercise intervention, have been shown to have an important impact on cardiometabolic risk. Regular exercise can help to reduce weight, reduce blood pressure, and improve lipid disorders, including raising HDL and lowering triglycerides [7,16–22]. Among the physiological systems that respond favorably to physical activity, it has been argued that one of the most demonstrable effects of regular exercise is its impact on insulin resistance [23,24]. A summary of key studies is shown in Table 1; notably, these studies are categorically consistent in demonstrating the benefits of being more physically active in terms of reducing risk for the metabolic syndrome.

Table 1. Sampling of studies assessing the impact of physical activity patterns or exercise intervention on the metabolic syndrome.

Observational Studies			
Author, Year; (Reference)	N (Men/Women), Mean Age	Assessment	Key Results
Thune, 1998; [25]	5220/5869 34.4 and 33.7 years, respectively	PA self-report	Higher PA associated with better lipid profile, overall metabolic risk profile over 7 years
Laaksonen, 2002; [26]	612 men 51.4 years	Assessment of LTPA over previous 12 months among high risk men; followed for 4 years	>3 h/week moderate to vigorous LTPA half as likely as sedentary men to have MetSyn Men in top 33% VO$_2$max 75% less likely than unfit men to develop MetSyn over 4 years
Sisson, 2010; [27]	697/749 47.5 years	Accelerometry	MetS prevalence decreased as steps/day increased; odds of having MetSyn were 10% lower for each additional 1000 steps/day

Table 1. *Cont.*

Observational Studies			
Author, Year; (Reference)	**N (Men/Women), Mean Age**	**Assessment**	**Key Results**
Healy, 2008; [28]	67/102 53.4 years	Accelerometer evaluation of time spent in sedentary, light, moderate-to-vigorous, and mean activity intensity in participants with diabetes and obesity	Moderate-to-vigorous activity associated with lower triglycerides. Sedentary time, light-intensity time, and exercise intensity associated with waist circumference and clustered metabolic risk
Ekelund, 2007; [29]	103/155 40.8 years	Accelerometry, exercise test, biometric measures on adults with a family history of type 2 diabetes	Total body movement inversely associated with triglycerides, insulin, HDL and clustered metabolic risk; moderate-and vigorous-intensity PA inversely associated with clustered metabolic risk

Exercise Intervention Studies			
Author, Year	**N**	**Intervention**	**Key Results**
Look AHEAD, 2013; [30]	3063/2082 58.8 years	Subjects with type 2 diabetes randomly assigned to intensive lifestyle intervention or diabetes support and education	Intervention group had greater reductions in weight loss, glycated hemoglobin and greater initial improvements in exercise capacity and all cardiovascular risk factors (except LDL)
Stewart, 2004; [31]	53/62 63.6 years	6 months of exercise training in subjects with or at high risk for MetSyn	Exercise group improved peak VO$_2$, muscle strength, and lean body mass; reductions in total and abdominal fat related to improved CVD risk
Katzmarzyk, 2003; [32]	288/333 31.6	20 weeks of supervised aerobic exercise training	Of 105 patients with MetSyn, 30.5% were no longer classified as having metabolic syndrome after exercise training
Balducci, 2008; [33]	329/234	Twice weekly aerobic & resistance training for 1 year	Exercise group improved fitness, HbA1c, and CVD risk profile
Diabetes Prevention Program Research Group, 2002; [34]	3234 50.6	Lifestyle intervention (150 min/week PA and nutritional counseling) vs. Metformin vs. placebo	Lifestyle intervention group achieved a 38% reversal of MetSyn and a 41% reduction of new onset MetSyn.

PA—physical activity; LTPA—leisure time physical activity; MetSyn—metabolic syndrome; HDL—high density lipoprotein; LDL—high density lipoprotein; CVD—cardiovascular disease; HbA1c—glycated hemoglobin.

2.1. Observational Studies Associating Physical Activity Patterns with Metabolic Risk

Observational or cross-sectional studies are inherently limited because they do not demonstrate cause and effect. In the current context, the weaknesses of these studies include the fact that intrinsically healthier individuals may be more likely to engage in physical activity, or that they may be genetically more fit irrespective of lifestyle or behavioral factors. Nevertheless, these studies have provided valuable information regarding patterns between physical activity habits, metabolic risk, and related conditions. Collectively, these studies suggest that more active individuals exhibit either a lower prevalence of risk factors for the metabolic syndrome, have a lower incidence of developing the metabolic syndrome over a given follow-up period, or both. While the levels of activity have been quantified and defined in different ways, these data support the concept that meeting the minimal guidelines on activity (i.e., 150 minutes per week of moderate intensity activity) is associated with a lower prevalence of the metabolic syndrome. In the following, a sampling of some of the key observational studies related to physical activity and the metabolic syndrome are outlined.

As part of the TROMSO study in Norway, Thune and colleagues [25] studied 5220 men and 5869 women who completed two physical activity surveys approximately 7 years apart. BMI and detailed lipid profiles were determined at both evaluations. There was a dose–response relationship between improved serum lipid levels, BMI, and higher levels of physical activity in both genders after adjustments for potential confounders. Differences in BMI and serum lipid levels between sedentary and sustained exercising groups were consistently more pronounced after 7 years than at baseline, especially in the oldest age group. The most dramatic differences in metabolic risk profiles occurred between the most active subjects compared to the least active subjects. An increase in leisure time activity over the 7 years improved metabolic profiles, whereas a decrease worsened them in both genders.

In a cross-sectional evaluation of physical activity and metabolic risk among individuals with a family history of Type 2 diabetes, Ekelund et al. [29] measured total body movement and five other subcomponents of physical activity by accelerometry in 258 at-risk adults. Body composition was determined using bioimpedance and waist circumference, and blood pressure, fasting triglycerides, HDL, glucose, and insulin were determined. In addition, continuously distributed clustered risk was calculated. Total body movement (counts/day) was significantly and independently associated with three of six risk factors (fasting triglycerides, insulin, and HDL) and with clustered metabolic risk after adjustment for age, gender, and obesity. Time spent at moderate- and vigorous-intensity physical activity was independently associated with clustered metabolic risk. Short (5- and 10-minute) bouts of activity, time spent sedentary, and time spent at light-intensity activity were not significantly related with clustered risk after adjustment for confounding factors. The association between total body movement and intermediary phenotypic risk factors for cardiovascular and metabolic disease along with clustered metabolic risk was independent of aerobic fitness and obesity. These investigators suggested that increasing the total amount of physical activity in sedentary and overweight individuals has beneficial effects on metabolic risk.

Laaksonen and colleagues [26] assessed 12-month leisure time physical activity (LTPA), VO_2max, and cardiovascular and metabolic risk factors among 612 middle-aged men without the metabolic syndrome at baseline. After 4 years of follow-up, 107 men had metabolic syndrome (using the WHO definition). Men engaging in 3 h/week of moderate or vigorous LTPA were half as likely as sedentary men to have the metabolic syndrome after adjustment for major confounders (age, BMI, smoking, alcohol, and socioeconomic status) or potentially mediating factors (insulin, glucose, lipids, and blood pressure). Vigorous LTPA had an even stronger inverse association with incidence of the metabolic syndrome among men who were unfit at baseline. Men in the upper tertile of VO_2max were 75% less likely than unfit men to develop the metabolic syndrome, even after adjustment for major confounders. Associations of LTPA and VO_2max with development of the metabolic syndrome were qualitatively similar. These results suggest that high-risk men engaging in commonly recommended levels of physical activity were less likely to develop the metabolic syndrome than sedentary men. CRF was also strongly protective, although possibly not independent of mediating factors.

2.2. Exercise Intervention Studies and the Metabolic Syndrome

Relative to cross-sectional studies, exercise and lifestyle intervention studies can provide more direct information on the cause and effect impact of physical activity, CRF, or both, on risk of the metabolic syndrome. While there is a lengthy history of studies applying exercise interventions to assess the effects of training on individual components of the metabolic syndrome (e.g., insulin resistance, blood pressure, abdominal adiposity), fewer studies have been specifically designed to examine the efficacy of exercise training on the clinical diagnosis or reversal of the metabolic syndrome. In recent years, a growing number of groups have conducted large, multicenter randomized trials of exercise training along with other lifestyle interventions among individuals with or at high risk for the metabolic syndrome.

Two large lifestyle intervention trials, the Finnish Diabetes Prevention Study (DPS) [35], and the US Diabetes Prevention Program (DPP) [36], were designed to either prevent type 2 diabetes in impaired glucose-tolerant subjects or reduce the prevalence of metabolic syndrome through changes in diet and physical activity. The DPS observed a 58% reduction in risk for the development of type 2 diabetes with lifestyle intervention, and the DPP demonstrated a reduced prevalence of the metabolic syndrome in the intervention group. Weight loss appeared to be a major determinant of both improvements in glucose tolerance and the reduction in metabolic syndrome prevalence, whereas physical activity and dietary composition contributed independently. A third trial performed in the Netherlands involved a lifestyle intervention designed to assess the impact of diet and physical activity intervention on glucose tolerance in impaired glucose-tolerant subjects (termed the Study of Lifestyle intervention and Impaired glucose tolerance Maastricht [SLIM] study) [37]. The SLIM study similarly reported a 58% reduction in diabetes risk after 3 years and a 47% reduction at the end of the intervention, despite a relatively modest weight reduction. A follow-up to the SLIM trial determined the effects of the exercise and lifestyle intervention on the incidence and prevalence of the metabolic syndrome during the active intervention and four years thereafter [38]. They observed that the prevalence of the metabolic syndrome was significantly lower in the intervention group (52.6%) compared to the control group (74.6%). In addition, among participants without the metabolic syndrome at baseline, cumulative incidence of the metabolic syndrome was 18.2% in the intervention group at the end of active intervention, compared to 73.7% in the control group. Four years after stopping active intervention, the reduced incidence of metabolic syndrome was maintained.

A landmark multicenter trial performed in the US, termed Action for Health in Diabetes (Look AHEAD) [30], assessed whether an intensive lifestyle intervention for weight loss would decrease cardiovascular morbidity and mortality in patients with Type 2 diabetes. In 16 study centers in the US, 5145 overweight or obese patients with type 2 diabetes were randomly assigned to participate in an intensive lifestyle intervention that promoted weight loss through decreased caloric intake and increased physical activity (intervention group) or to receive diabetes support and education (control group). The primary outcome was a composite of death from cardiovascular causes, nonfatal myocardial infarction, nonfatal stroke, or hospitalization for angina during a maximum follow-up of 13.5 years. The trial was stopped early on the basis of a futility analysis at a median follow-up of 9.6 years. Weight loss was greater in the intervention group than in the control group throughout the study (8.6% vs. 0.7% at 1 year; 6.0% vs. 3.5% at study end). The intensive lifestyle intervention also produced greater reductions in HbA1c and greater initial improvements in fitness and all cardiovascular risk factors, except for LDL cholesterol. The primary outcome occurred in 403 patients in the intervention group and in 418 in the control group (1.83 and 1.92 events per 100 person-years, respectively); these differences were not significant ($p = 0.51$).

While the Look AHEAD study did not reduce the rate of cardiovascular events in overweight or obese adults with type 2 diabetes, there were many notable benefits among subjects in the intervention group. These included the fact that modest weight loss occurred and was maintained over 10 years, clinically meaningful improvements in HbA1c which were greatest during the first year but were at least partly sustained throughout follow-up, fewer subjects needing treatment with insulin, partial remission of diabetes during the first 4 years of the trial vs. control subjects, reduced sleep apnea and depression, and improvements in quality of life, physical functioning, and mobility.

There are also numerous notable single-center trials that have assessed the impact of exercise intervention on metabolic risk. Stewart et al. [31] studied 51 men and 53 women with or at elevated risk for metabolic syndrome who underwent either a 6-month supervised exercise program or usual care. Exercise significantly increased aerobic and muscle fitness, lean mass, and HDL, and reduced total and abdominal fat. Reductions in total body and abdominal fat and increases in leanness, largely independent of weight loss, were associated with improved systolic and diastolic blood pressure, total cholesterol, very low-density lipoprotein cholesterol, triglycerides, lipoprotein(a), and insulin sensitivity. At baseline, 42.3% of participants had metabolic syndrome. At 6 months, nine exercisers (17.7%) and eight controls (15.1%) no longer had metabolic syndrome, whereas four controls (7.6%) and no exercisers developed it.

Katzmarzyk, et al. [32] studied the efficacy of exercise training in treating the metabolic syndrome among 621 participants from the HERITAGE Family Study, identified at baseline as sedentary but apparently healthy. Subjects underwent a 20-week program of exercise training consisting of 3 sessions/week of supervised cycle ergometer training. The presence of the metabolic syndrome and the cluster of associated risk factors were determined before and after the study period. Exercise training resulted in marked improvements in the metabolic profile of the participants, including triglycerides, HDL cholesterol, blood pressure, fasting plasma glucose, and waist circumference. Of the 105 participants with the metabolic syndrome at baseline, 30.5% (32 participants) were no longer classified as having the metabolic syndrome after training. There were no sex or race differences in the efficacy of exercise in treating the metabolic syndrome.

2.3. Meta-Analyses of Exercise and Cardiometabolic Risk

There have been many individual trials in the context of physical activity and the metabolic syndrome, and many have lacked adequate sample sizes. The metabolic syndrome is more complex than many other conditions because it involves the clustering of several risk factors, and has been defined in different ways. Some studies have reported a significant effect on one or several risk factors but a minimal effect on another. Meta-analyses have been particularly helpful in this area by combining results from different studies to obtain a better estimate of the overall effect of a particular intervention. There have been several notable meta-analyses in the area of physical activity and metabolic syndrome which are discussed in the following.

Wewege et al. [39] recently performed a meta-analysis examining the effect of aerobic, resistance and combined (aerobic and resistance) exercise on cardiovascular risk factors among individuals with the metabolic syndrome, but without a diagnosis of diabetes. Interestingly, this is an understudied group, yet it represents the majority of the metabolic syndrome population. Randomized controlled trials >4 weeks in duration that compared an exercise intervention to non-exercise control groups in patients with metabolic syndrome without diabetes were included. Eleven studies with 16 interventions were analyzed (12 aerobic, 4 resistance). Aerobic exercise significantly improved waist circumference, fasting glucose, HDL cholesterol, triglycerides, diastolic blood pressure, and cardiorespiratory fitness (by 4.2 mL/kg/min, $p < 0.01$), among other outcomes. No significant effects were determined following resistance exercise possibly due to limited data. Sub-analyses suggested that aerobic exercise that progressed to vigorous intensity, and conducted 3 days/week for ≥12 weeks, offered larger and more widespread improvements. While these results strongly support the use of aerobic exercise for patients with the metabolic syndrome who have not yet developed diabetes, they also suggest that more studies on resistance/combined exercise programs are required to improve the quality of evidence.

Naci and Ioannidis [40] performed a recent meta-analysis among 14,716 subjects randomized to either a physical activity intervention or usual care. While the analysis did not address metabolic syndrome per se, the results are remarkable in that they provided a direct comparison between exercise and drug therapies for diabetes and CVD risk. Among 57 trials comparing the effects of drug and physical activity interventions on health outcomes compared to usual care, they observed that exercise intervention was similar to drug interventions for the secondary prevention of prediabetes, cardiovascular disease (CVD) and mortality. Importantly, physical activity was markedly superior to drug treatment among patients with stroke. The extent to which standard pharmacologic treatment would complement exercise interventions in treating or preventing diabetes or other health outcomes is unknown since there are so few data on comparative effectiveness involving exercise. These results are striking given the investments made in drug interventions relative to the comparatively meager investments devoted to exercise and other preventive strategies.

Ostman and colleagues [41] performed a meta-analysis that included 16 studies with 23 intervention groups and a total of 77,000 patient-hours of exercise training. All studies included subjects with a clinical diagnosis of the metabolic syndrome at baseline, an intervention involving exercise vs. sedentary controls, and all studies included incidence of mortality and hospitalization. Exercise training duration ranged between 8 weeks and 1 year. In analyses comparing aerobic exercise training versus control groups, there were reductions in BMI, waist circumference, systolic blood pressure and diastolic blood pressure, fasting blood glucose, triglycerides and low-density lipoprotein. Peak VO_2 was significantly improved among those randomized to exercise (mean difference 3.0 mL/kg/min, $p < 0.001$). Similar changes were observed for studies using combined aerobic and resistance exercise.

2.4. Synopsis—Physical Activity and the Metabolic Syndrome

Higher levels of physical activity, whether through observational studies or as part of formal exercise intervention trials, generally have a favorable impact on the metabolic syndrome and its components. In some studies, the proportion of participants who meet the criteria for the metabolic syndrome is reduced with exercise intervention. In longitudinal studies, more active individuals have a lower incidence of the metabolic syndrome. In a limited number of studies in which the dose–response relationship has been assessed, the most active subjects tend to have the greatest reductions in metabolic risk. Although the dose of physical activity has varied in the different studies, achieving the minimal physical activity guidelines (at least 150 minutes per week of moderate-intensity activity or 75 minutes per week of vigorous intensity activity) has been consistently demonstrated to have significant benefits on metabolic risk. While there are comparatively few studies on the impact of strength training on cardiometabolic risk, higher levels of muscular strength are associated with lower risk for developing the metabolic syndrome. Thus, in addition to aerobic exercise, individuals should strive to achieve the minimal recommendations of at least 2 days per week of resistance training.

3. Cardiorespiratory Fitness and the Metabolic Syndrome

Some of the inconsistencies between metabolic syndrome incidence and self-reported physical activity status [26,42] may be explained by the subjectivity and inaccuracy of self-reported physical activity assessments [43]. In this regard, directly measured or estimated VO_2 max based on a standardized exercise treadmill or cycle ergometer represents an objective assessment of CRF, as subject bias in reporting physical activity is removed. Overall, such studies have been consistent in reporting a lower prevalence of metabolic syndrome in those with higher CRF among both men and women regardless of race and after adjustment for relevant confounders [44–48]. An overview of some of the key studies is provided in Table 2.

Table 2. Sampling of studies assessing the association between cardiorespiratory fitness and the metabolic syndrome.

Author, Year; (Reference)	N (Men/Women)	Key Results
Carnethon, 2003; [49]	4487 (2029/2458)	Only men and women in the highest 40% of maximal treadmill performance were protected against developing MetSyn.
Franks, 2004; [50]	847 men	A strong inverse association between physical activity and MetSyn. The magnitude of the association between physical activity and the MetSyn was >3-fold greater than for VO_2max.
LaMonte, 2005; [46]	10,498 (9007/1491)	An independent and progressive decline in the risk of developing MetSyn with higher CRF for men and women. Also, 20% to 26% lower risks occurred among participants with moderate CRF and 53% to 63% lower risks observed in highest CRF categories vs. the lowest CRF category.

Table 2. *Cont.*

Author, Year; (Reference)	N (Men/Women)	Key Results
Hassinen, 2008; [44]	1347 (671/676)	Men and women in the lowest third of VO_2max had 10.2 times (men) and 10.8 times (women) higher risk of having MetSyn than those in the highest VO_2max category.
Hassinen, 2010; [48]	1226 (589/637)	Risk of developing MetSyn within 2 years of follow-up was 44% lower for each 1-SD increase in VO_2 max. Each 1-SD higher VO_2 max from baseline resulted in 1.8 times higher likelihood to resolve MetSyn during 2 years of follow-up.
Earnest, 2013; [51]	38,659 (30,927/7732)	CRF demonstrated a strong inverse relationship with MetSyn in both genders. The association was strongest in those with lower waist circumference and fasting glucose, in both genders.
Adams-Campbell, 2016; [47]	170 women	CRF was inversely related to the prevalence of the metabolic syndrome in overweight/obese African-American postmenopausal women.
Ingle, 2017; [52]	9666 men	The likelihood of developing MetSyn was approximately 50% lower in fit men compared to unfit, independent of BMI particularly in men <50 years.
Kelly, 2018; [45]	3636 (2007/1629)	Significant, inverse and graded association between VO_2max and MetSyn. Highest fit had >20 times lower risk of having MetSyn compared to least-fit individuals. The difference in VO_2max between those with MetSyn and those without was ≈ 2.5 METs.

CRF—cardiorespiratory fitness; BMI—body mass index; MetSyn—metabolic syndrome; METS—metabolic equivalents.

In Finland, men and women in the lowest tertile of VO_2max had 10.2 and 10.8 times, respectively, higher risks of having metabolic syndrome than those in the highest VO_2max category [44]. Similar findings were reported by Kelley et al. [45] in middle-aged men and women in the US. Importantly, an inverse and graded association between CRF and the incidence of metabolic syndrome has been observed with relatively small changes in CRF (e.g., 2.5 metabolic equivalents) yielding significant reductions in risk. The risk of metabolic syndrome prevalence was more than 20 times less likely for individuals in the highest fit category compared to the least-fit individuals. Similarly, the risk of developing metabolic syndrome within 2 years of follow-up was reported to be 44% lower for each 1-SD increase in VO_2 max [48]. Individuals in the highest sex-specific fitness category were 68% less likely to develop metabolic syndrome. In a more recent Finnish study, each 1-SD higher change in VO_2 max from baseline was associated with a 1.8-fold higher likelihood of resolving metabolic syndrome during 2 years of follow-up [48].

An interaction between CRF risk of and metabolic syndrome has also been suggested by the Australian National Health Survey. An inverse association between CRF and the metabolic syndrome was observed in those with lower waist circumference and fasting glucose in both men and women [51]. However, the impact of CRF on metabolic syndrome was independent of obesity as defined by body mass index among 9666 middle-aged (48.7 ± 8.4 years) asymptomatic men [52]. The likelihood of developing metabolic syndrome was approximately 50% lower in fit men compared to unfit men (OR = 0.51, 95% CI 0.46 to 0.57), independent of BMI, particularly in men <50 years. There is also evidence to suggest that objectively measured energy expenditure is a stronger deterrent for the metabolic syndrome than measured VO_2 max. Franks and colleagues [50] reported that the magnitude of the association between physical activity and the metabolic syndrome was >3-fold greater than for VO_2max, suggesting that the risk of metabolic syndrome can be modulated by higher intensity activities as well as lower intensity aerobic activities (below the threshold required to increase aerobic capacity).

Some evidence also suggests that the CRF-metabolic syndrome risk association may be gender-specific. Hassinen et al. [48] observed that each 1-SD higher VO_2 max (6.1 mL/kg/min in men; 4.8 mL/kg/min in women) resulted in 56% and 35% decreased risks of developing metabolic syndrome over two years of follow-up in men and women, respectively. In men, a 4.8 mL/kg/min increase in VO_2 max resulted in a 56% decrease in risk [48]. However, gender differences in the association between CRF and incidence of metabolic syndrome were not supported by the same group in their previous study [44].

There are also indications that only high CRF may offer protection against the development of metabolic syndrome. Laaksonen et al. [26] reported 47% and 75% lower odds of developing metabolic syndrome among men in the middle and highest tertiles of measured VO_2max, respectively, compared to men in the lowest tertile. However, this association was no longer significant after adjustment for baseline metabolic risk factors. Similarly, Carnethon et al. [49] reported that only men and women in the highest 40% of maximal treadmill performance were protected against developing metabolic syndrome. In contrast, LaMonte et al. [46] reported an independent and progressive decline in the risk of developing metabolic syndrome with increased CRF for men and women. Specifically, they reported 20% to 26% lower risks among participants with moderate CRF levels and 53% to 63% lower risks in the highest CRF categories, when compared to those in the lowest CRF category.

Finally, in the Diabetes Prevention Program trial, 3234 subjects (53% with metabolic syndrome) at high risk for diabetes were randomized to a lifestyle intervention group or usual care [34]. Those in the lifestyle intervention group (aerobic exercise 150 minutes per week and nutritional counseling) achieved a 38% reversal of the metabolic syndrome and a 41% reduction of new onset of metabolic syndrome. In contrast, treatment with metformin only reduced new cases of metabolic syndrome by 17%. To prevent one case of diabetes during a period of three years, 6.9 persons would have had to participate in the lifestyle-intervention program, and 13.9 would have had to receive metformin. These findings suggest that a healthy lifestyle may be more effective in preventing metabolic syndrome than the anti-hyperglycemic agent metformin.

Synopsis—Cardiorespiratory Fitness and the Metabolic Syndrome

Although physical activity and CRF are often used interchangeably, it is important to recognize that they are different; physical activity is a behavior and CRF is an attribute. CRF is improved by activity, but it is influenced by other factors, including genetics. Nevertheless, most sedentary individuals will improve CRF by following the widely-recognized minimal guidelines on physical activity. Both CRF levels from observational studies and changes in CRF as a result of 3–12-month exercise interventions have consistently been shown to improve cardiometabolic risk. In some studies, a proportion of a study sample no longer meets the criteria for metabolic syndrome after an exercise intervention that increases CRF. Taken together, cross-sectional studies demonstrate that subjects in the highest-fit categories exhibit between 5- and 20-fold lower likelihood of having the metabolic syndrome vs. subjects in the least-fit groups. Longitudinally, subjects in the highest fit groups exhibit ≈40% to as much as 20-fold lower risks of developing the metabolic syndrome. Efforts to improve CRF should be part of standard therapy for individuals with or at high risk for the metabolic syndrome.

4. Mechanisms Underlying the Metabolic Syndrome and Implications for Physical Activity and Fitness

4.1. Pathophysiology of Metabolic Syndrome

The underlying cause(s) of the metabolic syndrome are unknown, but it is significantly influenced by the twin epidemics of diabetes and obesity. Indeed, metabolic syndrome shares diabetes-related insulin resistance (IR) and dysfunctional adipose fuel handling and central obesity as its core. However, despite the commonality of traits, many subjects with metabolic syndrome do not display IR [53] nor do all obese individuals have metabolic syndrome [54,55]. Thus, neither IR nor central obesity fully explains the pathophysiological features of metabolic syndrome and other factors implicated include inflammation, genetics, epigenetics, and circadian abnormalities. As will be discussed further, enhanced CRF modulates the negative impact of these causative drivers of metabolic syndrome.

4.2. Insulin Resistance

The concept of IR was introduced by Himmsworth in 1936 who showed that diabetes could be subdivided into two categories—insulin-sensitive and insulin-insensitive types [56]—and this was later confirmed by Yalow and Berson with the novel measurement of insulin itself [57]. Once clamp techniques were developed, it was established that IR predominated in type 2 diabetes [58,59] and that hyperinsulinemia was the best predictor of the development of type 2 diabetes in nondiabetic individuals [60]. Reaven coined the term Syndrome X, later renamed by others to metabolic syndrome, to describe the role of IR (i.e., hyperinsulinemia or impaired glucose tolerance) as the driver of atherosclerotic dyslipidemia, type 2 diabetes, and hypertension [61]. Indeed, elevations of insulin concentration were shown to prospectively precede the development of these metabolic disorders [62] and the role of IR in metabolic syndrome was shown to be related to low insulin sensitivity [63]. With an increasing degree of metabolic syndrome components (i.e., metabolic syndrome score), there is an increase in fasting glucose, insulin levels, and HOMA IR [64].

During physiological conditions, insulin binds to its receptor leading to tyrosine phosphorylation of downstream substrates including activation of the phosphoinositide 3-kinase (PI3K) pathway resulting in recruitment of GLUT4 to mediate glucose transport into muscle and adipose tissue where it is phosphorylated and either stored as glycogen or metabolized to produce ATP. However, when a state of compensatory hyperinsulinemia occurs in IR subjects, due to changes in insulin secretion and/or insulin clearance [65], the ensuing response includes mild forms of glucose intolerance, dyslipidemia (high triglycerides, low HDL, small dense LDL), and hypertension which is the pathophysiological construct of the insulin resistance syndrome developed by Reaven leading to increased risk of CVD, as well conditions such as stroke, polycystic ovary syndrome, non-alcoholic fatty liver disease, cancer, and sleep apnea [66]. Importantly, according to Reaven, the individual components of the IR syndrome can occur without IR, and the presence of IR does not have to lead to any of the components of the syndrome. Interestingly, although IR has been considered the central driver of type 2 diabetes and metabolic syndrome, an alternative argument places IR as an adaptive biomarker of poor metabolic health and insulin hyperresponsivness as the root cause [67].

The reason why IR leads to atherogenesis has been attributed to the activation by insulin of the mitogen activated protein (MAP) kinase pathway which, as opposed to the muted PI3K pathway, functions normally in IR. Subnormal PI3K-Akt activity leads to a reduction in endothelial nitric oxide formation and endothelial dysfunction, reduction in GLUT4 translocation, and decreased skeletal muscle and fat glucose uptake [68]. Concurrently, the persistence of MAP kinase activity results in augmented expression of endothelin-1 and endothelial adhesion molecules with vascular smooth muscle cell mitogenesis which leads to vascular abnormalities and increased atherosclerosis risk.

The skeletal muscle mass comprises approximately 40% of total body mass and is the primary source of insulin-mediated glucose uptake and fatty acid oxidation. The exposure to exercise evokes adaptation in skeletal muscle in a multitude of signaling pathways, the functional response to which is determined by training volume, mode of training, intensity and frequency. With persistent exercise exposure, there is mitochondrial biogenesis, fast-to-slow fiber-type transformation, changes in substrate metabolism, and angiogenesis. Moreover, a host of myokines are released from active muscles providing communication throughout the body. Enhanced fitness is associated with high levels of insulin sensitivity/insulin action. While glucose homeostasis at rest is insulin-sensitive, exercise with muscle contractions increases glucose uptake from the circulation that is not reliant on insulin. Indeed, GLUT-4 is responsive to both insulin and muscle contraction independently.

Whatever the role of IR, it is known that exercise augments insulin signaling independent of PI3K and when skeletal muscles are stimulated by contraction combined with insulin, glucose transport and GLUT4 translocation are enhanced. Thus, exercise provides a potent means to avert metabolic syndrome supported by the results of the Diabetes Prevention Program study [36], where exercise intervention decreased metabolic syndrome prevalence significantly compared to the control group throughout the intervention. Interestingly, although both aerobic and resistance training increase glucose transport and are often additive, these metabolic responses appear to be mediated by different mechanisms. In at least one study among nonobese young women, the investigators reported that insulin sensitivity increases in both aerobically-trained and resistance-trained women. However, when data were expressed per kg of free-fat mass (FFM) the improvement in glucose disposal persisted in endurance-trained women, whereas no significant change was noted in resistance-trained subjects or controls. This led to the conclusion that the increased glucose disposal associated with resistance exercise was the result of the increase in the quantity of lean body mass, without altering the intrinsic capacity of the muscle to respond to insulin. On the other hand, endurance training enhanced glucose disposal independent of changes in lean body mass or VO_2max, suggestive of an intrinsic change in the ability of the muscle to metabolize glucose [69].

4.3. Adipose Fuel Metabolism

The metabolic consequences related to an unhealthy lifestyle were proposed in 1923 by Kylin consisting of a syndrome of hypertension, hyperglycemia, hyperuricemia, and obesity [70]. "Androgenic obesity" contributing to diabetes and CVD was proposed later by Vague in 1940 [71]. The upper-body or abdominal obesity type with hyperinsulinemia, in particular, was proposed as the primary factor leading to metabolic syndrome and CVD independent of overall obesity [72–74]. Being a multifunctional organ providing cross-talk between various systems, including the immune and the cardiovascular systems, this type of abdominal obesity, being the most common manifestation of metabolic syndrome, has been viewed as a cellular biomarker of dysfunctional adipose tissue [55] or adiposopathy [75].

Insulin is the major regulator of fuel metabolism in adipocytes and is adversely impacted by excess caloric intake and inactivity. Hyperinsulinemia is well documented in individuals with obesity with or without IR and is related to increases in insulin secretion and decreases in insulin clearance rate [76]. It has been known for some time that insulin insensitivity can cause a distinct biochemical syndrome with elevated free fatty acids [77] and in metabolic syndrome-prone subjects, relative tissue hypoinsulinemia results in release of excess free fatty acids, mainly from visceral depots, resulting in increased liver synthesis VLDL, elevated triglycerides, increased HDL clearance and small dense LDL. Increased free fatty acid release also causes IR in the liver resulting in increased gluconeogenesis and hyperglycemia. These metabolic events result in adipocyte fuel malfunction manifested as adipocyte hypertrophy and ectopic lipid deposition in vital organs such as the liver, pancreas, muscle and heart. In the pancreas, lipid excess can lead to lipotoxicity which can promote endoplasmic reticulum stress-mediated β-cell death [78].

Adipose tissue also harbors fat-derived mesenchymal stem cells which experimentally have the capacity to modify mRNA expression contributing to IR [79]. Moreover, abdominal fat and fat-derived mesenchymal stem cells are responsive to physical activity; both high-intensity aerobic and resistance training decrease visceral fat effectively [80] while the molecular expression of fat-derived mesenchymal stem cells is significantly altered with exercise preventing adipogenesis [81].

4.4. Inflammation

Systemic inflammation has been strongly linked to CVD via multiple immune system biomarkers, factors also associated with metabolic syndrome. Thus, metabolic syndrome is associated with pro-inflammatory cytokines such as TNF, IL-beta, and is characterized by chronic systemic low-grade inflammation manifested by elevated CRP [82]. Chronic inflammation links metabolic syndrome to IR [83,84] and to CVD via promotion of vascular dysfunction [85]. Adipocyte hypertrophy, abnormal local blood flow, hypoxia, altered adipokine expression, and local infiltration of immune cells all conspire to adiposopathy which is infiltrated by macrophages, with elevated TNF and IL-6. Moreover, these macrophage-associated adipocytes are undergoing necrosis. A recent finding showed that the use of the anti-inflammatory agent colchicine significantly improved obesity-associated inflammatory variables in metabolic syndrome and appeared to be safe [86].

The degree of cardiorespiratory fitness in metabolic syndrome subjects has been shown to have inverse associations with CRP, IL-6, and IL-18, partially explained by the degree of abdominal obesity [87]. Using IL-18 as a biomarker of inflammation, aerobic exercise reduced inflammation which was not observed with resistance exercise despite a similar degree of loss of fat mass in metabolic syndrome subjects [88].

4.5. Genetics/Epigenetics

Inheritance plays a role in metabolic syndrome and its influence may range from 10% to 30% being strongest between waist circumference and IR, which has also been documented in twin studies [89]. Techniques such as linkage analysis, candidate gene approach, and genome-wide association (GWAS) studies have been applied to detect gene variants for metabolic syndrome focusing on loci for individual components such as obesity, dyslipidemia, hypertension, and diabetes [90]. For example, eight single nucleotide polymorphisms (SNPs) were associated with the dyslipidemia in metabolic syndrome [91]. In other studies, GWAS associations have shown that transcription factor 7-like 2 (TCF7L2), which is part of the Wnt signaling pathway, mediates metabolic syndrome trait susceptibility towards developing diabetes and dyslipidemia [92]. Another example is the caveolin-1 gene (CAV1) variant associated with IR which is also associated with metabolic syndrome, especially in non-obese subjects [93].

The concept of epigenetics, originally accredited to Waddington, has evolved to specify how gene activation or silencing influence gene expression without changing the DNA sequence itself and the epigenome include DNA methylation, histone modification, and various RNA-mediated processes. The epigenetic expression can be altered during development, during varying nutritional conditions, and by physical activity. One of the epigenetic mechanisms involves DNA methylation which results in a methyl group being attached to a cytosine pyrimidine ring and thereby influence gene expression especially when located in promotor regions. A burgeoning area of inquiry involves DNA methylation which has been reported to be related to several components of the metabolic syndrome [94] including an inverse association between levels of methylation and worsening of the metabolic syndrome [95]. Studies assessing global DNA methylation and also assessing methylation at specific genes related to lipid metabolism appear to be related to causation of the metabolic syndrome [96]. Epigenetic methylation changes related to physical activity have been reported to occur in the regions regulating peroxisome proliferator-activated receptor-1α, the master regulator of exercise-muscle activity, and also impact the adipose tissue response [97–99].

4.6. Circadian Disruption and Metabolic Syndrome

Disrupted diurnal rhythms due to excessive light or shift work can have profound and disruptive whole-body metabolic effects impacting most hormones that are normally governed by circadian rhythmicity so it is not surprising that these perturbations can lead to metabolic syndrome conditions with IR and obesity. Clock genes are expressed in adipose tissue and correlate to metabolic syndrome parameters [100]. A shortened sleep duration less than 6 hours has been associated with increased risk of metabolic syndrome and CVD [101] and meta analyses support these associations between sleep deprivation and risk for metabolic syndrome [102,103]. Moreover, the relationship of shortened sleep and metabolic syndrome may be dose related [104]. However, a normal sleep pattern decreases the risk of metabolic syndrome, albeit prolonged sleep appears to be neutral in this regard [105]. Regular exercise can re-set clock genes and have a salutary impact on clock time which might be another way to inhibit the metabolic syndrome [106,107]. A complementary medical strategy may be the use of a sympatholytic dopamine D2 receptor agonist to combat the circadian disruption and improve metabolic syndrome [108].

5. Summary

Both single center trials and recent meta-analyses suggest that exercise training, higher CRF, or both, improve factors that underlie the metabolic syndrome. Among subjects who meet the criteria for the metabolic syndrome, health outcomes are significantly improved by aerobic or resistance training, or their combination. In some individuals, an exercise program has been demonstrated to improve risk markers to an extent that they no longer meet the criteria for the metabolic syndrome. There are numerous physiological, lifestyle, and genetic factors that account for these salutary effects of physical activity or formal exercise programs. These include the impact of exercise on insulin resistance, adipose fuel metabolism, inflammation, and epigenetic factors. Physical activity interventions clearly have a favorable impact on metabolic disease and the burden it places not only on individuals but also on health care systems. Incorporating physical activity as an integral part of treatment strategies for the metabolic syndrome would appear to go a long way toward reducing the adverse health impact of this condition.

References

1. Riley, L.; Guthold, R.; Cowan, M.; Savin, S.; Bhatti, L.; Armstrong, T.; Bonita, R. The World Health Organization STEPwise Approach to Noncommunicable Disease Risk-Factor Surveillance: Methods, Challenges, and Opportunities. *Am. J. Public Health* **2016**, *106*, 74–78. [CrossRef] [PubMed]
2. Haller, H. Epidemiology and associated risk factors of hyperlipoproteinemia. *Zeitschrift für Sie Gesamte Innere Medizin und Ihre Grenzgebiete* **1977**, *32*, 124–128.
3. Grundy, S.M.; Cleeman, J.I.; Daniels, S.R.; Donato, K.A.; Eckel, R.H.; Franklin, B.A.; Gordon, D.J.; Krauss, R.M.; Savage, P.J.; Smith, S.C., Jr.; et al. American Heart Association; National Heart, Lung, and Blood Institute. Diagnosis and management of the metabolic syndrome: An American Heart Association/National Heart, Lung, and Blood Institute Scientific Statement. *Circulation* **2005**, *112*, 2735–2752. [CrossRef] [PubMed]
4. Sperling, L.S.; Mechanick, J.I.; Neeland, I.J.; Herrick, C.J.; Després, J.P.; Ndumele, C.E.; Vijayaraghavan, K.; Handelsman, Y.; Puckrein, G.A.; Araneta, M.R.; et al. The CardioMetabolic Health Alliance: Working toward a new care model for the metabolic syndrome. *J. Am. Coll. Cardiol.* **2015**, *66*, 1050–1067. [CrossRef] [PubMed]
5. Mottillo, S.; Filion, K.B.; Genest, J.; Joseph, L.; Pilote, L.; Poirier, P.; Rinfret, S.; Schiffrin, E.L.; Eisenberg, M.J. The metabolic syndrome and cardiovascular risk. A systematic review and meta-analysis. *J. Am. Coll. Cardiol.* **2010**, *56*, 1113–1132. [CrossRef] [PubMed]
6. DeBoer, M.D.; Filipp, S.L.; Gurka, M.J. Use of a metabolic syndrome severity z score to track risk during treatment of prediabetes: An analysis of the diabetes prevention program. *Diabetes Care* **2018**, *41*, dc181079. [CrossRef] [PubMed]
7. Pucci, G. Sex- and gender-related prevalence, cardiovascular risk and therapeutic approach in metabolic syndrome: A review of the literature. *Pharmacol. Res.* **2017**, *120*, 34–42. [CrossRef] [PubMed]
8. Myers, J.; McAuley, P.; Lavie, C.; Despres, J.P.; Arena, R.; Kokkinos, P. Physical activity and cardiorespiratory fitness as major markers of cardiovascular risk: Their independent and interwoven importance to health status. *Prog. Cardiovasc. Dis.* **2015**, *57*, 306–314. [CrossRef]
9. US Department of Health and Human Services. Physical Activity: Facts and Statistics. Available online: https://www.hhs.gov/fitness/resource-center/facts-and-statistics/index.html (accessed on 27 January 2019).
10. Chau, J.; Chey, T.; Burks-Young, S.; Engelen, L.; Bauman, A. Trends in prevalence of leisure time physical activity and inactivity: Results from Australian National Health Surveys 1989 to 2011. *Aust. N. Z. J. Public Health* **2017**, *41*, 617–624. [CrossRef]
11. Hallal, P.C.; Andersen, L.B.; Bull, F.C.; Guthold, R.; Haskell, W.; Ekelund, U. Global physical activity levels: Surveillance progress, pitfalls, and prospects. *Lancet* **2012**, *380*, 247–257. [CrossRef]
12. Duncan, G.E. Exercise, fitness, and cardiovascular disease risk in type 2 diabetes and the metabolic syndrome. *Curr. Diab. Rep.* **2006**, *6*, 29–35. [CrossRef] [PubMed]

13. Church, T. Exercise in obesity, metabolic syndrome, and diabetes. *Prog. Cardiovasc. Dis.* **2011**, *53*, 412–418. [CrossRef] [PubMed]

14. Zhang, D.; Liu, X.; Liu, Y.; Sun, X.; Wang, B.; Ren, Y.; Zhao, Y.; Zhou, J.; Han, C.; Yin, L.; et al. Leisure-time physical activity and incident metabolic syndrome: A systematic review and dose-response meta-analysis of cohort studies. *Metabolism* **2017**, *75*, 36–44. [CrossRef] [PubMed]

15. Strasser, B. Physical activity in obesity and metabolic syndrome. *Ann. N. Y. Acad. Sci.* **2013**, *1281*, 141–159. [CrossRef] [PubMed]

16. Bull, F.; Goenka, S.; Lambert, V.; Pratt, M. Physical Activity for the Prevention of Cardiometabolic Disease. In *Cardiovascular, Respiratory, and Related Disorders*, 3rd ed.; Prabhakaran, D., Anand, S., Gaziano, T.A., Mbanya, J.C., Wu, Y., Nugent, R., Eds.; The International Bank for Reconstruction and Development/The World Bank: Washington, DC, USA, 2017; Chapter 5.

17. Myers, J. The new AHA/ACC guidelines on cardiovascular risk: When will fitness get the recognition it deserves? *Mayo Clin. Proc.* **2014**, *89*, 722–726. [CrossRef] [PubMed]

18. Franklin, B.A. physical activity to combat chronic diseases and escalating health care costs: The unfilled prescription. *Curr. Sports Med. Rep.* **2008**, *7*, 122–125. [CrossRef] [PubMed]

19. Sallis, R.E.; Matuszak, J.M.; Baggish, A.L.; Franklin, B.A.; Chodzko-Zajko, W.; Fletcher, B.J.; Gregory, A.; Joy, E.; Matheson, G.; McBride, P.; et al. Call to Action on Making Physical Activity Assessment and Prescription a Medical Standard of Care. *Curr. Sports Med. Rep.* **2016**, *15*, 207–214. [CrossRef] [PubMed]

20. Berra, K.; Rippe, J.; Manson, J.E. Making Physical Activity Counseling a Priority in Clinical Practice: The Time for Action Is Now. *JAMA* **2015**, *314*, 2617–2618. [CrossRef] [PubMed]

21. Omura, J.D.; Bellissimo, M.P.; Watson, K.B.; Loustalot, F.; Fulton, J.E.; Carlson, S.E. Primary care providers' physical activity counseling and referral practices and barriers for cardiovascular disease prevention. *Prev. Med.* **2018**, *108*, 115–122. [CrossRef]

22. U.S. Department of Health and Human Services. *Physical Activity Guidelines for Americans*, 2nd ed.; U.S. Department of Health and Human Services: Washington, DC, USA, 2018.

23. Roberts, C.K.; Hevener, A.L.; Barnard, R.J. Metabolic syndrome and insulin resistance: Underlying causes and modification by exercise training. *Compr. Physiol.* **2013**, *3*, 1–58.

24. Henriksen, E.J. Effects of acute exercise and exercise training on insulin resistance. *J. Appl. Physiol.* **2002**, *93*, 788–796. [CrossRef] [PubMed]

25. Thune, I.; Njølstad, I.; Løchen, M.L.; Førde, O.H. Physical activity improves the metabolic risk profiles in men and women: The Tromsø Study. *Arch. Intern. Med.* **1998**, *158*, 1633–1640. [CrossRef] [PubMed]

26. Laaksonen, D.E.; Lakka, H.M.; Salonen, J.T.; Niskanen, L.K.; Rauramaa, R.; Lakka, T.A. Low levels of leisure-time physical activity and cardiorespiratory fitness predict development of the metabolic syndrome. *Diabetes Care* **2002**, *25*, 1612–1618. [CrossRef] [PubMed]

27. Sisson, S.B.; Camhi, S.M.; Church, T.S.; Tudor-Locke, C.; Johnson, W.D.; Katzmarzyk, P.T. Accelerometer-determined steps/day and metabolic syndrome. *Am. J. Prev. Med.* **2010**, *38*, 575–582. [CrossRef] [PubMed]

28. Healy, G.N.; Wijndaele, K.; Dunstan, D.W.; Shaw, J.E.; Salmon, J.; Zimmet, P.Z.; Owen, N. Objectively measured sedentary time, physical activity, and metabolic risk: The Australian Diabetes, Obesity and Lifestyle Study (AusDiab). *Diabetes Care* **2008**, *31*, 369–371. [CrossRef] [PubMed]

29. Ekelund, U.; Griffin, S.J.; Wareham, N.J. Physical activity and metabolic risk in individuals with a family history of type 2 diabetes. *Diabetes Care* **2007**, *30*, 337–342. [CrossRef] [PubMed]

30. Look AHEAD Research Group. Cardiovascular effects of intensive lifestyle intervention in type 2 diabetes. *N. Engl. J. Med.* **2013**, *369*, 145–154. [CrossRef]

31. Stewart, K.J.; Bacher, A.C.; Turner, K.; Lim, J.G.; Hees, P.S.; Shapiro, E.P.; Tayback, M.; Ouyang, P. Exercise and risk factors associated with metabolic syndrome in older adults. *Am. J. Prev. Med.* **2005**, *28*, 9–18. [CrossRef]

32. Katzmarzyk, P.T.; Leon, A.S.; Wilmore, J.H.; Skinner, J.S.; Rao, D.C.; Rankinen, T.; Bouchard, C. Targeting the metabolic syndrome with exercise: Evidence from the HERITAGE Family Study. *Med. Sci. Sports Exerc.* **2003**, *35*, 1703–1709. [CrossRef]

33. Balducci, S.; Zanuso, S.; Massarini, M.; Corigliano, G.; Nicolucci, A.; Missori, S.; Cavallo, S.; Cardelli, P.; Alessi, E.; Pugliese, G.; et al. The Italian Diabetes and Exercise Study (IDES): Design and methods for a prospective Italian multicentre trial of intensive lifestyle intervention in people with type 2 diabetes and the metabolic syndrome. *Nutr. Metab. Cardiovasc. Dis.* **2008**, *18*, 585–595. [CrossRef]

34. Diabetes Prevention Program Research Group. Reduction in the Incidence of Type 2 Diabetes with Lifestyle Intervention or Metformin. *N. Engl. J. Med.* **2002**, *346*, 393–403. [CrossRef] [PubMed]
35. Tuomilehto, J.; Lindstrom, J.; Eriksson, J.G.; Valle, T.T.; Hamalainen, H.; Ilanne-Parikka, P.; Keinänen-Kiukaanniemi, S.; Laakso, M.; Louheranta, A.; Rastas, M.; et al. Prevention of type 2 diabetes mellitus by changes in lifestyle among subjects with impaired glucose tolerance. *N. Engl. J. Med.* **2001**, *344*, 1343–1350. [CrossRef] [PubMed]
36. Orchard, T.J.; Temprosa, M.; Goldberg, R.; Haffner, S.; Ratner, R.; Marcovina, S.; Fowler, S. The effect of metformin and intensive lifestyle intervention on the metabolic syndrome: The Diabetes Prevention Program randomized trial. *Ann. Intern. Med.* **2005**, *142*, 611–619. [CrossRef] [PubMed]
37. Roumen, C.; Feskens, E.J.; Corpeleijn, E.; Mensink, M.; Saris, W.H.; Blaak, E.E. Predictors of lifestyle intervention outcome and dropout: The SLIM study. *Eur. J. Clin. Nutr.* **2011**, *65*, 1141–1147. [CrossRef] [PubMed]
38. Den Boer, A.T.; Herraets, I.J.; Stegen, J.; Roumen, C.; Corpeleijn, E.; Schaper, N.C.; Feskens, E.; Blaak, E.E. Prevention of the metabolic syndrome in IGT subjects in a lifestyle intervention: Results from the SLIM study. *Nutr. Metab. Cardiovasc. Dis.* **2013**, *23*, 1147–1153. [CrossRef] [PubMed]
39. Wewege, M.A.; Thom, J.M.; Rye, K.A.; Parmenter, B.J. Aerobic, resistance or combined training: A systematic review and meta-analysis of exercise to reduce cardiovascular risk in adults with metabolic syndrome. *Atherosclerosis* **2018**, *274*, 162–171. [CrossRef] [PubMed]
40. Naci, H.; Ioannidis, J.P. Comparative effectiveness of exercise and drug interventions on mortality outcomes: Metaepidemiological study. *BMJ* **2013**, *347*, f5577. [CrossRef] [PubMed]
41. Ostman, C.; Smart, N.A.; Morcos, D.; Duller, A.; Ridley, W.; Jewiss, D. The effect of exercise training on clinical outcomes in patients with the metabolic syndrome: A systematic review and meta-analysis. *Cardiovasc. Diabetol.* **2017**, *16*, 110. [CrossRef] [PubMed]
42. Palaniappan, L.; Carnethon, M.R.; Wang, Y.; Hanley, A.J.; Fortmann, S.P.; Haffner, S.M.; Wagenknecht, L. Predictors of the incident metabolic syndrome in adults: The Insulin Resistance Atherosclerosis Study. *Diabetes Care* **2004**, *27*, 788–793. [CrossRef] [PubMed]
43. LaMonte, M.J.; Ainsworth, B.E. Quantifying energy expenditure and physical activity in the context of dose response. *Med. Sci. Sports Exerc.* **2001**, *33*, S370–S378. [CrossRef]
44. Hassinen, M.; Lakka, T.; Savonen, K.; Litmanen, H.; Kiviaho, L.; Laaksonen, D.E.; Komulainen, P.; Rauramaa, R. Cardiorespiratory Fitness as a Feature of Metabolic Syndrome in Older Men and Women. *Diabetes Care* **2008**, *31*, 1242–1247. [CrossRef] [PubMed]
45. Kelley, E.; Imboden, M.T.; Harber, M.P.; Finch, H.; Kaminsky, L.A.; Whaley, M.H. Cardiorespiratory Fitness Is Inversely Associated with Clustering of Metabolic Syndrome Risk Factors: The Ball State Adult Fitness Program Longitudinal Lifestyle Study. *Mayo Clin. Proc. Innov. Qual. Outcomes* **2018**, *2*, 155–164. [CrossRef] [PubMed]
46. LaMonte, M.J.; Barlow, C.E.; Jurca, R.; James, B.; Kampert, J.B.; Church, T.S.; Blair, S.N. Cardiorespiratory fitness is inversely associated with the incidence of metabolic syndrome: A prospective study of men and women. *Circulation* **2005**, *112*, 505–512. [CrossRef] [PubMed]
47. Adams-Campbell, L.L.; Dash, C.; Kim, B.H.; Hicks, J.C.; Makambi, K.; Hagberg, J.M. Cardiorespiratory fitness and metabolic syndrome in postmenopausal African-American women. *Int. J. Sports Med.* **2016**, *37*, 261–266. [CrossRef] [PubMed]
48. Hassinen, M.; Lakka, T.; Hakola, L.; Savonen, K.; Komulainen, P.; Litmanen, H.; Kiviniemi, V.; Kouki, R.; Heikkilá, H.; Rauramaa, R. Cardiorespiratory fitness and metabolic syndrome in older men and women. *Diabetes Care* **2010**, *33*, 1655–1657. [CrossRef] [PubMed]
49. Carnethon, M.R.; Gidding, S.S.; Nehgme, R.; Sidney, S.; Jacobs, D.R., Jr.; Liu, K. Cardiorespiratory fitness in young adulthood and the development of cardiovascular disease risk factors. *JAMA* **2003**, *290*, 3092–3100. [CrossRef]
50. Franks, P.W.; Ekelund, U.; Brage, S.; Wong, M.-Y.; Wareham, N.J. Does the association of habitual activity with the metabolic syndrome differ by level of cardiorespiratory fitness? *Diabetes Care* **2004**, *27*, 1187–1193. [CrossRef] [PubMed]
51. Earnest, C.P.; Artero, C.G.; Sui, X.; Church, T.S.; Blair, S.N. Maximal estimated cardiorespiratory fitness, cardiometabolic risk factors, metabolic syndrome in the aerobics center longitudinal study. *Mayo Clin. Proc.* **2013**, *88*, 259–270. [CrossRef]

52. Ingle, L.; Mellis, M.; Brodie, D.; Sandercock, G.R. Associations between cardiorespiratory fitness and the metabolic syndrome in British men. *Heart* **2017**, *103*, 524–528. [CrossRef]

53. Cheal, K.L.; Abbasi, F.; Lamendola, C.; McLaughlin, T.; Reaven, G.M.; Ford, E.S. Relationship to insulin resistance of the adult treatment panel III diagnostic criteria for identification of the metabolic syndrome. *Diabetes* **2004**, *53*, 1195–2000. [CrossRef]

54. Meigs, J.B.; Wilson, P.W.; Fox, C.S.; Vasan, R.S.; Nathan, D.M.; Sullivan, L.M.; D'Agostino, R.B. Body mass index, metabolic syndrome, and risk of type 2 diabetes or cardiovascular disease. *J. Clin. Endocrinol. Metab.* **2006**, *91*, 2906–2912. [CrossRef] [PubMed]

55. Despres, J.P.; Lemieux, I. Abdominal obesity and metabolic syndrome. *Nature* **2006**, *444*, 881–887. [CrossRef] [PubMed]

56. Himsworth, H.P. Diabetes mellitus: Its differentiation into insulin sensitive and insulin insensitive types. *Lancet* **1936**, *1*, 127–130. [CrossRef]

57. Yalow, R.S.; Berson, S.A. Plasma insulin concentrations in nondiabetic and early diabetic subjects. Determinations by a new sensitive immuno-assay technique. *Diabetes* **1960**, *9*, 254–260. [CrossRef] [PubMed]

58. Ginsberg, H.; Olefsky, J.M.; Reaven, G.M. Further evidence that insulin resistance exists in patients with chemical diabetes. *Diabetes* **1974**, *23*, 674–678. [CrossRef] [PubMed]

59. DeFronzo, R.A.; Tobin, J.D.; Andres, R. Glucose clamp technique: A method for quantifying insulin secretion and resistance. *Am. J. Physiol.* **1979**, *237*, E214–E223. [CrossRef] [PubMed]

60. Lillioja, S.; Mott, D.M.; Spraul, M.; Ferraro, R.; Foley, J.E.; Ravussin, E.; Knowler, W.C.; Bennett, P.H.; Bogardus, C. Insulin resistance and insulin secretory dysfunction as precursors of non-insulin-dependent diabetes mellitus. Prospective studies of Pima Indians. *N. Engl. J. Med.* **1993**, *329*, 1988–1992. [CrossRef]

61. Reaven, G.M. Banting lecture 1988. Role of insulin resistance in human disease. *Diabetes* **1988**, *37*, 1595–1607. [CrossRef]

62. Haffner, S.M.; Valdez, R.A.; Hazuda, H.P.; Mitchell, B.D.; Morales, P.A.; Stern, M.P. Prospective analysis of the insulin-resistance syndrome (syndrome X). *Diabetes* **1992**, *41*, 715–722. [CrossRef]

63. Rewers, M.; Zaccaro, D.; D'Agostino, R.; Haffner, S.; Saad, M.F.; Selby, J.V.; Bergman, R.; Savage, P. Insulin sensitivity, insulinemia, and coronary artery disease: The Insulin Resistance Atherosclerosis Study. *Diabetes Care* **2004**, *27*, 781–787. [CrossRef]

64. Solymoss, B.C.; Bourassa, M.G.; Campeau, L.; Sniderman, A.; Marcil, M.; Lespérance, J.; Lévesque, S.; Varga, S. Effect of increasing metabolic syndrome score on atherosclerotic risk profile and coronary artery disease angiographic severity. *Am. J. Cardiol.* **2004**, *93*, 159–164. [CrossRef]

65. Jones, C.N.; Pei, D.; Staris, P.; Polonsky, K.S.; Chen, Y.D.; Reaven, G.M. Alterations in the glucose-stimulated insulin secretory dose-response curve and in insulin clearance in nondiabetic insulin-resistant individuals. *J. Clin. Endocrinol. Metab.* **1997**, *82*, 1834–1838. [CrossRef]

66. Samson, S.L.; Garber, A.J. Metabolic Syndrome. *Endocrinol. Metab. Clin. N. Am.* **2014**, *43*, 1–23. [CrossRef]

67. Nolan, C.J.; Prentki, M. Insulin resistance and insulin hypersecretion in the metabolic syndrome and type 2 diabetes: Time for a conceptual framework shift. *Diabetes Vasc. Dis. Res.* **2019**, *16*, 118–127. [CrossRef]

68. Sylow, L.; Kleinert, M.; Richter, E.A.; Jensen, T.E. Exercise-stimulated glucose uptake regulation and implications for glycaemic control. *Nat. Rev. Endocrinol.* **2017**, *13*, 133–148. [CrossRef]

69. Poehlman, E.T.; Dvorak, R.V.; DeNino, W.F.; Brochu, M.; Ades, P.A. Different mechanisms leading to the stimulation of muscle glucose transport: Effects of resistance training and endurance training on insulin sensitivity in nonobese, young women: A controlled randomized trial. *J. Clin. Endocrinol. Metab.* **2000**, *85*, 2463–2468.

70. Kylin, E. Studien über das Hypertonie-Hyperglykämie- Hyperurikämiesyndrom. *Zentralblatt für Innere Medizin* **1923**, *44*, 105–127.

71. Vague, J. The degree of masculine differentiation of obesities. *Am. J. Clin. Nutr.* **1956**, *4*, 20–34. [CrossRef]

72. Kaplan, N.M. The Deadly Quartet. Upper-Body Obesity, Glucose Intolerance, Hypertriglyceridemia, and Hypertension. *Arch. Intern. Med.* **1989**, *149*, 1514–1520. [CrossRef]

73. Després, J.P.; Lemieux, I.; Bergeron, J.; Pibarot, P.; Mathiu, P.; Larose, E.; Rodés-Cabau, J.; Bertrand, O.F.; Poirier, P. Abdominal obesity and the metabolic syndrome: Contribution to global cardiometabolic risk. *Arterioscler. Thromb. Vasc. Biol.* **2008**, *28*, 1039–1049. [CrossRef]

74. McLaughlin, T.; Lamendola, C.; Liu, A.; Abbasi, F. Preferential fat deposition in subcutaneous versus visceral depots is associated with insulin sensitivity. *J. Clin. Endocrinol. Metab.* **2011**, *96*, E1756–E1760. [CrossRef]

75. Bays, H.E. Adiposopathy: Is "sick fat" a cardiovascular disease? *J. Am. Coll. Cardiol.* **2011**, *57*, 2461–2473. [CrossRef]

76. Kim, M.K.; Reaven, G.M.; Chen, Y.D.; Kim, E.; Kim, S.H. Hyperinsulinemia in individuals with obesity: Role of insulin clearance. *Obesity* **2015**, *23*, 2430–2434. [CrossRef]

77. Randle, P.J.; Garland, P.B.; Hales, C.N.; Newsholme, E.A. The glucose fatty-acid cycle. Its role in insulin sensitivity and the metabolic disturbances of diabetes mellitus. *Lancet* **1963**, *1*, 785–789. [CrossRef]

78. Cnop, M.; Ladriere, L.; Hekerman, P.; Ortis, F.; Cardozo, A.K.; Dogusan, Z.; Flamez, D.; Boyce, M.; Yuan, J.; Eizirik, D.L. Selective inhibition of eukaryotic translation initiation factor 2 alpha dephosphorylation potentiates fatty acid-induced endoplasmic reticulum stress and causes pancreatic beta-cell dysfunction and apoptosis. *J. Biol. Chem.* **2007**, *282*, 3989–3997. [CrossRef]

79. Conley, S.M.; Zhu, X.Y.; Eirin, A.; Tang, H.; Lerman, A.; van Wijnen, A.J.; Lerman, L.O. Metabolic syndrome alters expression of insulin signaling-related genes in swine mesenchymal stem cells. *Gene* **2018**, *20*, 101–106. [CrossRef]

80. Dutheil, F.; Lac, G.; Lesourd, B.; Chapier, R.; Walther, G.; Vinet, A.; Sapin, V.; Verney, J.; Ouchchane, L.; Duclos, M.; et al. Different modalities of exercise to reduce visceral fat mass and cardiovascular risk in metabolic syndrome: The RESOLVE randomized trial. *Int. J. Cardiol.* **2013**, *168*, 3634–3642. [CrossRef]

81. Kundu, N.; Domingues, C.C.; Nylen, E.S.; Paal, E.; Kokkinos, P.; Sen, S. Endothelium-derived factors influence Differentiation of Fat-Derived Stromal Cells Post-Exercise in Subjects with Prediabetes. *Metab. Syndr. Relat. Disord.* **2019**. [CrossRef]

82. Lemieux, I.; Pascot, A.; Prud'homme, D.; Almeras, N.; Bogaty, P.; Nadeau, A.; Bergeron, J.; Despres, J.P. Elevated C-reactive protein: Another component of the atherothrombotic profile of abdominal obesity. *Arterioscler. Thromb. Vasc. Biol.* **2001**, *21*, 961–967. [CrossRef]

83. Festa, A.; D'Agostino, R., Jr.; Howard, G.; Mykkanen, L.; Tracy, R.P.; Haffner, S.M. Chronic subclinical inflammation as part of the insulin resistance syndrome: The Insulin Resistance Atherosclerosis Study (IRAS). *Circulation* **2000**, *102*, 42–47. [CrossRef]

84. Lee, W.Y.; Park, J.S.; Noh, S.Y.; Rhee, E.J.; Sung, K.C.; Kim, B.S.; Kang, J.H.; Kim, S.W.; Lee, M.H.; Park, J.R. C-reactive protein concentrations are related to insulin resistance and metabolic syndrome as defined by the ATP III report. *Int. J. Cardiol.* **2004**, *97*, 101–106. [CrossRef]

85. Ridker, P.M.; Buring, J.E.; Cook, N.R.; Rifai, N. C-reactive protein, the metabolic syndrome, and risk of incident cardiovascular events: An 8-year follow-up of 14 719 initially healthy American women. *Circulation* **2003**, *107*, 391–397. [CrossRef]

86. Demidowich, A.P.; Levine, J.A.; Onyekaba, G.I.; Khan, S.M.; Chen, K.Y.; Brady, S.M.; Broadney, M.M.; Yanovski, J.A. Effects of colchicine in adults with metabolic syndrome: A pilot randomized controlled trial. *Diabetes Obes. Metab.* **2019**, *21*, 1642–1651. [CrossRef]

87. Wedell-Neergaard, A.S.; Krogh-Madsen, R.; Petersen, G.L.; Hansen, Å.M.; Pedersen, B.K.; Lund, R.; Bruunsgaard, H. Cardiorespiratory fitness and the metabolic syndrome: Roles of inflammation and abdominal obesity. *PLoS ONE* **2018**, *13*, e0194991. [CrossRef]

88. Stensvold, D.; Slørdahl, S.A.; Wisløff, U. Effect of exercise training on inflammation status among people with metabolic syndrome. *Metab. Syndr. Relat. Disord.* **2012**, *10*, 267–272. [CrossRef]

89. Povel, C.M.; Boer, J.M.; Feskens, E.J. Shared genetic variance between the features of the metabolic syndrome: Heritability studies. *Obes. Rev.* **2011**, *12*, 952–957. [CrossRef]

90. Stancakova, A.; Laakso, M. Genetics of metabolic syndrome. *Rev. Endocr. Metab. Disord.* **2014**, *15*, 243–252. [CrossRef]

91. Povel, C.M.; Boer, J.M.; Reiling, E.; Feskens, E.J. Genetic variants and the metabolic syndrome: A systematic review. *Obes. Rev.* **2011**, *12*, 952–967. [CrossRef]

92. Palizban, A.; Rezaei, M.; Khanahmad, H.; Fazilati, M. Transcription factor 7-like 2 polymorphism and context-specific risk of metabolic syndrome, type 2 diabetes, and dyslipidemia. *J. Res. Med. Sci.* **2017**, *15*, 2–24. [CrossRef]

93. Baudrand, R.; Goodarzi, M.O.; Vaidya, A.; Underwood, P.C.; Williams, J.S.; Jeunemaitre, X.; Hopkins, P.N.; Brown, N.; Raby, B.A.; Lasky-Su, J.; et al. A prevalent caveolin-1 gene variant is associated with the metabolic syndrome in Caucasians and Hispanics. *Metabolism* **2015**, *64*, 1674–1681. [CrossRef]

94. Castellano-Castillo, D.; Moreno-Indias, I.; Fernández-García, J.C.; Alcaide-Torres, J.; Moreno-Santos, I.; Ocaña, L.; Gluckman, E.; Tinahones, F.; Queipo-Ortuño, M.I.; Cardona, F. Adipose tissue LPL methylation is associated with triglyceride concentrations in the metabolic syndrome. *Clin. Chem.* **2018**, *64*, 210–218. [CrossRef]

95. Turcot, V.; Tchernof, A.; Deshaies, Y.; Pérusse, L.; Bélisle, A.; Marceau, S.; Biron, S.; Lescelleur, O.; Biertho, L.; Vohl, M.C. LINE-1 methylation in visceral adipose tissue of severely obese individuals is associated with metabolic syndrome status and related phenotypes. *Clin. Epigenetics* **2012**, *4*, 10. [CrossRef]

96. Castellano-Castillo, D.; Moreno-Indias, I.; Sanchez-Alcoholado, L.; Ramos-Molina, B.; Alcaide-Torres, J.; Morcillo, S.; Ocaña-Wilhelmi, L.; Tinahones, F.; Queipo-Ortuño, M.I.; Cardona, F. Altered adipose tissue DNA methylation status in metabolic syndrome: Relationships between global DNA methylation and specific methylation at adipogenic, lipid metabolism and inflammatory candidate genes and metabolic variables. *J. Clin. Med.* **2019**, *8*, 87. [CrossRef]

97. Gidlund, E.K. Exercise and mitochondria. In *Cardiorespiratory Fitness in Cardiometabolic Diseases Prevention and Management in Clinical Practice*; Kokkinos, P., Narayan, P., Eds.; Springer: Basel, Switzerland, 2019.

98. Alibegovic, A.C.; Sonne, M.P.; Højbjerre, L.; Bork-Jensen, J.; Jacobsen, S.; Nilsson, E.; Færch, K.; Hiscock, N.; Mortensen, B.; Friedrichsen, M.; et al. Insulin resistance induced by physical inactivity is associated with multiple transcriptional changes in skeletal muscle in young men. *Am. J. Physiol. Endocrinol. Metab.* **2010**, *299*, 752–763. [CrossRef]

99. Ling, C.; Rönn, T. Epigenetics in human obesity and type 2 diabetes. *Cell Metab.* **2019**, *29*, 1–17. [CrossRef]

100. Gomez-Abellan, P.; Hernandez-Morante, J.J.; Lujan, J.A.; Madrid, J.A.; Garaulet, M. Clock genes are implicated in the human metabolic syndrome. *Int. J. Obes.* **2008**, *32*, 121–128. [CrossRef]

101. Chaput, J.P.; McNeil, J.; Després, J.P.; Bouchard, C.; Tremblay, A. Short sleep duration is associated with an increased risk of developing features of the metabolic syndrome in adults. *Prev. Med.* **2013**, *57*, 872–877. [CrossRef]

102. Xi, B.; He, D.; Zhang, M.; Xue, J.; Zhou, D. Short sleep duration predicts risk of metabolic syndrome: A systematic review and meta-analysis. *Sleep Med. Rev.* **2014**, *18*, 293–297. [CrossRef]

103. Lian, Y.; Yuan, Q.; Wang, G.; Tang, F. Association between sleep quality and metabolic syndrome: A systematic review and meta-analysis. *Psychiatry Res.* **2019**, *274*, 66–74. [CrossRef]

104. Iftikhar, I.H.; Donley, M.A.; Mindel, J.; Pleister, A.; Soriano, S.; Magalang, U.J. Sleep duration and metabolic syndrome. An updated dose-risk meta-analysis. *Ann. Am. Thorac. Soc.* **2015**, *12*, 1364–1372. [CrossRef]

105. Chaput, J.P.; McNeil, J.; Després, J.P.; Bouchard, C.; Tremblay, A. Seven to eight hours of sleep a night is associated with a lower prevalence of the metabolic syndrome and reduced overall cardiometabolic risk in adults. *PLoS ONE* **2013**, *8*, e72832. [CrossRef]

106. Dollet, L.; Zierath, J.R. Interplay between diet, exercise and the molecular circadian clock in orchestrating metabolic adaptations of adipose tissue. *J. Physiol.* **2019**, *597*, 1439–1450. [CrossRef]

107. Gabriel, B.M.; Zierath, J.R. Circadian rhythms and exercise—Re-setting the clock in metabolic disease. *Nat. Rev. Endocrinol.* **2019**, *15*, 197–206. [CrossRef]

108. Chamarthi, B.; Gaziano, J.M.; Blonde, L.; Vinik, A.; Scranton, R.E.; Ezrokhi, M.; Rutty, D.; Cincotta, A.H. Timed Bromocriptine-QR therapy reduces progression of cardiovascular disease and dysglycemia in subjects with well-controlled type 2 diabetes mellitus. *J. Diabetes Res.* **2015**, *2015*, 157698. [CrossRef]

15

Dietary Fat Intake and Metabolic Syndrome in Older Adults

Alicia Julibert [1], Maria del Mar Bibiloni [1], David Mateos [1], Escarlata Angullo [1,2] and Josep A. Tur [1,*]

[1]   Research Group on Community Nutrition & Oxidative Stress, University of Balearic Islands, IDISBA & CIBEROBN, 07122 Palma de Mallorca, Spain

[2]   Escola Graduada Primary Health Care Center, IBSalut, 07001 Palma de Mallorca, Spain

*   Correspondence: pep.tur@uib.es

Abstract: Background: Metabolic Syndrome (MetS) is associated with higher rates of cardiovascular disease (CVD), type 2 diabetes mellitus, and cancer worldwide. Objective: To assess fat intake in older adults with or without MetS. Design: Cross-sectional nutritional survey in older adults living in the Balearic Islands ($n = 477$, 48% women, 55–80 years old) with no previous CVD. Methods: Assessment of fat (total fat, MUFA, PUFA, SFA, TFA, linoleic acid, α-linolenic acid, marine and non-marine ω-3 FA, animal fat and vegetable fat, cholesterol) and macronutrient intake using a validated food frequency questionnaire, and its comparison with recommendations of the US Institute of Medicine (IOM) and the Spanish Society of Community Nutrition (SENC). Results: Participants with MetS showed higher BMI, lower physical activity, higher total fat and MUFA intake, and lower intake of energy, carbohydrates, and fiber than participants without MetS. Men and women with MetS were below the Acceptable Macronutrient Distribution Range (AMDR) proposed by IOM for carbohydrates and above the AMDR for total fat and MUFAs, and women were below the AMDR proposed for α-linolenic acid (ALA) compared with participants without MetS. Conclusions: Subjects with MetS were less likely to meet IOM and SENC recommendations for fat and macronutrient intakes as compared to non-MetS subjects.

Keywords: older adults; macronutrient intake; dietary intake; fat intake; metabolic syndrome

1. Introduction

Metabolic syndrome (MetS) is a clinical condition characterized by several metabolic risk factors [1,2] associated with higher prevalence of cardiovascular disease (CVD), type 2 diabetes (T2DM), and cancer worldwide [3]. These factors involve abdominal obesity, blood pressure, glycaemia, triglyceridemia (TG), and high-density lipoprotein cholesterol (HDL-c) [1].

The prevalence of MetS has been increasing over the years and is now reaching epidemic proportions [4]. In Western countries, the prevalence of MetS is approximately one-fifth of the adult population and increases with age. However, the prevalence of MetS will vary according to the population studied, age, gender, race, and ethnicity, as well as the definition applied [5,6].

MetS is also influenced by nutrient intake, alcohol consumption, physical exercise, or smoking [3]. Unhealthy eating patterns and lifestyle, such as malnutrition and inactivity, can worsen the clinical status, with accumulation of body fat and alteration of the parameters that characterize MetS [7].

As shown in the ANIBES study, the macronutrient distribution is worsening and somewhat moving away from the recommendations and traditional Mediterranean dietary pattern, although the negative changes are less pronounced as age increases [8]. Age, sex, lower levels of education, economic status, smoking status, and alcohol intake predict lower dietary variety. There is evidence that older Spanish adults with MetS had a high risk of inadequate nutrient intake [9].

Eating patterns and their food and nutrient characteristics are the primary emphasis of the recommendations of U.S. Dietary Guidelines 2015–2020 [10]. Accordingly, therehas been a focus on the roles of macronutrients (carbohydrates, fat, and proteins) [11–17] and dietary patterns [7,18–20] on MetS.

Therefore, taking into consideration the scientific evidence on nutrients in the development of MetS, this study aimed to assess fat intake in older adults with or without MetS.

2. Materials and Methods

2.1. Design and Participants

The sample had477 participants (48% women; aged 55–80 years old)with no previously documented CVD that were engaged in social and municipal clubs, health centers, and sport clubs ofacross-sectional study conducted in the Balearic Islands. The age range was chosen since they are at high risk of suffering non communicable disease, the association of MetS with CVD, and because the increasing prevalence of MetS with age is known [21]. Exclusion criteria included being institutionalized, suffering from a physical or mental illness thatlimited their participation in physical fitness or their ability to respond to questionnaires, chronic alcoholism or drug addiction, and intake of drugs for clinical research over the past year.

The study protocols followed the Declaration of Helsinki ethical standards, and were approved by the Ethics Committee of Research of Balearic Islands (refs. CEIC-IB2251/14PI and CEIC-IB1295/09PI). All participants provided informed written consent.

2.2. Anthropometric Measurements

Anthropometric variables were measured by trained personnel to minimize the inter-observer coefficients of variation. Weight and height were measured with high-quality electronic calibrated scales and a wall-mounted stadiometer, respectively. Height was determined using a mobile anthropometer (Seca 213, SECA Deutschland, Hamburg, Germany) to the nearest millimeter, with the participant's head maintained in the Frankfort Horizontal Plane position. Body weight and body fat were determined using a Segmental Body Composition Analyzer (Tanita BC-418, Tanita, Tokyo, Japan). The participants were weighed in bare feet and light clothes (0.6 kg was subtracted for their clothing). Body mass index (BMI) was calculated as weight in kilograms divided by the square of height in meters (kg/m^2). Waist circumference (WC) was measured half-way between the last rib and the iliac crest by using an anthropometric tape. Blood pressure was measured using a validated semi-automatic oscillometer (Omron HEM-705CP, Hoofddorp, The Netherlands) after 5 min of rest inbetween measurements while the participant was in a seated position. All anthropometric variables were determined in duplicate, except for blood pressure (in triplicate).

2.3. Blood Collection and Analysis

Blood samples were collected after an overnight fast and biochemical analyses were performed on fasting plasma glucose, total cholesterol, HDL-c, and TG concentrations in local laboratories using standard enzymatic methods. Participants were classified as "with MetS" ($n = 333$) and "without MetS" ($n = 144$) according to the updated harmonized definition of the International Diabetes Federation and the American Heart Association and National Heart, Lung, and Blood Institute [2].

2.4. Dietary Intake Assessment

Licensed dieticians administered a semiquantitative, 137-item food frequency questionnaire (FFQ), repeatedly validated in Spain [22]. For each item, a typical portion size was included and consumption frequencies were registered in 9 categories that ranged from "never or almost never" to "≥6 times/day". Energy and nutrient intakes were calculated as frequency multiplied by nutrient composition of specified portion size for each food item, using a self-made computerized program based on available information in the Spanish food composition tables by Moreiras et al. [23]. When foods in the Spanish food composition tables were not available, the BEDCA food database was used in order to complete missing information [24]. Dietary intake of energy, carbohydrates (CHOs), proteins, total fat, monounsaturated fatty acids (MUFAs), polyunsaturatedfatty acids (PUFAs) and SFAs, trans-fatty acid (TFA), linoleic acid (LA), α-linolenic acid (ALA), marine and non-marine ω-3 fatty acid (ω-3 FA), animal fat and vegetable fat, cholesterol, and fiber were estimated. The vegetable fat included vegetables, fruits, nuts, legumes, total cereals, olives, oils, cookies, fritters, cocoa powder, mustard, ketchup, fried tomato, sugar, marmalade, and snacks. The animal fat included total dairy products, total meat, total fish, pizza, butter, lard, bakery goods, nougat, ready-to-eat meals, salad cream, and honey. The fat quality index (FQI) was also calculated as previously described [25]. Briefly, the FQI was calculated using the ratio (MUFA + PUFA)/(SFA + TFA) as a continuous variable.

Macronutrients and diff

erent fat intakes were compared with Institute of Medicine (IOM) and Spanish Society of Community Nutrition (SENC) recommendations. The dietary references intakes (DRIs) values proposed by IOM [26] were used, which are quantitative estimates of nutrient intakes to assess and plan diets for healthy people, including the Acceptable Macronutrient Distribution Range (AMDR) values. The prevalence of inadequate macronutrient intake according to the 2020 Nutritional Objectives for Spanish Population proposed by SENC [27] was used.

2.5. Socioeconomic and Lifestyle Determinants

Sociodemographic and lifestyle characteristics were collected from each participant. Educational level was ranked into primary school, secondary school, and university. Physical activity was measured using the validated Spanish version of the Minnesota Leisure Time Physical Activity Questionnaire [28,29]; it was taken by interview with trained research assistants and measured leisure time physical activities (LTPA), including household activities, over the previous 12 months. The Minnesota questionnaire was used to estimate physical activity levels by using metabolic equivalents of tasks (METs) [30]. METs are calculated by multiplying the intensity (showed by the MET-score) and the duration spent on that activity (measured in minutes). The MET-score can be derived from tables (the Compendium of Physical Activities) [31] that show the intensity of the activity relative to resting (METhours/week) spent on physical activity refer to the energy that is spent on activities, over and above existing levels of resting energy expenditure. Finally, information related to individual medical history, current medication use, and smoking status were also obtained.

2.6. Statistical Analyses

Analyses were performed with the SPSS statistical software package version 25.0 (SPSS Inc., Chicago, IL, USA). All analyses were stratified by sex and MetS status. Data are shown as mean, standard deviation (SD), or median and interquartile range (IQR). Normality of data was assessed using Kolmogorov–Smirnov test. Difference in medians between two comparison groups were tested by the Mann-Whitney U-test when variables were not normally distributed, and difference in means between the two comparison groups were tested by unpaired Students' t-test when variables were normally distributed. Differences in prevalence of MetS or not among participants were examined using χ^2 (all p values are two-tailed). Logistic regression analyses with the calculation of corresponding odds ratio (OR) and the 95% confidence interval (95% Confidence Interval, CI) were also used to assess the association between pathological features of MetS and macronutrients, specific types of fat, and dietary intake. Results were adjusted for sex, age (continuous variable), BMI (continuous variable), energy intake (continuous variable), and total physical activity (continuous variable, expressed as METmin/hour) to control for potential confounders. Results were considered statistically significant if p-value (2 tailed) <0.05.

3. Results

Comparison of socioeconomic and lifestyle characteristics between the two study groups stratified by sex are shown in Table 1. Participants with MetS showed higher BMI and lower total physical activity than participants without MetS. As expected, the groups differed in all MetS components, except for blood pressure in women. A higher percentage of patients with MetS showed pathological cut-off values than patients without MetS in all MetS components.

Male MetS patients with high blood pressure plus hyperglycemia plus high abdominal fat comprised 64.5% of the total MetS population; those with high blood pressure plus hypertriglyceridemia plus low HDL-c comprised 42.6% of the MetS population. Female MetS patients with high blood pressure plus hyperglycemia plus high abdominal fat comprised 59.3% of the total MetS population; those with high blood pressure plus hypertriglyceridemia plus low HDL-c comprised 38.7% of the MetS population.

Comparisons of nutrient intakes and food consumption between the two study groups stratified by sex are shown in Tables 2 and 3, respectively. Participants with MetS showed higher total fat and MUFA intake but lower intake of energy, carbohydrates, and fiber than those without MetS ($p < 0.05$). Participants with MetS also showed higher FQI than non-MetS participants. Women with MetS reported higher intake of proteins but lower intake of TFA, ω-3 FA, LA, ALA, and marine and non-marine ω-3 FA than women without MetS. Participants with MetS reported lower consumption of fruits, potatoes, total cereals, whole grain bread, and rice and pasta than participants without MetS. Men with MetS reported lower consumption of ready to-eat-meals than those without MetS. On the other hand, women reported lower consumption of bakery goods and alcohol than those without MetS.

Table 4 shows that participants with MetS, for both men and women, were more likely to be below the AMDR proposed by IOM for carbohydrates and ALA (except for men) and more likely to be above the AMDR for total fat and MUFAs than participants without MetS. Similar results were obtained when the 2020 Nutritional Objectives for the Spanish population were assessed (Table 5). Participants with MetS were also more likely to be below the acceptable nutritional range for carbohydrates and more likely to be above the acceptable nutritional range for total fat and MUFAs than participants without MetS. Finally, participants with MetS were more likely to be below the 2020 Nutritional Objectives for the Spanish population for TFA but also for total fiber, such as in fruits and vegetables.

Multivariate adjusted odds ratio (OR) for the association between pathological features of the MetS components and dietary macronutrient intake in participants with and without MetS showed, after adjustment for potential confounders (i.e., age, sex, BMI, energy and physical activity), that hypertension (equal or higher pathological cut-off value was OR reference: 1.00) is related with lower intake of PUFA (OR: 0.95; 95% CI: 0.91–0.98), SFA (OR: 0.95; 95% CI: 0.92–0.99), TFA (OR: 0.95; 95% CI: 0.91–0.99), LA (OR: 0.94; 95% CI: 0.90–0.98), and ALA (OR: 0.95; 95% CI: 0.91–0.99). However, abdominal obesity (equal or higher pathological cut-off value was OR reference: 1.00) was associated with high PUFA intake (OR: 1.10; 95% CI: 1.01–1.19), LA (OR: 0.12; 95% CI: 1.02–1.23) and vegetable fat (OR: 1.05; 95% CI: 1.01–1.08). No other relationships were found between other pathological components of MetS and dietary macronutrient intake.

Table 1. Socioeconomicand lifestyle characteristics of participants "with Metabolic Syndrome" (n = 333) and "without Metabolic Syndrome" (n = 144) stratified by sex.

	Men					Women				
	Without MetS (n = 63)		With MetS (n = 183)		p-Value *	Without MetS (n = 81)		With MetS (n = 150)		p-Value *
	Mean ± SD	Median (IQR)	Mean ± SD	Median (IQR)		Mean ± SD	Median (IQR)	Mean ± SD	Median (IQR)	
Age (y)	63.8 ± 5.9	64.0 (59.0, 67.0)	64.1 ± 5.9	64.0 (59.0, 69.0)	0.544	66.8 ± 5.0	66.0 (63.0, 70.0)	65.9 ± 4.5	66.0 (62.0, 69.0)	0.340
BMI (kg/m²)	27.0 ± 3.2	27.5 (24.9, 28.7)	32.0 ± 3.6	31.9 (29.0, 34.5)	<0.001	25.3 ± 3.3	25.6 (22.9, 27.4)	32.8 ± 4.2	32.7 (30.1, 36.1)	<0.001
Current smoking habit (%)										
Yes		6.3		14.8	0.081		6.2		12.8	0.119
No		93.7		85.2			93.8		87.2	
Education (%)					0.660					0.595
Primary		39.7		37.1			53.1		60.0	
Secondary		39.7		36.5			30.9		26.9	
University or graduate		20.6		26.4			16.0		13.1	
Total physica lactivity(n) ‡		63		158			81		131	
Total physical activity (MET·hour/week) †	123 ± 208	84 (60, 117)	61 ± 50	46 (24, 85)	<0.001	88 ± 34	84 (63, 107)	60 ± 46	46 (26, 89)	<0.001
MetScomponents										
High blood pressure										
Systolic blood pressure (mmHg)	137.0 ± 19.0	134.5 (124, 143)	141.0 ± 16.9	141 (129.7, 148.5)	0.038	135.9 ± 15.8	136 (125.8, 146.3)	138.4 ± 17.3	137.6 (126.7, 148.6)	0.280
Diastolic blood pressure (mmHg)	81.5 ± 9.4	81.5 (74.5, 88.5)	82.8 ± 9.5	83 (75.7, 89.5)	0.362	79.9 ± 9.0	80.5 (74.3, 86.3)	79.6 ± 9.8	79.7 (74.6, 85.3)	0.828
(%) ‡		76.2		95.6	<0.001 §		69.1		88.0	<0.001 §
Hyperglycaemia (mg/dL)	98.3 ± 32.2	97 (71, 119)	119.9 ± 39.0	110 (100, 127)	<0.001	89.0 ± 8.0	89 (83, 94)	110.5 ± 23.4	104 (95, 120)	<0.001
(%) ‡		27.0		81.4	<0.001 §		3.7		48.0	<0.001 §
Hypertriglyceridemia (mg/dL)	96.2 ± 9.2	95 (93, 100)	155.6 ± 77.1	133 (96, 198)	<0.001	84.5 ± 27.2	80 (64, 100)	135.3 ± 55.5	125 (91, 169.8)	<0.001
(%) ‡		9.5		53.6	<0.001 §		11.0		51.6	<0.001 §
Low HDL-cholesterol (mg/dL)	51.5 ± 9.9	50 (45, 55)	41.2 ± 10.0	40 (35, 46)	<0.001	63.3 ± 11.9	63 (55.5, 71)	49.1 ± 10.7	48 (42, 54.5)	<0.001
(%) ‡		11.1		53.0	<0.001 §		22.2		58.0	<0.001 §
Abdominal obesity (cm)	92.9 ± 10.1	94 (87.7, 99.2)	112.1 ± 10.3	111.1 (103.9, 120.5)	<0.001	79.9 ± 7.7	80 (75.4, 85.4)	104.6 ± 11.1	105.5 (97.0, 112.3)	<0.001
(%) ‡		12.7		86.3	<0.001 §		11.1		96.0	<0.001 §

Abbreviations: BMI, body mass index; FA, fatty acids; FQI, fat quality index; IQR, interquartile range; MetS, Metabolic Syndrome; MET, metabolic equivalent of task; MUFAs, monounsaturated fatty acids; PUFAs, polyunsaturated fatty acids; SD, standard deviation; SFAs, saturated fatty acids.* Differences in means between participants without and with MetS were tested by unpaired Students' t-test. † Participants who did not respond to the physical activity questionnaires were excluded from the analysis (i.e., 25 men and 19 women). ‡ Percentage (%) of patients without and with MetS were tested by χ². § Differences between participants without and and with MetS.

Table 2. Nutrient intake in participants "with Metabolic Syndrome" ($n = 333$) and "without Metabolic Syndrome" ($n = 144$) stratified by sex.

	Men					Women				
	Without MetS ($n = 63$)		With MetS ($n = 183$)		p-Value*	Without MetS ($n = 81$)		With MetS ($n = 150$)		p-Value*
	Mean ±SD	Median (IQR)	Mean ±SD	Median (IQR)		Mean ±SD	Median (IQR)	Mean ±SD	Median (IQR)	
Energy intake (kcal/day)	2872 ± 738	2858 (2315, 3282)	2641 ± 689	2561 (2153, 3071)	0.019	2366 ± 698	2323 (1881, 2697)	2071 ± 543	1952 (1713, 2448)	<0.001
Carbohydrate intake (% total E)	44.7 ± 6.2	44.7 (41.3, 48.3)	40.0 ± 6.8	40.7 (34.9, 45.2)	<0.001	44.6 ± 5.2	44.3 (40.7, 47.1)	41.0 ± 6.9	40.9 (36.4, 45.5)	<0.001
Protein intake (% total E)	15.9 ± 2.4	15.6 (14.3, 17.6)	16.3 ± 3.1	15.9 (14.3, 17.7)	0.599	16.9 ± 3.0	16.4 (14.9, 18.5)	18.0 ± 3.2	18.0 (15.7, 20.4)	0.010
Fat intake (% total E)	36.2 ± 6.1	35.6 (31.6, 40.2)	38.9 ± 7.0	38.6 (34.0, 44.0)	0.008	37.6 ± 5.7	37.8 (32.8, 41.3)	40.9 ± 7.6	40.7 (35.5, 46.1)	<0.001
PUFA (% total E)	7.6 ± 3.4	6.3 (5.3, 9.1)	7.5 ± 3.0	6.7 (5.5, 8.8)	0.673	8.0 ± 3.6	6.6 (5.8, 8.9)	8.1 ± 4.1	6.7 (5.6, 9.2)	0.941
MUFA (% total E)	17.5 ± 4.3	16.8 (14.5, 19.7)	19.3 ± 5.0	18.8 (15.9, 22.2)	0.007	18.9 ± 4.4	18.3 (15.5, 21.1)	21.1 ± 5.9	20.3 (17.1, 24.6)	0.003
SFA (% total E)	11.7 ± 3.5	10.9 (9.6, 12.9)	12.0 ± 3.3	11.4 (9.6, 13.3)	0.517	12.5 ± 3.6	11.6 (9.9, 14.4)	12.5 ± 4.0	11.6 (10.1, 13.8)	0.975
Trans FA (g/d)	8.1 ± 8.9	4.7 (2.9, 7.2)	6.8 ± 7.5	3.8 (2.3, 6.5)	0.123	7.8 ± 8.5	4.9 (2.8, 10.3)	6.4 ± 8.5	3.0 (1.5, 5.4)	0.005
Linoleic acid (g/d)	16.2 ± 10.5	12.5 (8.8, 21.2)	14.5 ± 8.9	11.2 (8.5, 18.8)	0.298	14.7 ± 9.8	11.7 (8.7, 16.8)	12.9 ± 9.6	10.0 (6.5, 16.3)	0.034
ω-3 FA (g/d)	26.0 ± 36.0	9.2 (8.9, 18.9)	21.2 ± 29.8	9.2 (1.2, 18.2)	0.135	26.5 ± 34.5	9.4 (8.7, 35.2)	21.8 ± 34.0	8.9 (1.0, 17.9)	0.003
Linolenic acid (g/d)	7.0 ± 9.0	2.8 (2.5, 5.5)	5.8 ± 7.5	2.8 (0.8, 5.1)	0.168	7.1 ± 8.6	3.1 (2.4, 9.2)	5.8 ± 8.5	2.6 (0.6, 4.9)	0.003
Marine ω-3 FA (g/d)	12.7 ± 18.0	4.4 (4.2, 9.1)	10.3 ± 14.9	4.3 (0.3, 8.9)	0.111	13.0 ± 17.3	4.5 (4.1, 17.4)	10.7 ± 17.0	4.2 (0.3, 8.8)	0.009
Non-marine ω-3 FA (g/d)	13.2 ± 18.0	4.9 (4.5, 10)	10.9 ± 14.9	4.9 (0.9, 9.4)	0.161	13.5 ± 17.3	5.1 (4.5, 17.9)	11.1 ± 17.0	4.6 (0.7, 9.2)	0.002
Animal fat (g/d)	49.8 ± 18.2	46.1 (38.5, 59.7)	48.3 ± 19.6	43.7 (34.8, 59.2)	0.307	41.5 ± 23.1	38.6 (27.3, 50.0)	36.0 ± 13.2	35.0 (26.2, 44.1)	0.091
Vegetable fat (g/d)	65.7 ± 23.4	62.3 (45.2, 85.4)	64.9 ± 22.8	62.8 (48.1, 79.9)	0.799	57.7 ± 19.9	56.1 (41.8, 69.2)	58.3 ± 23.9	56.6 (41.9, 70.4)	0.987
FQI score	1.9 ± 0.5	1.7 (1.6, 2.1)	2.0 ± 0.4	1.9 (1.7, 2.3)	0.048	1.8 ± 0.4	1.8 (1.6, 2.0)	2.1 ± 0.5	2.0 (1.7, 2.4)	<0.001
Cholesterol (mg/d)	362 ± 105	358 (289, 423)	348 ± 115	334 (274, 399)	0.146	303 ± 122	286 (243, 349)	288 ± 79	283 (250, 355)	0.819
Fiber intake (g/d)	42.2 ± 17.0	38.2 (28.2, 52.0)	32.9 ± 13.1	31.2 (22.6, 39.5)	<0.001	38.6 ± 16.7	34.0 (28.9, 45.3)	31.2 ± 14.9	27.3 (20.9, 36.2)	<0.001

Abbreviations: E, energy; FA, fatty acids; FQI, fat quality index; IQR, interquartile range; MetS, Metabolic Syndrome; MUFAs, monounsaturated fatty acids; PUFAs, polyunsaturated fatty acids; SD, standard deviation; SFAs, saturated fatty acids. * Difference in means between participants without and with MetS were tested by unpaired Students' t-test.

Table 3. Food consumption in participants "with Metabolic Syndrome" (n = 333) and "without Metabolic Syndrome" (n = 144) stratified by sex.

	Men					Women				
	Without MetS (n = 63)		With MetS (n = 183)		p-Value	Without MetS (n = 81)		With MetS (n = 150)		p-Value *
	Mean ±SD	Median (IQR)	Mean ±SD	Median (IQR)		Mean ±SD	Median (IQR)	Mean ±SD	Median (IQR)	
Fruits (g/day)	487 ± 205	495 (344, 627)	402 ± 229	364 (220, 546)	0.002	576 ± 218	553 (419, 697)	394 ± 214	352 (242, 499)	<0.001
Vegetables (g/day)	346 ± 147	341 (232, 426)	311 ± 157	284 (192, 415)	0.075	357 ± 151	334 (258, 431)	343 ± 159	327 (242, 420)	0.407
Potatoes (g/day)	96.7 ± 45.8	95.7 (57.1, 149.8)	70.2 ± 45.2	56.0 (31.4, 97.4)	<0.001	77.6 ± 45.0	85.7 (38.6, 107.1)	67.3 ± 57.9	49.5 (28.0, 94.1)	0.013
Legumes (g/day)	20.5 ± 14.7	16.6 (12.0, 25.1)	18.9 ± 12.9	16.1 (12.1, 24.8)	0.901	18.0 ± 12.2	16.0 (12.0, 21.1)	17.8 ± 12.3	16.1 (12.0, 21.6)	0.582
Olives and EVOO (g/day)	34.7 ± 34.0	28.3 (10.0, 46.4)	39.3 ± 28.2	32.0 (21.0, 50.0)	0.070	24.7 ± 16.5	25.0 (12.4, 32.1)	29.8 ± 24.0	28.3 (10.9, 46.0)	0.289
Other olives oils	14.3 ± 16.7	10.0 (0.0, 25.0)	13.0 ± 16.4	4.2 (0.0, 25.0)	0.563	15.9 ± 15.4	10.0 (0.0, 25.0)	15.1 ± 14.8	10.0 (0.0, 25.0)	0.724
Other oils and fats	4.4 ± 9.2	1.3 (0.0, 4.3)	4.9 ± 8.9	0.8 (0.0, 5.0)	0.856	4.7 ± 6.8	2.1 (0.7, 5.8)	3.9 ± 6.6	0.8 (0.0, 5.0)	0.112
Nuts (g/day)	15.8 ± 17.3	8.6 (4.0, 25.7)	13.3 ± 13.3	8.4 (4.0, 21.0)	0.594	14.7 ± 13.6	8.6 (4.3, 25.7)	11.7 ± 13.5	7.2 (2.0, 16.7)	0.023
Totalfish (g/day)	96.3 ± 36.2	88.1 (68.1, 120.5)	87.7 ± 45.2	80.3 (56.6, 111.3)	0.049	87.4 ± 37.5	80.7 (60.3, 107.4)	88.1 ± 42.2	80.7 (56.6, 115.1)	0.925
White fish	25.4 ± 19.7	21 (10, 21)	26.3 ± 22.4	21.0 (10.1, 21.4)	0.620	28.0 ± 21.6	21.4 (10.0, 42.9)	28.3 ± 22.9	21.0 (10.1, 63.0)	0.362
Bluefish	21.9 ± 19.9	18.6 (8.7, 18.6)	17.2 ± 16.8	8.7 (8.7, 18.2)	0.121	18.1 ± 17.0	18.6 (8.7, 18.6)	20.2 ± 18.7	18.2 (8.7, 18.6)	0.769
Seafood	35.6 ± 14.6	30.7 (26.7, 45.9)	31.1 ± 23.7	30.8 (17.4, 35.2)	0.096	31.6 ± 17.8	30.7 (26.7, 33.0)	28.9 ± 22.3	30.7 (13.4, 31.9)	0.985
Canned fish/seafood	11.7 ± 10.5	7.1 (3.3, 21.4)	11.0 ± 9.6	7.0 (3.4, 21.0)	0.215	8.3 ± 7.4	6.7 (3.3, 12.4)	9.4 ± 8.5	7.0 (3.4, 13.0)	0.115
Total cereal (g/day)	229.3 ± 131.7	222.8 (131.4, 251.6)	135.9 ± 131.3	135.9 (91.8, 217.7)	<0.001	149 ± 82	126 (95, 222)	122.8 ± 69.8	102.4 (79.7, 164.3)	0.004
Whole grain bread	105.2 ± 122.3	75.0 (5.0, 187.5)	61.4 ± 73.8	31.5 (5.0, 75.0)	0.012	66.7 ± 60.0	75.0 (32.1, 75.0)	57.1 ± 63.5	31.5 (5.0, 75.0)	0.019
Refined grain bread	85.3 ± 108.0	32.1 (5.0, 187.5)	66.6 ± 83.1	31.5 (5.0, 75.0)	0.329	47.2 ± 71.1	10.7 (0.0, 75.0)	39.3 ± 53.6	31.5 (0.0, 75.0)	0.895
Rice and pasta	34.5 ± 14.7	34.3 (17.1, 51.4)	27.6 ± 18.2	25.2 (12.4, 34.3)	<0.001	28.7 ± 17.5	17.1 (17.1, 34.3)	23.1 ± 15.1	17.0 (12.4, 33.6)	0.001
Total dairy products (g/day)	295 ± 168	289 (215, 342)	303 ± 216	269 (181, 363)	0.612	312 ± 214	282 (150, 394)	264 ± 164	246 (148, 342)	0.131
Dairy esserts	31.9 ± 34.6	15.3 (6.7, 51.2)	33.6 ± 47.2	15.3 (6.7, 43.0)	0.930	19.9 ± 27.9	8.7 (6.7, 24.1)	18.4 ± 27.9	6.7 (0.0, 23.4)	0.814
Cheese	32.9 ± 26.9	24.8 (21.4, 44.5)	32.1 ± 31.2	24.4 (14.0, 42.9)	0.395	33.1 ± 23.2	28.1 (19.6, 48.0)	29.3 ± 22.3	24.4 (10.4, 42.0)	0.179
Skimmed dairy	84.8 ± 137.6	8.3 (0.0, 125.0)	115 ± 202	52.5 (0.0, 156.0)	0.215	141.6 ± 194.8	53.6 (0.0, 209.5)	114.4 ± 136.5	52.5 (0.0, 200.0)	0.529
Whole-fat dairy	144.1 ± 141.3	125.0 (8.3, 208.3)	120 ± 141	84.0 (0.0, 200.0)	0.090	112.5 ± 158.6	17.9 (0.0, 200.0)	100 ± 140	17.5 (0.0, 200.0)	0.765
Total meat (g/day)	152.0 ± 61.1	137 (112, 202)	166.2 ± 71.7	154 (117, 204)	0.247	130 ± 61.7	118 (93, 165)	140 ± 56.6	139 (104, 172)	0.076
Processed meat	40.7 ± 27.0	34.0 (27.0, 52.0)	46.9 ± 34.7	39.1 (21.0, 62.0)	0.433	31.4 ± 21.4	30.0 (18.2, 39.5)	34.0 ± 28.3	28.7 (16.7, 42.7)	0.869
Other meats,	108.4 ± 48.8	104.3 (71.4, 135.7)	116 ± 57	107 (76, 149)	0.500	97.2 ± 51.6	87.6 (64.8, 122.9)	103.8 ± 46.3	103.7 (74.9, 135.8)	0.172
Bakery godos (g/day)	60.4 ± 44.5	51.2 (26.7, 72.4)	52.1 ± 45.0	44.5 (20.6, 66.7)	0.101	51.0 ± 30.2	46.5 (26.5, 74.2)	37.2 ± 30.6	31.0 (10.4, 53.7)	<0.001
Ready-to-eat-meals	35.0 ± 34.2	26.2 (13.6, 37.6)	27.8 ± 40.3	15.4 (9.4, 30.0)	0.003	19.9 ± 18.7	15.3 (4.3, 26.2)	20.5 ± 23.3	15.4 (2.0, 26.4)	0.357
Alcohol (g/day)	230 ± 183	198 (82, 337)	291 ± 322	200 (76, 367)	0.753	109 ± 128	47.1 (0.0, 170)	70 ± 101	28.8 (0.0, 100.0)	0.032

Abbreviations: EVOO, extra virgin olive oil; IQR, interquartile range; MetS, Metabolic Syndrome; SD, standard deviation. * Difference in means between participants without and with MetS were tested by unpaired Students' t-test.

Table 4. Percentage of participants "with Metabolic Syndrome" and "without Metabolic Syndrome" below, inside, and above Acceptable Macronutrient Distribution Range (AMDR) proposed by the Institute of Medicine.

Variable	AMDR	Group	% below	% inside	% above	p *
All						
Carbohydrate	45–65%	Without MetS	55.6	44.4	0.0	<0.001
		With MetS	72.7	27.3	0.0	
Protein	10–35%	Without MetS	0.0	100.0	0.0	0.510
		With MetS	0.3	99.7	0.0	
Total fat	20–35%	Without MetS	0.0	39.6	60.4	0.001
		With MetS	0.0	24.9	75.1	
MUFAs	>20%	Without MetS	72.2	-	27.8	0.001
		With MetS	55.6	-	44.4	
LA	5–10%	Without MetS	66.7	20.1	13.2	0.159
		With MetS	64.9	26.4	8.7	
ALA	0.6–1.2%	Without MetS	21.5	29.2	49.3	0.005
		With MetS	36.3	21.0	42.6	
Men						
Carbohydrate	45–65%	Without MetS	52.4	47.6	0.0	0.003
		With MetS	72.7	27.3	0.0	
Protein	10–35%	Without MetS	0.0	100.0	0.0	0.557
		With MetS	0.5	99.5	0.0	
Total fat	20–35%	Without MetS	0.0	46.0	54.0	0.008
		With MetS	0.0	27.9	72.1	
MUFAs	>20%	Without MetS	77.8	-	22.2	0.025
		With MetS	62.3	-	37.7	
LA	5–10%	Without MetS	65.1	22.2	12.7	0.276
		With MetS	66.7	26.8	6.6	
ALA	0.6–1.2%	Without MetS	22.2	38.1	39.7	0.119
		With MetS	35.0	27.3	37.7	
Women						
Carbohydrate	45–65%	Without MetS	58.0	42.0	0.0	0.023
		With MetS	72.7	27.3	0.0	
Protein	10–35%	Without MetS	0.0	100.0	0.0	1.000
		With MetS	0.0	100.0	0.0	
Total fat	20–35%	Without MetS	0.0	34.6	65.4	0.029
		With MetS	0.0	21.3	78.7	
MUFAs	>20%	Without MetS	67.9	-	32.1	0.003
		With MetS	47.3	-	52.7	
LA	5–10%	Without MetS	67.9	18.5	13.6	0.427
		With MetS	62.7	26.0	11.3	
ALA	0.6–1.2%	Without MetS	21.0	22.2	56.8	0.019
		With Met	38.0	13.3	48.7	

Abbreviations: ALA, α-linolenic acid; LA, linoleic acid; MetS, metabolic syndrome; MUFAs, monounsaturated fatty acids. * The differences in prevalence across the two comparison groups was examined using χ^2.

Table 5. Percentage of participants "with Metabolic Syndrome" and "without Metabolic Syndrome" below, inside, and above the 2020 Nutritional Objectives for the Spanish Population proposed by the Spanish Society of Community Nutrition.

Variable	Nutritional Objectives	Group	% Below	% Inside	% Above	p *
Carbohydrate	50–55%	Without MetS	83.3	12.5	4.2	0.004
		With MetS	93.1	5.7	1.2	
Protein	10–20%	Without MetS	0.0	100.0	0.0	1.000
		With MetS	0.0	100.0	0.0	
Total fat	30–35%	Without MetS	9.7	29.9	60.4	0.001
		With MetS	9.3	15.6	75.1	
MUFAs	20%	Without MetS	72.2	-	27.8	0.001
		With MetS	55.6	-	44.4	
PUFAs	5%	Without MetS	14.6	-	85.4	0.774
		With MetS	15.6	-	84.4	
LA	3%	Without MetS	18.1	-	81.9	0.217
		With MetS	23.1	-	76.9	
ALA	1–2%	Without MetS	42.4	30.6	27.1	0.417
		With MetS	48.6	28.5	22.8	
SFA	7–8%	Without MetS	2.8	3.5	93.8	0.952
		With MetS	3.3	3.6	93.1	
Trans FA	<1%	Without MetS	21.5	-	78.5	0.001
		With MetS	36.6	-	63.4	
DHA	300 mg	Without MetS	100.0	-	0.0	1.000
		With MetS	100.0	-	0.0	
Total fiber	M: 35 g/d F: 25 g/d	Without MetS	27.8	-	72.2	<0.001
		With MetS	52.0	-	48.0	
Cholesterol	<300 mg/d	Without MetS	41.0	-	59.0	0.123
		With MetS	48.6	-	51.4	
Fruits	>300 g/d	Without MetS	11.1	-	88.9	<0.001
		With MetS	35.4	-	64.6	
Vegetables	>250g/d	Without MetS	24.3	-	75.7	0.032
		With MetS	34.2	-	65.8	
Sugar foods	<6%	Without MetS	0.7	-	99.3	0.905
		With MetS	0.6	-	99.4	

Abbreviations: ALA, α-linolenic acid; DHA, docosahexaenoic acid; FA, fatty acid; LA, linoleic acid; MetS, metabolic syndrome; MUFA, monounsaturated fatty acids; PUFAs, polyunsaturated fatty acids; SFAs, saturated fatty acids. * Differences in prevalence between groups were assessed by χ^2.

4. Discussion

Subjects with MetS and without MetS showed differences for energy and macronutrient intake, as well as for intake of specific fat subtypes.

Energy and nutrient intake in MetS subjects revealed a diet lower in calories and carbohydrates, but higher in total fat and MUFA than those without MetS. Carbohydrate intake of MetS subjects was below the recommended limits (45–65% of total energy intake) and total fat intake of the same subjects was above the recommended limits (20–35% of total energy intake). Women with MetS showed more energy intake from protein than those without MetS (18% vs. 16.9%, respectively) ($p < 0.01$), but both were within recommended ranges [26,27]. A similar nutrient distribution among Spanish population with MetS [32] and healthy adults has been previously shown [8]. Differences were also previously observed between subjects with and without MetS for total energy intake, sugar intake, dietary glycemic load, percentage of dietary protein, PUFA, and fiber intake [33].

Despite women with MetS reporting lower consumption of bakery goods than those without MetS, differences in sugary food intake (bakery goods, dairy desserts, beverages, fruit juices, breakfast cereals, marmalade, ice creams, chocolate, and ready-to-eat meals) between subjects with and without MetS were not found in our study when the 2020 Nutritional Objectives for the Spanish population were assessed. Total sugar intake was also quantified in the ANIBES study: results were higher in children (17.18%) and adolescents (16.33%) and markedly lower in adults (15.34%) and older adults (12.97%) [8]. The inhabitants of Northern Spain, especially men, consumed more sugar and sweets than adult from other Spanish areas [32]. Conversely, the World Health Organization (WHO) recommended <10% of energy intake be provided by sugars [34], whereas <5% has been recommended in the United Kingdom [35]. It is well known that simple sugar intake is associated with significantly higher risk of developing MetS, including increased blood pressure, central obesity, and serum TG and glucose levels [36–38]. Frequent consumption of sugar-containing foods can also increase the risk of dental caries [39].

This study also demonstrated an association of gender and fat intake for MetS risk. Women showed an inverse association between fat intake and MetS, irrespective of fatty acid type. Women consumed less ω-3 and ω-6 FA, which could be related to the lower consumption of nuts observed in this group. Previously, Bibiloni et al. [40] showed that nut consumers were less likely to be below the estimated average requirement (EAR) for some nutrients and above the adequate intake (AI) for others than non-nut consumers. Other studies showed that European Food Safety Authority (EFSA) recommendations for intake of different types of ω-3 and ω-6 FA, such as LA, ALA, and eicosapentaenoic acid (EPA) + DHA, were not met in around half, one-quarter, and three-quarters of the European countries, respectively [41]. The most recent reviews also concluded that in half of the countries worldwide, the reported average PUFA intake was lower than the recommended range of 6–11% of energy [42–44]. In addition, the ω-3 and ω-6 FA intake was inversely associated with MetS prevalence in females [45]. In our study, total PUFA and specific types of PUFA (LA or ALA) intake were inversely associated with high blood pressure and positively associated with abdominal obesity. Evidence from observational and intervention studies supports the benefits of both ω-3 and ω-6 PUFA in reducing MetS [37,46–49], although other studies showed conflicting results [49–51]. Particularly, the adequate intake of MUFA and PUFAs in the PREvención con DIeta MEDiterránea (PREDIMED) study, mainly due to a high consumption of nuts and olive oil, has been previously associated with better adherence to the Mediterranean diet (MedDiet) [40] and to lower risk of CVD [52]. Moreover, other dietary patterns (Dietary Approaches to Stop Hypertension (DASH), new Nordic and vegetarian diets) have also been proposed as alternatives to the MedDiet for preventing MetS [5].

It is also worth noting that no differences were observed between subjects with and without MetS for SFA and animal fat, although participants without MetS showed higher consumption of bakery goods than those with MetS. Moreover, an association between pathological features of MetS and dietary macronutrient intake showed that hypertensionwas inversely associated with SFA. Contrarily to our results, a positive association between SFA intake and MetS components has been observed in most studies [46,50,53–56], although other studies pointed to a lack of association [49,57]. On the other hand, increased vegetable fat intake was positively associated with abdominal obesity; certain vegetable products may also have high saturated fat contents, such as coconut oil and palm kernel oil, along withmany prepared foods [10,58]. Moreover, most of the countries reported an average higher SFA intake than the recommended maximum of 10% of energy [42–44]. A prospective study with an older adult population at high risk of cardiovascular disease also observed an average higher SFA intake (10.3%) [59]. However, there is evidence that the intake of these fats is lower in the adults and older adults in the Mediterranean population, who consume low amounts of processed food; olive oil and meat ranked as the primary individual contributors [8].

Moreover, our findings show that women with MetS consumed more energy from TFA than those without MetS (6.4% versus 7.8%, respectively) ($p < 0.005$). Accordingly, TFA intake was inversely associated with hypertension. In a previous study, plasma TFA concentrations were significantly associated with MetS prevalence and its individual components, except for blood pressure [60]. In another study, the reduction in TFA intake over 1 year was significantly associated with a reduction in low-density lipoprotein particle number (LDL-P), a novel marker of CVD risk [61]. Actually, the 2015–2020 U.S. Dietary Guidelines for Americans and the IOM both recommend that individuals should limit TFA intake as much as possible to avoid their adverse effects on health [62].

Otherwise, the current findings showed that participants with MetS consumed less dietary fiber than the recommended dietary allowances (35 g for males and 25 g for females of this age group), which may be linked to low consumption of fruits and vegetables in our population study. This outcome is according tothe outcomes of a previous meta-analysis that provided a potential link between dietary fiber consumption and MetS risk factors [63]. Previous studies also showed a protective effect of fruit intake on MetS development [17,64–66], as well as a protective role on CVD development [67].

Finally, our results also show higher BMI and lower total physical activity in participants with MetS ($p < 0.001$), which is in agreement with a previous study that also showed higher level of physical activity in the control group compared to the MetS group, although this difference disappeared when the subjects were separated by sex and adjusted for total energy intake [16]. Another previous study showed that participants with lower levels of physical activity, being overweight and obese, were associated with higher risk of CVD. Accordingly, the impact of physical activity on CVD might outweigh that of BMI among middle-aged and elderly participants [68]. There is evidence that interventions including regular physical activity practice in patients with MetS improves MetS risk factors [69–75], indicating that maintaining a good physical condition would be essential for a healthy status.

Strengths and Limitations of the Study

This study has several strengths. First, to our knowledge our study provides data on the intake of macronutrients and different types of fat in older adults with MetS or without it, which has been scarcelyreported previously. Our research also provides information about dietary fat intake in comparison to national and international recommendations, which may provide references for future public policies.

Some methodological limitations should be acknowledged. First, the cross-sectional study nature; thus, causal inferences cannot be drawn. Second, the relatively small sample size, specifically in the non-MetS group; for this reason, these findings cannot be generalized to the broader community based on this study alone. Third, the FFQ, the source of information to assess dietary fat intake, could overestimate the intake of certain food groups, even thosethat have been validated. In our study, a trained dietician conducted the interviews to collect the food frequency data; it is hoped that this approach (as compared with self-administration) reduced any potential misclassification bias. Another limitation of this study was that the used food composition databases showed missing or uncalculated data forseveral fats and fatty acid contents; these missing data are lower than 5% of all analyzed foods (for total fat, SFA, MUFA, PUFA, and cholesterol contents) and lower than 10% of foods (LA, ALA, trans-fat, EPA, DHA, and DPA are mainly from marine species and may change according to season, source, such as wild or from a fish farm, and cooking method) [76].

5. Conclusions

Subjects with MetS were less likely to meet IOM and SENC recommendations for fat and macronutrient intake as compared to non-MetS subjects. A healthy lifestyle is critical to prevent or delay the onset of MetS in older adults and to prevent CVD in those with existing MetS. Thus, healthy diet and lifestyle patternscan be recommended for all people with MetS and should emphasize the consumption of a variety of legumes, cereals (whole grains), fruits, vegetables, fish, and nuts, which have a high nutrient content and are more likely to meet dietary recommendations. This study also raises the possibility that future recommendations and educational campaigns should be most effective in preventing MetS via lifestyle changes.

Author Contributions: M.d.M.B. and J.A.T. designed the study and wrote the protocol. A.J., D.M., and E.A. collected data, conducted literature searches, and provided summaries of previous research studies. M.D.M.B. conducted the statistical analysis. M.D.M.B., A.J., and J.A.T. wrote the first draft of the manuscript. All read and approved the final manuscript.

Acknowledgments: This study was supported by the official funding agency for biomedical research of the Spanish Government, Institute of Health Carlos III (ISCIII) through the Fondo de Investigación para la Salud (FIS), which is co-funded by the European Regional Development Fund (Projects 11/01791, 14/00636, and 17/01827, Red Predimed-RETIC RD06/0045/1004, and CIBEROBN CB12/03/30038), Fundació La Marató TV3 (Spain) project ref. 201630.10, Grant of support to research groups no. 35/2011 and Grant no. AAEE097/2017 (Balearic Islands Gov.), and E.U. Cost ACTION CA16112. The funders had no role in study design, data collection and analysis, decision to publish, or preparation of the manuscript.

References

1. Grundy, S.M.; Hansen, B.; Smith, S.C., Jr.; Cleeman, J.I.; Kahn, R.A.; American Heart Association; National Heart, Lung, and Blood Institute; American Diabetes Association. Clinical management of metabolic syndrome: Report of the American Heart Association/National Heart, Lung, and Blood Institute/American Diabetes Association conference on scientific issues related to management. *Circulation* **2004**, *109*, 551–556. [CrossRef] [PubMed]

2. Alberti, K.G.; Eckel, R.H.; Grundy, S.M.; Zimmet, P.Z.; Cleeman, J.I.; Donato, K.A.; Fruchart, J.C.; James, W.P.; Loria, C.M.; Smith, S.C., Jr.; et al. Harmonizing the metabolic syndrome: A joint interim statement of the International Diabetes Federation Task Force on Epidemiology and Prevention. *Circulation* **2009**, *120*, 1640–1645. [CrossRef] [PubMed]

3. O'Neill, S.; O'Driscoll, L. Metabolic syndrome: A closer look at the growing epidemic and its associated pathologies. *Obes. Rev.* **2015**, *16*, 1–12. [CrossRef] [PubMed]

4. Beltran-Sanchez, H.; Harhay, M.O.; Harhay, M.M.; McElligott, S. Prevalence and trends of metabolic syndrome in the adult U.S. population, 1999–2010. *J. Am. Coll. E703Cardiol.* **2013**, *62*, 697–703. [CrossRef] [PubMed]

5. Pérez-Martínez, P.; Mikhailidis, D.P.; Athyros, V.G.; Bullo, M.; Couture, P.; Covas, M.I.; de Koning, L.; Delgado-Lista, J.; Díaz-López, A.; Drevon, C.A.; et al. Lifestyle recommendations for the prevention and management of metabolic syndrome: An international panel recommendation. *Nutr. Rev.* **2017**, *75*, 307–326. [CrossRef] [PubMed]

6. De Carvalho-Vidigal, F.; Bressan, J.; Babio, N.; Salas-Salvadó, J. Prevalence of metabolic syndrome in Brazilian adults: A systematic review. *BMC Public Health* **2013**, *13*, 1198. [CrossRef] [PubMed]

7. Godos, J.; Zappalà, G.; Bernardini, S.; Giambini, I.; Bes-Rastrollo, M.; Martinez-Gonzalez, M. Adherence to the Mediterranean diet is inversely associated with metabolic syndrome occurrence: A meta-analysis of observational studies. *Int. J. Food Sci. Nutr.* **2017**, *68*, 138–148. [CrossRef]

8. Ruiz, E.; Ávila, J.M.; Valero, T.; Del Pozo, S.; Rodriguez, P.; Aranceta-Bartrina, J.; Gil, Á.; González-Gross, M.; Ortega, R.M.; Serra-Majem, L.; et al. Macronutrient Distribution and Dietary Sources in the Spanish Population: Findings from the ANIBES Study. *Nutrients* **2016**, *8*, 177. [CrossRef]

9.   Cano-Ibáñez, N.; Gea, A.; Martínez-González, M.A.; Salas-Salvadó, J.; Corella, D.; Zomeño, M.D.;
     Romaguera, D.; Vioque, J.; Aros, F.; Wärnberg, J.; et al. Dietary Diversity and Nutritional Adequacy among
     an Older Spanish Population with Metabolic Syndrome in the PREDIMED-PlusStudy: A Cross-Sectional
     Analysis. *Nutrients* **2019**, *11*, 958. [CrossRef]
10. U.S. Department of Health and Human Services; U.S. Department of Agriculture. *2015–2020 Dietary
     Guidelines for Americans*, 8th ed.; Government Printing Office: Washington, DC, USA, 2015.
11. McKeown, N.M.; Meigs, J.B.; Liu, S.; Saltzman, E.; Wilson, P.W.; Jacques, P.F. Carbohydrate Nutrition, Insulin
     Resistance, and the Prevalence of the Metabolic Syndrome in the Framingham Offspring Cohort. *Diabetes
     Care* **2004**, *27*, 538–546. [CrossRef]
12. Freire, R.D.; Cardoso, M.A.; Gimeno, S.G.; Ferreira, S.R. for the Japanese-Brazilian Diabetes Study Group
     Dietary Fat Is Associated With Metabolic Syndrome in Japanese Brazilians. *Diabetes Care* **2005**, *28*, 1779–1785.
     [CrossRef] [PubMed]
13. Bruscato, N.M.; Vieira, J.L.D.C.; Nascimento, N.M.R.D.; Canto, M.E.P.; Stobbe, J.C.; Gottlieb, M.G.;
     Wagner, M.B.; Dalacorte, R.R. Dietary intake is not associated to the metabolic syndrome in elderly
     women. *North. Am. J. Med. Sci.* **2010**, *2*, 182–188.
14. Guo, X.F.; Li, X.; Shi, M.; Li, D. n-3 Polyunsaturated Fatty Acids and Metabolic Syndrome Risk: A
     Meta-Analysis. *Nutr.* **2017**, *9*, 703. [CrossRef] [PubMed]
15. da Cunha, A.T.; Pereira, H.T.; de Aquino, S.L.; Sales, C.H.; Sena-Evangelista, K.C.; Lima, J.G.; Lima, S.C.;
     Pedrosa, L.F. Inadequacies in the habitual nutrient intakes of patients with metabolic syndrome: A
     cross-sectional study. *Diabetol. Metab. Syndr.* **2016**, *8*, 32. [CrossRef] [PubMed]
16. Al-Daghri, N.M.; Khan, N.; Alkharfy, K.M.; Al-Attas, O.S.; Alokail, M.S.; Alfawaz, H.A.; Alothman, A.;
     Vanhoutte, P.M. Selected Dietary Nutrients and the Prevalence of Metabolic Syndrome in Adult Males and
     Females in Saudi Arabia: A Pilot Study. *Nutrients* **2013**, *5*, 4587–4604. [CrossRef] [PubMed]
17. de Oliveira, E.P.; McLellan, K.C.; Vaz de Arruda Silveira, L.; Burini, R.C. Dietary factors associated with
     metabolic syndrome in Brazilian adults. *Nutr. J.* **2012**, *11*, 3. [CrossRef] [PubMed]
18. Zhao, M.; Chiriboga, D.; Olendzki, B.; Xie, B.; Li, Y.; McGonigal, L.J.; Maldonado-Contreras, A.; Ma, Y.
     Substantial Increase in Compliance with Saturated Fatty Acid Intake Recommendations after One Year
     Following the American Heart Association Diet. *Nutrients* **2018**, *10*, 1486. [CrossRef] [PubMed]
19. Zhang, L.; Pagoto, S.; May, C.; Olendzki, B.; Tucker, L.K.; Ruiz, C.; Cao, Y.; Ma, Y. Effect of AHA dietary
     counselling on added sugar intake among participants with metabolic syndrome. *Eur. J. Nutr.* **2018**, *57*,
     1073–1082. [CrossRef] [PubMed]
20. Rodríguez-Monforte, M.; Sánchez, E.; Barrio, F.; Costa, B.; Flores-Mateo, G. Metabolic syndrome and dietary
     patterns: A systematic review and meta-analysis of observational studies. *Eur. J. Nutr.* **2017**, *56*, 925–947.
     [CrossRef]
21. Amor, A.J.; Masana, L.; Soriguer, F.; Goday, A.; Calle-Pascual, A.; Gaztambide, S.; Rojo-Martínez, G.;
     Valdés, S.; Gomis, R.; Ortega, E.; et al. Estimating Cardiovascular Risk in Spain by the European Guidelines
     on Cardiovascular Disease Prevention in Clinical Practice. *Rev. Esp. Cardiol. (Engl. Ed).* **2015**, *68*, 417–425.
     [CrossRef]
22. Fernandez-Ballart, J.D.; Piñol, J.L.; Zazpe, I.; Corella, D.; Carrasco, P.; Toledo, E.; Perez-Bauer, M.;
     Martínez-González, M.Á.; Salas-Salvadó, J.; Martín-Moreno, J.M. Relative validity of a semi-quantitative
     food-frequency questionnaire in an elderly Mediterranean population of Spain. *Br. J. Nutr.* **2010**, *103*,
     1808–1816. [CrossRef]
23. Moreiras, O.; Carbajal, A.; Cabrera, L.; Cuadrado, C. *Tablas de Composición de Alimentos*, 17th ed.; Food
     Composition Tables; Piramide: Madrid, Spain, 2015.
24. BEDCA: Base de Datos Española de Composición de Alimentos. Available online: http://www.bedca.net/
     (accessed on 10 February 2019).
25. Sánchez-Tainta, A.; Zazpe, I.; Bes-Rastrollo, M.; Salas-Salvadó, J.; Bullo, M.; Sorlí, J.V.; Corella, D.; Covas, M.I.;
     Arós, F.; Gutierrez-Bedmar, M. Nutritional adequacy according to carbohydrates and fat quality. *Eur. J. Nutr.*
     2016, *55*, 93–106. [CrossRef] [PubMed]
26. The National Academies of Sciences Engineering Medicine; Institute of Medicine; Food and Nutrition
     Board. Dietary Reference Intakes (DRIs): Acceptable Macronutrient Distribution Ranges. Available online:
     http://nationalacademies.org/HMD/Activities/Nutrition/SummaryDRIs/DRI-Tables.aspx (accessed on 11
     April 2019).

27.   SENC. Objetivosnutricionales para la población española. Consenso de la Sociedad Española de NutriciónComunitaria 2011. *Rev. Esp. Nutr. Com.* **2011**, *17*, 178–199.

28.   Elosua, R.; García, M.; Aguilar, A.; Molina, L.; Covas, M.I.; Marrugat, J. Validation of the Minnesota Leisure Time Physical Activity Questionnaire in Spanish Women. *Med. Sci. Sports Exerc.* **2000**, *32*, 1431–1437. [CrossRef]

29.   Elosua, R.; Marrugat, J.; Molina, L.; Pons, S.; Pujol, E. Validation of the Minnesota Leisure Time Physical Activity Questionnaire in Spanish Men. *Am. J. Epidemiol.* **1994**, *139*, 1197–1209. [CrossRef] [PubMed]

30.   Conway, J.M.; Seale, J.L.; Jacobs, D.R.; Irwin, M.L.; Ainsworth, B.E. Comparison of energy expenditure estimates from doubly labeled water, a physical activity questionnaire, and physical activity records1–3. *Am. J. Clin. Nutr.* **2002**, *75*, 519–525. [CrossRef]

31.   Ainsworth, B.E.; Haskell, W.L.; Whitt, M.C.; Irwin, M.L.; Swartz, A.M.; Strath, S.J.; O'brien, W.L.; Bassett, D.R.; Schmitz, K.H.; Emplaincourt, P.O.; et al. Compendium of Physical Activities: An update of activity codes and MET intensities. *Med. Sci. Sports Exerc.* **2000**, *32*, S498–S516. [CrossRef] [PubMed]

32.   Cano-Ibáñez, N.; Bueno-Cavanillas, A.; Martínez-González, M.A.; Corella, D.; Salas-Salvadó, J.; Zomeño, M.D.; García-de-la-Hera, M.; Romaguera, D.; Martínez, J.A.; Barón-López, F.J.; et al. Dietary Intake in Population with Metabolic Syndrome: Is the Prevalence of Inadequate Intake Influenced by Geographical Area? Cross-Sectional Analysis from PREDIMED-Plus Study. *Nutrients* **2018**, *10*, 1661. [CrossRef]

33.   Cabello-Saavedra, E.; Bes-Rastrollo, M.; Martínez, J.A.; Díez-Espino, J.; Buil-Cosiales, P.; Serrano-Martínez, M.; Martinez-Gonzalez, M.A. Macronutrient Intake and Metabolic Syndrome in Subjects at High Cardiovascular Risk. *Ann. Nutr. Metab.* **2010**, *56*, 152–159. [CrossRef]

34.   WHO. Sugars Intake for Adults and Children-Guideline. 2015. Available online: http://www.who.int/nutrition/publications/guidelines/sugars_intake/en/ (accessed on 31 May 2019).

35.   Tedstone, A.; Targett, V.; Allen, R. Public Health England-Sugar Reduction. The Evidence for Action. Available online: https://www.gov.uk/government/publications/sugar-reduction-from-evidence-into-action (accessed on 31 May 2019).

36.   Barrio-Lopez, M.T.; Martinez-Gonzalez, M.A.; Fernández-Montero, A.; Beunza, J.J.; Zazpe, I.; Bes-Rastrollo, M. Prospective study of changes in sugar-sweetened beverage consumption and the incidence of the metabolic syndrome and its components: The SUN cohort. *Br. J. Nutr.* **2013**, *110*, 1722–1731. [CrossRef]

37.   Chan, T.F.; Lin, W.T.; Huang, H.L.; Lee, C.Y.; Wu, P.W.; Chiu, Y.W.; Huang, C.C.; Tsai, S.; Lin, C.L.; Lee, C.H. Consumption of sugar-sweetened beverages is associated with components of the metabolic syndrome in adolescents. *Nutrients* **2014**, *6*, 2088–2103. [CrossRef] [PubMed]

38.   Abdelmagid, S.A.; Clarke, S.E.; Roke, K.; Nielsen, D.E.; Badawi, A.; El-Sohemy, A.; Mutch, D.M.; Ma, D.W. Ethnicity, sex, FADS genetic variation, and hormonal contraceptive use influencedelta-5- and delta-6-desaturaseindices and plasma docosahexaenoic acid concentration in young Canadian adults: A cross-sectional study. *Nutr. Metab. (Lond).* **2015**, *12*, 14. [CrossRef] [PubMed]

39.   Burt, A.B.; Pai, S. Sugar consumption and caries risk: A systematic review. *J. Dent. Educ.* **2001**, *65*, 1017–1023. [PubMed]

40.   Bibiloni, M.D.M.; Julibert, A.; Bouzas, C.; Martínez-González, M.A.; Corella, D.; Salas-Salvadó, J.; Zomeño, M.D.; Vioque, J.; Romaguera, D.; Martínez, J.A.; et al. Nut Consumptions as a Marker of Higher Diet Quality in a Mediterranean Population at High Cardiovascular Risk. *Nutrients* **2019**, *11*, 754. [CrossRef] [PubMed]

41.   Sioen, I.; van Lieshout, L.; Eilander, A.; Fleith, M.; Lohner, S.; Szommer, A.; Petisca, C.; Eussen, S.; Forsyth, S.; Calder, P.C.; et al. Systematic Review on N-3 and N-6 Polyunsaturated Fatty Acid Intake in European Countries in Light of the Current Recommendations - Focus on Specific Population Groups. *Ann. Nutr. Metab.* **2017**, *70*, 39–50. [CrossRef] [PubMed]

42.   Harika, R.K.; Eilander, A.; Alssema, M.; Osendarp, S.J.; Zock, P.L. Intake of Fatty Acids in General Populations Worldwide Does Not Meet Dietary Recommendations to Prevent Coronary Heart Disease: A Systematic Review of Data from 40 Countries. *Ann. Nutr. Metab.* **2013**, *63*, 229–238. [CrossRef] [PubMed]

43.   Micha, R.; Khatibzadeh, S.; Shi, P.; Fahimi, S.; Lim, S.; Andrews, K.G.; Engell, R.E.; Powles, J.; Ezzati, M.; Mozaffarian, D.; et al. Global, regional, and national consumption levels of dietary fats and oils in 1990 and 2010: A systematic analysis including 266 country-specific nutrition surveys. *BMJ.* **2014**, *348*, g2272. [CrossRef] [PubMed]

44. Eilander, A.; Harika, R.K.; Zock, P.L. Intake and sources of dietary fatty acids in Europe: Are current population intakes of fats aligned with dietary recommendations? *Eur. J. Lipid Sci. Technol.* **2015**, *117*, 1370–1377. [CrossRef]

45. Park, S.; Ahn, J.; Kim, N.S.; Lee, B.K. High carbohydrate diets are positively associated with the risk of metabolic syndrome irrespective to fatty acid composition in women: The NHANES 2007–2014. *Int. J. Food Sci. Nutr.* **2017**, *68*, 479–487. [CrossRef] [PubMed]

46. Shab-Bidar, S.; Hosseini-Esfahani, F.; Mirmiran, P.; Hosseinpour-Niazi, S.; Azizi, F. Metabolic syndrome profiles, obesity measures and intake of dietary fatty acids in adults: Tehran Lipid and Glucose Study. *J. Hum. Nutr. Diet* **2014**, *27*, 98–108. [CrossRef]

47. Baik, I.; Abbott, R.D.; Curb, J.D.; Shin, C. Intake of Fish and n-3 Fatty Acids and Future Risk of Metabolic Syndrome. *J. Am. Diet. Assoc.* **2010**, *110*, 1018–1026. [CrossRef]

48. Babio, N.; Toledo, E.; Estruch, R.; Ros, E.; Martínez-González, M.A.; Castañer, O.; Bulló, M.; Corella, D.; Arós, F.; Gómez-Gracia, E.; et al. Mediterranean diets and metabolic syndrome status in the PREDIMED randomized trial. *CMAJ* **2014**, *186*, E649–E657. [CrossRef] [PubMed]

49. Ahola, A.J.; Harjutsalo, V.; Thorn, L.M.; Freese, R.; Forsblom, C.; Mäkimattila, S.; Groop, P.-H. The association between macronutrient intake and the metabolic syndrome and its components in type 1 diabetes. *Br. J. Nutr.* **2017**, *117*, 450–456. [CrossRef]

50. Ebbesson, S.O.E.; Tejero, M.E.; Nobmann, E.D.; Lopez-Alvarenga, J.C.; Ebbesson, L.; Romenesko, T.; Carter, E.A.; Resnick, H.E.; Devereux, R.B.; Maccluer, J.W.; et al. Fatty acid consumption and metabolic syndrome components: The GOCADAN study. *J. Cardio. Metab. Syndr.* **2007**, *2*, 244–249. [CrossRef]

51. Lana, L.Y.; Petrone, A.B.; Pankow, J.S.; Arnett, D.K.; North, K.E.; Ellison, R.C.; Hunt, S.C.; Djoussé, L. Association of dietary omega-3 fatty acids with prevalence of metabolic syndrome: The National Heart, Lung, and Blood Institute Family Heart Study. *Clin. Nutr.* **2013**, *32*, 966–969.

52. PREDIMED Study Investigators; Guasch-Ferré, M.; Babio, N.; Martínez-González, A.M.; Corella, D.; Ros, E.; Martín-Peláez, S.; Estruch, R.; Arós, F.; Gómez-Gracia, E.; et al. Dietary fat intake and risk of cardiovascular disease and all-cause mortality in a population at high risk of cardiovascular disease. *Am. J. Clin. Nutr.* **2015**, *102*, 1563–1573.

53. Hekmatdoost, A.; Mirmiran, P.; Hosseini-Esfahani, F.; Azizi, F. Dietary fatty acid composition and metabolic syndrome in Tehranian adults. *Nutrition* **2011**, *27*, 1002–1007. [CrossRef] [PubMed]

54. Hosseinpour-Niazi, S.; Mirmiran, P.; Fallah-Ghohroudi, A.; Azizi, F. Combined effect of unsaturated fatty acids and saturated fatty acids on the metabolic syndrome: Tehran lipid and glucose study. *J. Health Popul. Nutr.* **2015**, *33*. [CrossRef]

55. Noel, S.E.; Newby, P.K.; Ordovas, J.M.; Tucker, K.L. Adherence to an (n-3) fatty acid/fish intake pattern is inversely associated with metabolic syndrome among Puerto Rican adults in the Greater Boston area. *J. Nutr.* **2010**, *14*, 1846–1854. [CrossRef]

56. Yubero-Serrano, E.M.; Delgado-Lista, J.; Tierney, A.C.; Perez-Martinez, P.; Garcia-Rios, A.; Alcala-Diaz, J.F.; Castaño, J.P.; Tinahones, F.J.; Drevon, C.A.; Defoort, C.; et al. Insulin resistance determines a differential response to changes in dietary fat modification on metabolic syndrome risk factors: The LIPGENE study. *Am. J. Clin. Nutr.* **2015**, *102*, 1509–1517. [CrossRef]

57. Siri-Tarino, P.W.; Sun, Q.; Hu, F.B.; Krauss, R.M. Meta-analysis of prospective cohort studies evaluating the association of saturated fat with cardiovascular disease12345. *Am. J. Clin. Nutr.* **2010**, *91*, 535–546. [CrossRef] [PubMed]

58. Eckel, R.H.; Jakicic, J.M.; Ard, J.D.; de Jesus, J.M.; Houston, M.N.; Hubbard, V.S.; Lee, I.M.; Lichtenstein, A.H.; Loria, C.M.; Millen, B.E.; et al. American College of Cardiology/American Heart Association Task Force on Practice Guidelines.2013 AHA/ACC guideline on lifestyle management to reduce cardiovascular risk: A report of the American College of Cardiology/American Heart Association Task Force on Practice Guidelines. *J. Am. Coll. Cardiol.* **2014**, *63*, 2960–2984.

59. Beulen, Y.; Martínez-González, M.A.; van de Rest, O.; Salas-Salvadó, J.; Sorlí, J.V.; Gómez-Gracia, E.; Fiol, M.; Estruch, R.; Santos-Lozano, J.M.; Schröder, H.; et al. Quality of Dietary Fat Intake and Body Weight and Obesity in a Mediterranean Population: Secondary Analyses within the PREDIMED Trial. *Nutrients* **2018**, *10*, 2011. [CrossRef] [PubMed]

60. Zhang, Z.; Gillespie, C.; Yang, Q. Plasma trans-fatty acid concentrations continue to be associated with metabolic syndrome among US adults after reductions in trans-fatty acid intake. *Nutr. Res.* **2017**, *43*, 51–59. [CrossRef]

61. Garshick, M.; Mochari-Greenberger, H.; Mosca, L. Reduction in dietary trans fat intake is associated with decreased LDL particle number in a primary prevention population. *Nutr. Metab. Cardiovasc. Dis.* **2014**, *24*, 100–106. [CrossRef] [PubMed]

62. Institute of Medicine (U.S.). *Panel on Macronutrients. Dietary Reference Intakes for Energy, Carbohydrate, Fiber, Fat, Fatty Acids, Cholesterol, Protein, and Amino Acids*; National Academies Press: Washington, DC, USA, 2005.

63. Chen, J.P.; Chen, G.C.; Wang, X.P.; Qin, L.; Bai, Y. Dietary Fiber and Metabolic Syndrome: A Meta-Analysis and Review of Related Mechanisms. *Nutrients* **2017**, *10*, 24. [CrossRef]

64. Steemburgo, T.; Dall'Alba, V.; Almeida, J.C.; Zelmanovitz, T.; Gross, J.L.; de Azevedo, M.J. Intake of soluble fibers has a protective role for the presence of metabolic syndrome in patients with type 2 diabetes. *Eur. J. Clin. Nutr.* **2009**, *63*, 127–133. [CrossRef] [PubMed]

65. Esmaillzadeh, A.; Kimiagar, M.; Mehrabi, Y.; Azadbakht, L.; Hu, F.B.; Willett, W.C. Fruit and vegetable intakes, C-reactive protein, and the metabolic syndrome. *Am. J. Clin. Nutr.* **2006**, *84*, 1489–1497. [CrossRef]

66. Shin, A.; Lim, S.Y.; Sung, J.; Shin, H.R.; Kim, J. Dietary Intake, Eating Habits, and Metabolic Syndrome in Korean Men. *J. Am. Diet. Assoc.* **2009**, *109*, 633–640. [CrossRef]

67. Zhu, Y.; Bo, Y.; Liu, Y. Dietary total fat, fatty acids intake, and risk of cardiovascular disease: A dose-response meta-analysis of cohort studies. *Lipids Health Dis.* **2019**, *18*, 91. [CrossRef]

68. Koolhaas, C.M.; Dhana, K.; Schoufour, J.D.; Ikram, M.A.; Kavousi, M.; Franco, O.H. Impact of physical activity on the association of overweight and obesity with cardiovascular disease: The Rotterdam Study. *Eur. J. Prev. Cardiol.* **2017**, *24*, 934–941. [CrossRef] [PubMed]

69. Esposito, K.; Marfella, R.; Ciotola, M. Effect of a Mediterranean-style diet on endothelial dysfunction and markers of vascular inflammation in the metabolic syndrome. A randomized trial. *ACC Curr. J. Rev.* **2004**, *13*, 16–17. [CrossRef]

70. Warburton, D.E.; Nicol, C.W.; Bredin, S.S. Health benefits of physical activity: The evidence. *Can. Med. Assoc. J.* **2006**, *174*, 801–809. [CrossRef]

71. Aizawa, K.; Shoemaker, J.K.; Overend, T.J.; Petrella, R.J. Effects of lifestyle modification on central artery stiffness in metabolic syndrome subjects with pre-hypertension and/or pre-diabetes. *Diabetes Res. Clin. Pr.* **2009**, *83*, 249–256. [CrossRef]

72. Fernández, J.M.; Rosado-Álvarez, D.; Da Silva Grigoletto, M.E.; Rangel-Zúñiga, O.A.; Landaeta-Díaz, L.L.; Caballero-Villarraso, J.; López-Miranda, J.; Pérez-Jiménez, F.; Fuentes-Jiménez, F. Moderate-to-high-intensity training and a hypocaloric Mediterranean diet enhance endothelial progenitor cells and fitness in subjects with the metabolic syndrome. *Clin. Sci. (Lond).* **2012**, *123*, 361–373. [CrossRef]

73. Gremeaux, V.; Drigny, J.; Nigam, A.; Juneau, M.; Guilbeault, V.; Latour, E.; Gayda, M. Long-term Lifestyle Intervention with Optimized High-Intensity Interval Training Improves Body Composition, Cardiometabolic Risk, and Exercise Parameters in Patients with Abdominal Obesity. *Am. J. Phys. Med. Rehabil.* **2012**, *91*, 941–950. [CrossRef] [PubMed]

74. Gomez-Huelgas, R.; Jansen-Chaparro, S.; Baca-Osorio, A.; Mancera-Romero, J.; Tinahones, F.; Bernal-Lopez, M. Effects of a long-term lifestyle intervention program with Mediterranean diet and exercise for the management of patients with metabolic syndrome in a primary care setting. *Eur. J. Intern. Med.* **2015**, *26*, 317–323. [CrossRef]

75. Lee, G.; Choi, H.Y.; Yang, S.J. Effects of Dietary and Physical Activity Interventions on Metabolic Syndrome: A Meta-analysis. *J. Korean Acad. Nurs.* **2015**, *45*, 483. [CrossRef] [PubMed]

76. FESNAD. Dietary Reference Intakes (DRI) for the Spanish Population—2010. *Act. Diet.* **2010**, *14*, 196–197.

Permissions

All chapters in this book were first published by MDPI; hereby published with permission under the Creative Commons Attribution License or equivalent. Every chapter published in this book has been scrutinized by our experts. Their significance has been extensively debated. The topics covered herein carry significant findings which will fuel the growth of the discipline. They may even be implemented as practical applications or may be referred to as a beginning point for another development.

The contributors of this book come from diverse backgrounds, making this book a truly international effort. This book will bring forth new frontiers with its revolutionizing research information and detailed analysis of the nascent developments around the world.

We would like to thank all the contributing authors for lending their expertise to make the book truly unique. They have played a crucial role in the development of this book. Without their invaluable contributions this book wouldn't have been possible. They have made vital efforts to compile up to date information on the varied aspects of this subject to make this book a valuable addition to the collection of many professionals and students.

This book was conceptualized with the vision of imparting up-to-date information and advanced data in this field. To ensure the same, a matchless editorial board was set up. Every individual on the board went through rigorous rounds of assessment to prove their worth. After which they invested a large part of their time researching and compiling the most relevant data for our readers.

The editorial board has been involved in producing this book since its inception. They have spent rigorous hours researching and exploring the diverse topics which have resulted in the successful publishing of this book. They have passed on their knowledge of decades through this book. To expedite this challenging task, the publisher supported the team at every step. A small team of assistant editors was also appointed to further simplify the editing procedure and attain best results for the readers.

Apart from the editorial board, the designing team has also invested a significant amount of their time in understanding the subject and creating the most relevant covers. They scrutinized every image to scout for the most suitable representation of the subject and create an appropriate cover for the book.

The publishing team has been an ardent support to the editorial, designing and production team. Their endless efforts to recruit the best for this project, has resulted in the accomplishment of this book. They are a veteran in the field of academics and their pool of knowledge is as vast as their experience in printing. Their expertise and guidance has proved useful at every step. Their uncompromising quality standards have made this book an exceptional effort. Their encouragement from time to time has been an inspiration for everyone.

The publisher and the editorial board hope that this book will prove to be a valuable piece of knowledge for researchers, students, practitioners and scholars across the globe.

List of Contributors

Sara Castro-Barquero, Ramon Estruch and Rosa Casas
Department of Medicine, Faculty of Medicine and Life Sciences, University of Barcelona, 08036 Barcelona, Spain
Institut d'Investigacions Biomèdiques August Pi I Sunyer (IDIBAPS), 08036 Barcelona, Spain
Centro de Investigación Biomédica en Red, Fisiopatología de la Obesidad y la Nutrición (CIBEROBN), Instituto de Salud Carlos III, 28029 Madrid, Spain

Ana María Ruiz-León
Institut d'Investigacions Biomèdiques August Pi I Sunyer (IDIBAPS), 08036 Barcelona, Spain
Centro de Investigación Biomédica en Red, Fisiopatología de la Obesidad y la Nutrición (CIBEROBN), Instituto de Salud Carlos III, 28029 Madrid, Spain

Maria Sierra-Pérez
Department of Medicine, Faculty of Medicine and Life Sciences, University of Barcelona, 08036 Barcelona, Spain

Yunjeong Yi and Jiyeon An
Department of Nursing, Kyungin Women's University, Incheon 21041, Korea

Janne Hukkanen
Research Unit of Internal Medicine, Biocenter Oulu, Medical Research Center Oulu, University of Oulu and Oulu University Hospital, FI-90014 Oulu, Finland

Jukka Hakkola
Research Unit of Biomedicine, Biocenter Oulu, Medical Research Center Oulu, University of Oulu and Oulu University Hospital, FI-90014 Oulu, Finland

Anne-Laure Borel
Department of Endocrinology, Diabetes and Nutrition, Grenoble Alpes University Hospital, 38043 Grenoble, France
"Hypoxia, Pathophysiology" (HP2) Laboratory INSERM U1042, Grenoble Alpes University, 38043 Grenoble, France

Leila Cheikh Ismail
Department of Clinical Nutrition and Dietetics, College of Health Sciences, University of Sharjah, Sharjah 27272, UAE
Nuffield Department of Women's & Reproductive Health, University of Oxford, Oxford OX1 2JD, UK
Research Institute of Medical and Health Sciences (RIMHS), University of Sharjah, Sharjah 27272, UAE

Tareq M. Osaili
Department of Clinical Nutrition and Dietetics, College of Health Sciences, University of Sharjah, Sharjah 27272, UAE
Research Institute of Medical and Health Sciences (RIMHS), University of Sharjah, Sharjah 27272, UAE
Department of Nutrition and Food Technology, Faculty of Agriculture, Jordan University of Science and Technology, Irbid 22110, Jordan

Maysm N. Mohamad, Amjad H. Jarrar, Habiba I. Ali and Ayesha S. Al Dhaheri
Department of Nutrition and Health, College of Medicine and Health Sciences, United Arab Emirates University, Al Ain 15551, UAE

Amina Al Marzouqi
Department of Health Services Administration, College of Health Sciences, University of Sharjah, Sharjah 27272, UAE

Dima O. Abu Jamous
Research Institute of Medical and Health Sciences (RIMHS), University of Sharjah, Sharjah 27272, UAE

Emmanuella Magriplis
Department of Food Science and Human Nutrition, Agricultural University of Athens, Iera Odos 75, 11855 Athens, Greece

Haleama Al Sabbah
College of Natural and Health Sciences, Zayed University, Dubai 19282, UAE

Hayder Hasan, Mona Hashim and Reyad R. Shaker Obaid
Department of Clinical Nutrition and Dietetics, College of Health Sciences, University of Sharjah, Sharjah 27272, UAE
Research Institute of Medical and Health Sciences (RIMHS), University of Sharjah, Sharjah 27272, UAE

Latifa M. R. AlMarzooqi
Nutrition Section, Ministry of Health and Prevention, Dubai 1853, UAE

Lily Stojanovska
Department of Nutrition and Health, College of Medicine and Health Sciences, United Arab Emirates University, Al Ain 15551, UAE
Institute for Health and Sport, Victoria University, Melbourne 14428, Australia

Sheima T. Saleh
Department of Clinical Nutrition and Dietetics, College of Health Sciences, University of Sharjah, Sharjah 27272, UAE

Robinson Ramírez-Vélez
Department of Health Sciences, Public University of Navarra, Navarrabiomed-Biomedical Research Centre, IDISNA-Navarra's Health Research Institute, C/ irunlarrea 3, Complejo Hospitalario de Navarra, 31008 Pamplona, Navarra, Spain

Miguel Ángel Pérez-Sousa
Faculty of Sport Sciences, University of Huelva, Avenida de las Fuerzas Armadas s/n, 21007 Huelva, Spain

Mikel Izquierdo
Department of Health Sciences, Public University of Navarra, Navarrabiomed-Biomedical Research Centre, IDISNA-Navarra's Health Research Institute, C/ irunlarrea 3, Complejo Hospitalario de Navarra, 31008 Pamplona, Navarra, Spain
Centro de Investigación Biomédica en Red de Fragilidad y Envejecimiento Saludable (CIBERFES), Instituto de Salud Carlos III, 28029 Madrid, Spain

Carlos A. Cano-Gutierrez
Hospital Universitario San Ignacio – Aging Institute, Pontificia Universidad Javeriana, Bogotá 110111, Colombia

Emilio González-Jiménez, Jacqueline Schmidt-RioValle and María Correa-Rodrígue
Department of Nursing, Faculty of Health Sciences, University of Granada, Av. Ilustración, 60, 18016 Granada, Spain

Katherine González-Ruíz
Grupo de Ejercicio Físico y Deportes, Vicerrectoría de Investigaciones, Facultad de Salud, Universidad Manuela Beltrán, Bogotá 110231, DC, Colombia

Maria Romanidou and Grigorios Tripsianis
Department of Medical Statistics, Medical Faculty, Democritus University of Thrace, 68100 Alexandroupolis, Greece

Maria Soledad Hershey
Department of Preventive Medicine and Public Health, Navarra Institute for Health Research, University of Navarra, 31008 Pamplona, Spain

Mercedes Sotos-Prieto
Department of Environmental Health, T.H. Chan School of Public Health, Harvard University, Boston, MA 02215, USA
Department of Preventive Medicine and Public Health, School of Medicine, Universidad Autónoma de Madrid, IdiPaz (Instituto de Investigación Sanitaria Hospital Universitario La Paz), Calle del Arzobispo Morcillo 4, 28029 Madrid, Spain
Biomedical Research Network Centre of Epidemiology and Public Health (CIBERESP), Carlos III Health Institute, 28029 Madrid, Spain

Costas Christophi
Department of Environmental Health, T.H. Chan School of Public Health, Harvard University, Boston, MA 02215, USA
Cyprus International Institute for Environmental and Public Health, Cyprus University of Technology, 30 Archbishop Kyprianou Str., Lemesos 3036, Cyprus

Steven Moffatt
National Institute for Public Safety Health, IN 324 E New York Street, Indianapolis, IN 46204, USA

Theodoros C. Constantinidis
Laboratory of Hygiene and Environmental Protection, Medical School, Democritus University of Thrace, 68100 Alexandroupolis, Greece

Stefanos N. Kales
Department of Environmental Health, T.H. Chan School of Public Health, Harvard University, Boston, MA 02215, USA
Occupational Medicine, Cambridge Health Alliance/ Harvard Medical School, Cambridge, MA 02319, USA

Scott A. Lear
Faculty of Health Sciences, Simon Fraser University, Burnaby, BC V5A 1S6, Canada
Division of Cardiology, Providence Health Care, Vancouver, BC V6Z 1Y6, Canada

Danijela Gasevic
School of Public Health and Preventive Medicine, Monash University, Melbourne, VIC 3004, Australia
Usher Institute, University of Edinburgh, Edinburgh EH8 9AG, UK

Siti Raihanah Shafie, Stephen Wanyonyi and Sunil K. Panchal
Functional Foods Research Group, University of Southern Queensland, Toowoomba, QLD 4350, Australia

Lindsay Brown
Functional Foods Research Group, University of Southern Queensland, Toowoomba, QLD 4350, Australia
School of Health and Wellbeing, University of Southern Queensland, Toowoomba, QLD 4350, Australia

Kaiser Wani, Sobhy M. Yakout, Mohammed Ghouse Ahmed Ansari, Shaun Sabico, Syed Danish Hussain, Majed S. Alokail and Nasser M. Al-Daghri
Chair for Biomarkers of Chronic Diseases, Department of Biochemistry, College of Science, King Saud University, Riyadh 11451, Saudi Arabia

Eman Sheshah
Diabetes Care Center, King Salman Bin Abdulaziz Hospital, Riyadh 12769, Saudi Arabia

Naji J. Aljohani
Specialized Diabetes and Endocrine Center, King Fahad Medical City, Riyadh 12231, Saudi Arabia

Yousef Al-Saleh
Chair for Biomarkers of Chronic Diseases, Department of Biochemistry, College of Science, King Saud University, Riyadh 11451, Saudi Arabia
College of Medicine, King Saud bin Abdulaziz University for Health Sciences, Riyadh 22490, Saudi Arabia
King Abdullah International Medical Research Center, Riyadh 11481, Saudi Arabia
Department of Medicine, Ministry of the National Guard—Health Affairs, Riyadh 14611, Saudi Arabia

Jean-Yves Reginster
Chair for Biomarkers of Chronic Diseases, Department of Biochemistry, College of Science, King Saud University, Riyadh 11451, Saudi Arabia
Department of Public Health, Epidemiology and Health Economics, University of Liège, 4000 Liège, Belgium

Maria Garralda-Del-Villar
Department of Occupational Medicine, University of Navarra, 31008 Pamplona, Navarra, Spain

Silvia Carlos-Chillerón and Alfredo Gea
Department of Preventive Medicine and Public Health, University of Navarra, 31008 Pamplona, Navarra, Spain
IDISNA, Navarra Health Research Institute, 31008 Pamplona, Navarra, Spain

Jesus Diaz-Gutierrez and Liz Ruiz-Estigarribia
Department of Preventive Medicine and Public Health, University of Navarra, 31008 Pamplona, Navarra, Spain

Miguel Ruiz-Canela and Maira Bes-Rastrollo
Department of Preventive Medicine and Public Health, University of Navarra, 31008 Pamplona, Navarra, Spain
IDISNA, Navarra Health Research Institute, 31008 Pamplona, Navarra, Spain
CIBER Fisiopatología de la Obesidad y Nutrición (CIBER Obn), Instituto de Salud Carlos III, 28029 Madrid, Spain

Miguel Angel Martínez-González
Department of Preventive Medicine and Public Health, University of Navarra, 31008 Pamplona, Navarra, Spain
IDISNA, Navarra Health Research Institute, 31008 Pamplona, Navarra, Spain
CIBER Fisiopatología de la Obesidad y Nutrición (CIBER Obn), Instituto de Salud Carlos III, 28029 Madrid, Spain
Department of Nutrition, Harvard T.H. Chan School of Public Health, Boston, MA 20115, USA

Alejandro Fernández-Montero
Department of Occupational Medicine, University of Navarra, 31008 Pamplona, Navarra, Spain
IDISNA, Navarra Health Research Institute, 31008 Pamplona, Navarra, Spain
Department of Environmental Health, Harvard T.H. Chan School of Public Health, Boston, MA 20115, USA

Jacopo Troisi
Department of Medicine and Surgery and Dentistry, "Scuola Medica Salernitana", Pediatrics Section University of Salerno, 84081 Baronissi (Salerno), Italy
Theoreo srl, Via degli Ulivi 3, 84090 Montecorvino Pugliano (SA), Italy
European Biomedical Research Institute of Salerno (EBRIS), Via S. de Renzi, 3, 84125 Salerno, Italy
Hosmotic srl, Via R. Bosco 178, 80069 Vico Equense (NA), Italy

Federica Belmonte, Antonella Bisogno, Luca Pierri, Antonella Di Nuzzi, Laura Di Michele, Anna Pia Delli Bovi and Salvatore Guercio Nuzio
Department of Medicine and Surgery and Dentistry, "Scuola Medica Salernitana", Pediatrics Section University of Salerno, 84081 Baronissi (Salerno), Italy

Angelo Colucci
Department of Medicine and Surgery and Dentistry, "Scuola Medica Salernitana", Pediatrics Section University of Salerno, 84081 Baronissi (Salerno), Italy Theoreo srl, Via degli Ulivi 3, 84090 Montecorvino Pugliano (SA), Italy

Pierpaolo Cavallo
Department of Physics, University of Salerno, 84084 Fisciano (Salerno), Italy

Claudia Mandato
Department of Pediatrics, Children's Hospital Santobono-Pausilipon, 80129 Naples, Italy

Pietro Vajro
Department of Medicine and Surgery and Dentistry, "Scuola Medica Salernitana", Pediatrics Section University of Salerno, 84081 Baronissi (Salerno), Italy European Laboratory of Food Induced Intestinal Disease (ELFID), University of Naples Federico II, 80100 Naples, Italy

Vasanti S. Malik
Department of Nutritional Sciences, Faculty of Medicine, University of Toronto, 1 King's College Circle, Toronto, ON M5S 1A8, Canada
Department of Nutrition, Harvard T.H. Chan School of Public Health, 665 Huntington Avenue, Boston, MA 02115, USA

Frank B. Hu
Department of Nutrition, Harvard T.H. Chan School of Public Health, 665 Huntington Avenue, Boston, MA 02115, USA

Department of Epidemiology, Harvard T.H. School of Public Health, Boston, MA 02115, USA
Channing Division of Network Medicine, Brigham and Women's Hospital and Harvard Medical School, Boston, MA 02115, USA

Giovanni Scala
Hosmotic srl, Via R. Bosco 178, 80069 Vico Equense (NA), Italy

Jonathan Myers
Cardiology Division, Veterans Affairs Palo Alto Health Care System and Stanford University, Stanford, CA 94304, USA

Peter Kokkinos
Cardiology Division, Washington DC Veterans Affairs Medical Center and Rutgers University, Washington, DC 20422, USA

Eric Nyelin
Endocrinology Division, Washington DC Veterans Affairs Medical Center, Washington, DC 20422, USA

Alicia Julibert, Maria del Mar Bibiloni, David Mateos and Josep A. Tur
Research Group on Community Nutrition & Oxidative Stress, University of Balearic Islands, IDISBA & CIBEROBN, 07122 Palma de Mallorca, Spain

Escarlata Angullo
Research Group on Community Nutrition & Oxidative Stress, University of Balearic Islands, IDISBA & CIBEROBN, 07122 Palma de Mallorca, Spain
Escola Graduada Primary Health Care Center, IBSalut, 07001 Palma de Mallorca, Spain

Index

Printed in the USA
CPSIA information can be obtained
at www.ICGtesting.com
JSHW051412091023
49903JS00006B/394

9 781646 465934